Epidermolysis Bullosa: Part I – Pathogenesis and Clinical Features

Guest Editor

DÉDÉE F. MURRELL, MA, BMBCh, FAAD, MD

DERMATOLOGIC CLINICS

www.derm.theclinics.com

Consulting Editor
BRUCE H. THIERS, MD

January 2010 • Volume 28 • Number 1

SAUNDERS an imprint of ELSEVIER, Inc.

W.B. SAUNDERS COMPANY
A Division of Elsevier Inc.

1600 John F. Kennedy Boulevard • Suite 1800 • Philadelphia, PA 19103-2899

http://www.theclinics.com

DERMATOLOGIC CLINICS Volume 28, Number 1
January 2010 ISSN 0733-8635, ISBN-13: 978-1-4377-1812-6

Editor: Carla Holloway

Dermatologic Clinics (ISSN 0733-8635) is published quarterly by Elsevier Inc., 360 Park Avenue South, New York, NY 10010-1710. Months of publication are January, April, July, and October. Business and editorial offices: 1600 John F. Kennedy Blvd., Suite 1800, Philadelphia, PA 19103-2899. Customer service office: 11830 Westline Drive, St. Louis, MO 63146. Periodicals postage paid at New York, NY, and additional mailing offices. Subscription prices are USD 296.00 per year for US individuals, USD 431.00 per year for US institutions, USD 347.00 per year for Canadian individuals, USD 516.00 per year for Canadian institutions, USD 406.00 per year for international individuals, USD 516.00 per year for international institutions, USD 141.00 per year for US students/residents, and USD 204.00 per year for Canadian and international students/residents. International air speed delivery is included in all *Clinics* subscription prices. All prices are subject to change without notice. **POSTMASTER:** Send address changes to *Dermatologic Clinics*, Elsevier Health Sciences Division, Subscription Customer Service, 3251 Riverport Lane, Maryland Heights, MO 63043. **Customer Service: 1-800-654-2452 (U.S. and Canada); 314-447-8871 (outside U.S. and Canada). Fax: 314-447-8029. E-mail: journalscustomerservice-usa@elsevier.com (for print support); journalsonlinesupport-usa@elsevier.com (for online support).**

Reprints. For copies of 100 or more, of articles in this publication, please contact the Commercial Reprints Department, Elsevier Inc., 360 Park Avenue South, New York, New York 10010-1710. Tel.: (212) 633-3813; Fax: (212) 462-1935; Email: reprints@elsevier.com.

The *Dermatologic Clinics* is covered in *MEDLINE/PubMed (Index Medicus)*, *Current Contents/Clinical Medicine*, *Excerpta Medica*, *Chemical Abstracts*, and *ISI/BIOMED*.

Printed and bound in the United Kingdom
Transferred to Digital Print 2011

Contributors

CONSULTING EDITOR

BRUCE H. THIERS, MD
Professor and Chair, Department of Dermatology,
Medical University of South Carolina, Charleston,
South Carolina

GUEST EDITOR

DÉDÉE F. MURRELL, MA, BMBCh, FAAD, MD
Professor and Head, Department of Dermatology,
St George Hospital, University of New South
Wales, Kogarah, Sydney, New South Wales,
Australia

AUTHORS

JOHANN W. BAUER, MD
Professor of Dermatology and Venerology,
Division of Molecular Dermatology;
EB House Austria, Department of Dermatology,
General Hospital Salzburg, Paracelsus Medical
University Salzburg, Salzburg, Austria

MARIA C. BOLLING, MD
Department of Dermatology, University
Medical Centre Groningen, Groningen,
The Netherlands

LEENA BRUCKNER-TUDERMAN, MD
Department of Dermatology, University Medical
Center Freiburg, Freiburg, Germany

DÉBORA CADORE DE FARIAS, MD
Department of Dermatology, Santa Casa de São
Paulo Hospital, João Moura Street, Jardim
América, São Paulo, Brazil

DANIELE CASTIGLIA, PhD
Team Leader, Laboratory of Molecular and Cell
Biology, IDI-IRCCS, Rome, Italy

HYE JIN CHUNG, MD, MS
Postdoctoral Research Fellow, Department of
Dermatology and Cutaneous Biology, Jefferson
Medical College, Jefferson Institute of Molecular
Medicine, Thomas Jefferson University,
Philadelphia, Pennsylvania

HEATHER IRINA COHN, BS, MD
PhD Candidate and Post-doctoral Fellow in
Dermatology, Department of Dermatology and
Cutaneous Biology, Jefferson Medical College,
Thomas Jefferson University, Philadelphia,
Pennsylvania; Department of Dermatology,
St George Hospital, Kogarah, Sydney,
New South Wales, Australia

MINAS T. CORONEO, MS, FRANZCO
Department of Ophthalmology, Prince
of Wales Hospital, Randwick, New South Wales,
Australia; University of New South Wales,
Randwick, Sydney, New South Wales, Australia

ANJA DIEM, MD
EB House Austria, Department of Dermatology,
General Hospital Salzburg, Paracelsus Medical
University Salzburg, Salzburg, Austria

MARIA-ANNA M.A. D'SOUZA, BSc, MSc
Children's Centre for Burns Research, The
University of Queensland, Queensland
Children's Medical Research Institute,
Royal Children's Hospital, Herston, Brisbane,
Queensland, Australia

BRUNA DUQUE-ESTRADA, MD
Instituto de Dermatologia Prof. Rubem David
Azulay, Rio de Janeiro, Brazil

EDWIN C. FIGUEIRA, MBBS, MS (Ophth)
Department of Ophthalmology, Prince of Wales
Hospital, Randwick, New South Wales, Australia

JOHN W. FREW, MBBS
Faculty of Medicine, University of New South
Wales, Sydney, Australia; Intern, Department
of Dermatology, St George Hospital, University
of New South Wales Medical School, Sydney,
Australia

KEVIN J. HAMILL, PhD
Department of Cell and Molecular Biology,
Feinberg School of Medicine, Northwestern
University, Chicago, Illinois

CRISTINA HAS, MD
Department of Dermatology, University Medical
Center Freiburg, Freiburg, Germany

HELMUT HINTNER, MD
Professor and Chair, Department of Dermatology,
Paracelsus Medical University Salzburg, Salzburg,
Austria

JONATHAN C.R. JONES, PhD
Professor of Cell and Molecular Biology, Medicine,
and Dermatology, Feinberg School of Medicine,
Northwestern University, Chicago, Illinois

MARCEL F. JONKMAN, MD, PhD
Department of Dermatology, University Medical
Centre Groningen, Groningen, The Netherlands

JOHANNES S. KERN, MD
Department of Dermatology, University Medical
Center Freiburg, Freiburg, Germany

ROY M. KIMBLE, MBBS, MD, FRCS
Professor and Head of Burns and Trauma,
Children's Centre for Burns Research, The
University of Queensland, Queensland Children's
Medical Research Institute, Royal Children's
Hospital, Herston, Brisbane, Queensland,
Australia

MYUNG S. KO, BA
Program in Epithelial Biology; MD Candidate;
Department of Dermatology, Stanford University
School of Medicine, Stanford, California

JOEY E. LAI-CHEONG, MBBS, MRCP (UK)
Division of Genetics and Molecular Medicine,
St John's Institute of Dermatology, King's College
London, Guy's Hospital, London, United Kingdom

MARTIN LAIMER, MD
Division of Molecular Dermatology, Department
of Dermatology, General Hospital Salzburg,
Paracelsus Medical University Salzburg, Salzburg,
Austria

CHRISTOPH MICHAEL LANSCHUETZER, MD
Division of Molecular Dermatology, Department
of Dermatology, General Hospital Salzburg,
Paracelsus Medical University Salzburg, Salzburg,
Austria

M. PETER MARINKOVICH, MD
Program in Epithelial Biology; Associate
Professor, Department of Dermatology, Stanford
University School of Medicine, Stanford;
Dermatology Service, Palo Alto VA Medical
Center, Palo Alto, California

JOHN A. McGRATH, MD, FRCP
Division of Genetics and Molecular Medicine,
St John's Institute of Dermatology, King's College
London, Guy's Hospital, London, United Kingdom

JAMES R. McMILLAN, BSc, MSc, PhD
Head of Burns Laboratory Research, Children's
Centre for Burns Research, The University of
Queensland, Queensland Children's Medical
Research Institute, Royal Children's Hospital,
Herston, Brisbane, Queensland, Australia

JEMIMA E. MELLERIO, MD, FRCP
St John's Institute of Dermatology, The Guy's and
St Thomas's NHS Foundation Trust, London,
United Kingdom

DÉDÉE F. MURRELL, MA, BMBCh, FAAD, MD
Professor and Head, Department of Dermatology,
St George Hospital, University of New South
Wales, Kogarah, Sydney, New South Wales,
Australia

KEN NATSUGA, MD
PhD Course Student, Department of Dermatology,
Hokkaido University Graduate School of Medicine,
Sapporo, Japan

ELKE NISCHLER, MD
Department of Dermatology, Paracelsus Medical
University Salzburg, Austria

WATARU NISHIE, MD, PhD
Part-time Lecturer, Department of Dermatology,
Hokkaido University Graduate School of Medicine,
Sapporo, Japan

EDEL A. O'TOOLE, MB, PhD, FRCP, FRCPI
Professor, Centre for Cutaneous Research, Blizard
Institute of Cell and Molecular Science, Barts and
the London School of Medicine and Dentistry,
Queen Mary, University of London, Whitechapel,
London, United Kingdom

AMY S. PALLER, MD
Professor and Chairman, Dermatology; Professor
of Pediatrics, Feinberg School of Medicine,
Northwestern University, Chicago, Illinois

GÜNTHER A. REZNICZEK, PhD
Department of Biochemistry and Cell Biology,
Max F. Perutz Laboratories, University of Vienna,
Vienna, Austria

HIROSHI SHIMIZU, MD, PhD
Professor and Chairman, Department of
Dermatology, Hokkaido University Graduate
School of Medicine, Sapporo, Japan

SATORU SHINKUMA, MD
PhD Course Student, Department of Dermatology,
Hokkaido University Graduate School of Medicine,
Sapporo, Japan

ANDREW P. SOUTH, PhD
Centre for Oncology and Molecular Medicine,
Ninewell's Hospital and Medical School, Dundee,
United Kingdom

ELI SPRECHER, MD, PhD
Department of Dermatology, Tel Aviv Sourasky
Medical Center, Tel Aviv, Israel

ANTONELLA TOSTI, MD
Department of Dermatology, University of
Bologna, Bologna, Italy

JOUNI UITTO, MD, PhD
Professor and Chair, Department of Dermatology
and Cutaneous Biology, Jefferson Medical
College, Jefferson Institute of Molecular Medicine,
Thomas Jefferson University, Philadelphia,
Pennsylvania

GERNOT WALKO, PhD
Department of Biochemistry and Cell Biology,
Max F. Perutz Laboratories, University of Vienna,
Vienna, Austria

GERHARD WICHE, PhD
Department of Biochemistry and Cell Biology,
Max F. Perutz Laboratories, University of Vienna,
Vienna, Austria

J. TIMOTHY WRIGHT, DDS, MS
Distinguished Professor and Chair, Department
of Pediatric Dentistry, School of Dentistry,
The University of North Carolina, Chapel Hill,
North Carolina

KIM B. YANCEY, MD
Professor and Chair, Department of Dermatology,
University of Texas Southwestern Medical Center
at Dallas, Dallas, Texas

GIOVANNA ZAMBRUNO, MD
Director, Laboratory of Molecular and Cell Biology,
IDI-IRCCS, Rome, Italy

Contents

PATHOGENESIS

> The dermal-epidermal basement membrane zone is an important epithelial and stromal interface, consisting of an intricately organized collection of intracellular, transmembrane, and extracellular matrix proteins. The basement membrane zone has several main functions including acting as a permeability barrier, forming an adhesive interface between epithelial cells and the underlying matrix, and controlling cellular organization and differentiation. This article identifies key molecular players of the dermal-epidermal membrane zone, and highlights recent research studies that have identified structural and functional roles of these components in the context of various blistering, neoplastic, and developmental syndromes.

> A mutation is an event that produces heritable changes in the DNA. There are many different types of mutations, including point mutations (changes that imply loss, duplication, or alterations of small DNA segments, often involving a single or a few nucleotides) and major DNA changes (loss, duplication, or rearrangements of entire genes or of gene segments). This article reviews how different types of mutation may result in defective gene expression.

> The prevalence of epidermolysis bullosa simplex (EBS) is estimated to be approximately 6 to 30 per 1 million live births. The disease is usually caused by missense mutations in *KRT5* and *KRT14*, encoding keratins mostly expressed in the epidermal basal layer. Major advances in understanding of the molecular basis of EBS and other keratin disorders have led to the development of DNA-based prenatal testing.

> Plectin is an important organizer of the keratin filament cytoskeleton in basal keratinocytes. It is essential for anchoring these filaments to the extracellular matrix via hemidesmosomal integrins. Loss of plectin or incorrect function of the protein due to mutations in its gene can lead to various forms of the skin blistering disease, epidermolysis bullosa simplex. Severity and subtype of the disease is dependent on the specific mutation and can be associated with (late-onset) muscular dystrophy or pyloric atresia. Mouse models mimicking the human phenotypes allow detailed study of plectin function.

Epidermolysis bullosa (EB) with pyloric atresia (PA) is a rare form of EB. This article describes the clinical and pathologic features and molecular genetics of EB-PA, the mutations in the $\alpha_6\beta_4$ integrin and plectin genes that cause EB-PA, and the clinical implications of molecular genetics on EB-PA.

Junctional epidermolysis bullosa type Herlitz (JEB-H) is the autosomal recessively inherited, more severe variant of "lucidolytic" JEB. Characterized by generalized, extensive mucocutaneous blistering at birth and early lethality, this devastating condition is most often caused by homozygous null mutations in the genes *LAMA3*, *LAMB3*, or *LAMC2*, each encoding for 1 of the 3 chains of the heterotrimer laminin-332. The JEB-H subtype usually presents as a severe and clinically diverse variant of the EB group of mechanobullous genodermatoses. This article outlines the epidemiology, presentation, and diagnosis of JEB-H. Morbidity and mortality are high, necessitating optimized protocols for early (including prenatal) diagnosis and palliative care. Gene therapy remains the most promising perspective.

Collagen XVII has been identified as having a role in inherited junctional epidermolysis bullosa non-Herlitz (JEB-other, MIM #226650). The role of collagen XVII in both autoimmune and genetic blistering disorders demonstrates its relevance to dermal-epidermal adhesion. Collagen XVII is a major structural component of the hemidesmosome (HD), a highly specialized multiprotein complex that mediates the anchorage of basal epithelial cells to the underlying basement membrane in stratified, pseudostratified, and transitional epithelia. This article examines the genetic and pathological features of collagen XVII.

Non-Herlitz junctional epidermolysis bullosa (nH JEB) is characterized by generalized blisters that predominate in sites exposed to friction, trauma, or heat. Whereas infants and children with nH JEB often appear to resemble patients with other forms of EB, adults with this disorder typically display atrophic scars, hypopigmentation, or hyperpigmentation at sites of healed blisters as well as incomplete alopecia, dystrophic nails, mucous membrane involvement, and dental abnormalities. Mild (or severe) disease early in life may be characterized by the opposite phenotype in adults with nH JEB. Although nH JEB is generally less severe than Herlitz disease, fatalities (especially in neonates) are not uncommon among patients with the former diagnosis.

The laminins are a secreted family of heterotrimeric molecules essential for basement membrane formation, structure, and function. It is now well established that the α3 subunit of laminins-332, -321, and -311 plays an important role in mediating epidermal-dermal integrity and is essential for the skin to withstand mechanical stresses. These laminins also regulate cell migration and mechanosignal transduction. This article provides an overview of the gene, transcripts, and protein structures of laminin α3. Also discussed are the proposed functions for the α3 subunit–containing laminins.

Laryngo-onycho-cutaneous (LOC) syndrome was reclassified as a subtype of junctional epidermolysis bullosa (JEB) based on clinical features similar to JEB and its association, in the majority of patients from the Punjab, with a unique mutation affecting the N terminus of the α3 chain of LM332. Although LOC syndrome is now a subtype of JEB(JEB-LOC) JEB-LOC has a distinct clinicopathologic appearance and molecular fingerprint. The intricacies of the JEB-LOC subtype are discussed in this article with regard to disease presentation, pathogenesis, management, and prognosis.

Type VII collagen is a major component of the anchoring fibrils of the dermal-epidermal adhesion on the dermal side at the lamina densa/papillary dermis interface. Dystrophic epidermolysis bullosa (DEB) emerged as a candidate for type VII collagen mutations because anchoring fibrils were shown to be morphologically altered, reduced in number, or completely absent in patients with different forms of DEB. Circulating autoantibodies recognize type VII collagen epitopes in epidermolysis bullosa acquisita. The suggestion that type VII collagen is required for human epidermal tumorigenesis relates to the increasing numbers of life-threatening complications associated with developing squamous cell carcinomas because of the extended life span of affected individuals with recessive DEB.

Dystrophic epidermolysis bullosa (DEB) is relatively well understood. Potential therapies are in development. This article describes the pathogenesis and clinical features of DEB. It also describes therapeutic options and the future of molecular therapies.

Kindler syndrome is caused by genetic defects in the focal contact–associated protein, fermitin family homologue 1 (FFH1), encoded by the gene FERMT1 (known as KIND1). Defects in FFH1 lead to abnormal integrin activation and loss of keratinocyte epidermal adhesion to the underlying basal lamina, disruption in normal cell cyto-skeleton within keratinocytes, and altered signaling pathways, leading to increased extracellular matrix production. Null mutations in FERMT1 result in skin blistering from birth and early childhood progressive poikiloderma, mucosal fragility, and increased risk of cancer. The complete range of FFH1 functions in skin and other epithelia has yet to be determined.

Kindler syndrome (MIM173650) is an autosomal recessive genodermatosis charac-terized by poikiloderma, trauma-induced skin blistering, mucosal inflammation, and photosensitivity. Loss-of-function mutations in the *FERMT1* gene are the cause of Kindler syndrome. Kindler syndrome is categorized as a subtype of epidermolysis bullosa (EB). During infancy and childhood, there is clinical overlap between Kindler syndrome and dystrophic EB. Unlike other forms of EB, Kindler syndrome is charac-terized by impaired actin cytoskeleton-extracellular matrix interactions and a variable plane of blister formation at or close to the dermal-epidermal junction. This article reviews clinicopathologic and molecular features of Kindler syndrome and dis-cusses patient management.

Pathogenic mutations have now been described in ten different desmosomal pro-teins: plakophilin 1 (PKP1) and 2 (PKP2); desmoplakin; plakoglobin; desmoglein 1, 2, and 4; desmocollin 2, and 3 corneodesmosin. Nevertheless, the first report of an inherited desmosomal gene disorder, published in 1997, involved loss-of-func-tion mutations on both alleles of *PKP1*, the PKP1 gene. Loss of PKP1 expression in human skin leads to skin erosions and crusting, notably with perioral fissuring as well as palmoplantar hyperkeratosis with painful cracking of the skin. Other more variable features include abnormalities of ectodermal development with growth delay, hypotrichosis or alopecia, hypohidrosis, and nail dystrophy. In con-trast to some other inherited disorders of desmosomes, there is no cardiac pathol-ogy in individuals with *PKP1* mutations since it is not expressed in the heart. The collection of clinical features in individuals with *PKP1* mutations has been termed *ec-todermal dysplasia–skin fragility (ED-SF) syndrome*. This genodermatosis is classi-fied as a suprabasal form of epidermolysis bullosa simplex and thus far there have been 10 published cases. Skin biopsy shows acanthosis, acantholysis, and a reduced number of small, poorly formed desmosomes. Loss of PKP1 expression results in an integral weakness within the desmosomal plaque, leading to desmo-somal detachment and cell-cell separation. Thus, the clinicopathologic features at-test to the significant role of PKP1 in stabilization of desmosome structure and function, predominantly in the spinous layers of the epidermis. This article reviews the clinical, structural, and molecular pathology of this genetic disorder of desmosomes.

Lethal acantholytic epidermolysis bullosa (LAEB) is an autosomal recessive disorder caused by mutations in the gene encoding the desmosomal protein, desmoplakin (DSP). It is recognized as a distinct form of suprabasal epidermolysis bullosa sim-plex, although only a single case has been reported. The phenotype comprises severe fragility of skin and mucous membranes with marked transcutaneous fluid loss. Other features include total alopecia, neonatal teeth, and anonychia. Skin biopsy reveals abnormal desmosomes with suprabasal clefting and acantholysis and disconnection of keratin intermediate filaments from desmosomes. The DSP abnormalities present in the affected individual involved expression of truncated DSP polypeptides that lacked the tail domain of the protein. This part of DSP has a vital role in binding to keratin filaments. The affected neonate died after 10 days because of heart failure with evidence of loss of epithelial integrity in the skin, lung, gastrointestinal tract, and bladder. This article provides a clinicopathologic overview of this unique desmosomal genodermatosis, set in the context of other *DSP* gene mutations, both dominant and recessive, that can cause a spectrum of skin, hair, and heart abnormalities.

For more than 2 decades, animal models have been used to clarify the pathogenic mechanisms of human diseases and develop new therapeutics for these diseases. Several therapies for human diseases have become available through trials using animal models. Epidermolysis bullosa (EB) is one of the most severe inherited skin disorders, whose effective treatments have not been fully available. EB is characterized by abnormalities of the proteins that consist of the dermoepidermal junction. EB has been classified into three major subtypes according to the level of skin cleavage: EB simplex, junctional EB, and dystrophic EB. To date, 13 genes have been shown to cause EB phenotype. After the discovery of the causative genes responsible for each EB subtype, many researchers have tried to develop EB animal models by genetically manipulating the corresponding genes.

Eye involvement in inherited epidermolysis bullosa (EB) can occur as a spectrum of symptoms and signs. This article describes these signs and symptoms. It also offers options for treatment.

Nail abnormalities are a common feature in most subtypes of epidermolysis bullosa (EB), and they recently have been included among the criteria for scoring EB severity. Trauma undoubtedly contributes to the development of nail dystrophy, and for this reason the great toenails often are affected more severely. The nail abnormalities may be the first or the only symptom of EB. Nail abnormalities observed in EB are not specific or pathognomonic, as they result from nail bed and matrix scarring. The spectrum of clinical severity is large, and nail abnormalities may cause severe disability or just be a mild cosmetic problem. This article reviews the nail abnormalities observed in EB.

The craniofacial and oral manifestations of the different epidermolysis bullosa (EB) types vary markedly in character and severity depending largely on the EB type.

The tissues affected and the phenotypes displayed are closely related to the specific abnormal or absent proteins resulting from the causative genetic mutations for these disorders. In this article, the major oral manifestations are reviewed for different EB subtypes and are related to the causative genetic mutations and gene expression.

Hair abnormalities observed in epidermolysis bullosa (EB) are of variable severity and include mild hair shaft abnormalities, patchy cicatricial alopecia, cicatricial alopecia with a male pattern distribution, and alopecia universalis. Alopecia is usually secondary to blistering, and scalp areas more exposed to friction, such as the occipital area, are involved more frequently. This article reviews the hair abnormalities reported in the different subtypes of EB.

Patients with recessive dystrophic epidermolysis bullosa develop numerous life-threatening skin cancers. The reasons for this remain unclear. Parallels exist with other scarring skin conditions, such as Marjolin ulcer. We summarize observational and experimental data and discuss proposed theories for the development of such aggressive skin cancers. A context-driven situation seems to be emerging, but more focused research is required to elucidate the pathogenesis of epidermolysis bullosa–associated squamous cell carcinoma.

Epidermolysis bullosa (EB) nevi are large, eruptive, asymmetrical, often irregularly pigmented melanocytic lesions. Such nevi may give rise to small satellite nevi surrounding the primary nevus, and thus frequently manifest clinical features suggestive of melanoma. They usually arise in sites of previous bullae or erosions. At least twice a year all persisting wounds and EB nevi should be evaluated with a low threshold for histopathologic examination if warranted. Our practice is to punch biopsy EB nevi showing dermoscopic features of concern as well as dermoscopically featureless lesions. Given the skin fragility and potentially impaired wound healing in EB patients, we avoid prophylactic total excision of large EB nevi, but rather use the dermoscope to select appropriate sites for punch biopsies within giant EB nevi.

Quality of life (QOL) evaluation in epidermolysis bullosa (EB) has important applications in clinical management, patient advocacy, clinical research, and the development of new treatments. Several new quantitative and qualitative QOL measurement tools were developed recently, providing insight into the impact EB has on individuals and their family members. Selection of the most appropriate QOL tool for patients who have EB depends on not only the type of information required but also the general or specific cohort being examined. EB-specific quantitative tools possess the highest level of content validity and statistical accuracy. However, generic dermatologic tools may also be appropriate in some circumstances. Overall, QOL evaluation in EB is still a developing area of research that may help improve patient management and assess emerging treatment modalities for their efficacy in improving the QOL of patients with EB.

Dermatologic Clinics

THE CLINICS ARE NOW AVAILABLE ONLINE!

Access your subscription at:
www.theclinics.com

Preface

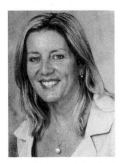

Dédée F. Murrell, MA, BMBCh, FAAD, MD
Guest Editor

When invited by Bruce Thiers to edit a special issue of *Dermatologic Clinics* on epidermolysis bullosa (EB), I was delighted and honored to accept.

Apart from two previous textbooks devoted to EB, no other single source accessible to dermatologists gave an overview of the latest information on this complex subject.

Unlike a textbook, where the chapters may be over 1 or 2 years out of date by the time the book is published, these articles have been written in the last 9 months and by respected leaders in specific aspects of EB. The issue has been organized to pair articles by leading scientists about the biology of the gene and protein of a particular form of EB, with articles by leading EB clinicians on the clinical aspects of that form of EB and explanations about the genotype-to-phenotype correlation. Unlike chapters in a textbook, these articles can be found on MEDLINE and PubMed and are accessible online. Also, the individual issues of the journal may be purchased for much less than either a textbook or the articles individually.

With so much to include about EB, it was decided to cover pathogenesis and an overview of clinical features of EB in the first issue. This issue starts with two articles that are the key to understanding EB. One is an excellent overview, by Myung Ko and Peter Marinkovich, on the basement membrane structure. This is followed by an article, by Daniele Castiglia and Giovanna Zambruno, on how different types of mutations in any gene lead to certain effects in the proteins. The articles that follow cover each type of EB going from the superficial layers of the skin to deeper layers. Each article relates the clinical abnormalities to the underlying gene and protein defects. These articles are written by such well-known EB experts as Johann Bauer, Leena Bruckner-Tuderman, Anja Diem, Kevin Hamill, Cristina Has, Helmut Hintner, Jonathan Jones, Marcel Jonkman, Joey Lai-Cheong, Martin Laimer, Christoph Lanschuetzer, John McGrath, Jemima Mellerio, James McMillan, Amy Paller, Eli Sprecher, Jouni Uitto, Gerhard Wiche, and Kim Yancey. Other writers include relative newcomers within their groups, who we hope will continue this work. After discussion of commoner forms of EB, rare and newly included forms of EB that were added to the 2008 Consensus are covered. Unusual for a clinician's journal is the article by Hiroshi Shimizu's group an the animal models of EB as a basis for understanding pathogenesis and testing new treatments.

The clinical features include topics that had not been written about much before, such as hair and nail manifestations, by Antonella Tosti; quality-of-life studies, by John Frew; ophthalmic manifestations, by Minas Coroneo with Edwin Figueira; and oral manifestations, by J. Timothy Wright. Some special problems are also addressed. These include squamous cell carcinomas, by Andy South and Edel O'Toole; and EB naevi, by Helmut Hintner's group from Salzburg.

The second issue will cover diagnosis and management of EB in detail.

The contributors deserve many thanks for their time and effort in writing these articles at relatively short notice and in a succinct manner with excellent color photographs and figures.

I hope these two issues will be educational not only for dermatologists but for all clinicians who

Dermatol Clin 28 (2010) xv–xvi
doi:10.1016/j.det.2009.10.025

derm.theclinics.com

interact with patients with EB, as well as for scientists, for family members, and for the patients themselves. Understanding what is so far known about a disease leads to improved clinical practice, better research, and improved compliance with therapy.

Dédée F. Murrell, MA, BMBCh, FAAD, MD
Department of Dermatology, St George Hospital
University of NSW, Gray Street, Kogarah
Sydney, NSW 2217, Australia

E-mail address:
d.murrell@unsw.edu.au

Role of Dermal-Epidermal Basement Membrane Zone in Skin, Cancer, and Developmental Disorders

Myung S. Ko, BA[a], M. Peter Marinkovich, MD[a,b,c,*]

KEYWORDS

- Basement membrane zone • Laminin • Integrin • Keratin
- Collagen • Epidermolysis bullosa • Blistering disorder

The dermal-epidermal basement membrane zone (BMZ) is an important epithelial and stromal interface, consisting of an intricately organized collection of intracellular, transmembrane, and extracellular matrix proteins. The BMZ has several main functions: acting as a permeability barrier, forming an adhesive interface between epithelial cells and the underlying matrix, and controlling cell organization and differentiation.

The BMZ of the skin contains a number of specialized adhesive structures, which help to promote tissue integrity in the face of disruptive external forces. At the superior aspect of the dermal-epidermal BMZ, intermediate filaments composed of keratins 5 and 14 insert on keratin linker proteins plectin and BPAG1 (BP230) as shown in **Fig. 1**. BPAG1 and plectin in turn form an intricate and precise interaction with two transmembrane BMZ molecules $\alpha 6\beta 4$ integrin and type XVII collagen (BP180/BPAG2). Collectively BPAG1, plectin, $\alpha 6\beta 4$ integrin, and type XVII collagen comprise the electron-dense condensations of the keratinocyte plasma membrane as seen ultrastructurally by electron microscopy, which are termed "hemidesmosomes."

Jutting out below the hemidesmosome are small threadlike structures termed "anchoring filaments." Anchoring filaments consist of or associate with type XVII collagen; $\alpha 6\beta 4$ integrin; and two extracellular proteins, laminin-332 and laminin-311. These laminins assemble with other molecules including laminin-511, type IV collagen, and nidogen to form an electron-dense central structure of the BMZ termed the "lamina densa." Finally, extending out perpendicularly as banded projections from the lamina densa are the anchoring fibrils. These structures contain polymeric associations of type VII collagen molecules, which intertwine between dermal interstitial collagen fibrils, joining the lamina densa to the papillary dermis. The dermal-epidermal BMZ serves to link the cytoskeleton of the basal epidermis, with the extensive network of interstitial collagen fibrils in the papillary dermis.

LAMININS OF THE DERMAL-EPIDERMAL BMZ

The laminin family of glycoproteins is a major constituent of the BMZ, providing a critical role in

[a] Program in Epithelial Biology, Stanford University School of Medicine, 269 Campus Drive, Stanford, CA 94305, USA
[b] Department of Dermatology, Stanford University School of Medicine, 269 Campus Drive, Room 2145, Stanford, CA 94305, USA
[c] Dermatology Service, Palo Alto VA Medical Center, Palo Alto, CA 94304, USA
* Corresponding author. Department of Dermatology, Stanford University School of Medicine, 269 Campus Drive, Room 2145, Stanford, CA 94305.
E-mail address: mpm@stanford.edu (M.P. Marinkovich).

Dermatol Clin 28 (2010) 1–16
doi:10.1016/j.det.2009.10.001
0733-8635/09/$ – see front matter. Published by Elsevier Inc.

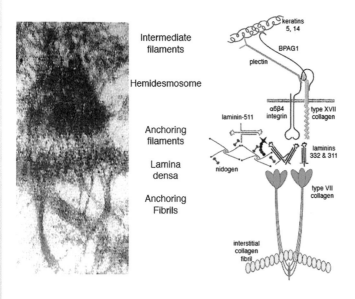

Fig. 1. Structural organization of the dermal-epidermal basement membrane zone. (*Left panel*) Appearance of the dermal-epidermal BMZ as seen by transmission electron microscopy, showing the ultrastructural entities listed immediately to the right of the micrograph. (*Right panel*) Major components of the dermal-epidermal basement membrane and their basic relationships to each other.

providing structure to the extracellular matrix anchorage for cells and tissues. The 16 known laminin isoforms are composed of three chains (α, β, and γ) bound by disulfide bonds.[1,2] To date, five α, four β, and three γ chains have been identified to create the laminin isoforms in humans.[3] The laminin trimer resembles a cross-like structure with a large globular domain (LG domain) at the base of the cross. The LG domain is the C-terminal domain, and has been shown to function as the principal site for the interaction of laminins with various cell surface receptors. The N-terminal domain is an important mediator for the interaction of laminin with the other matrix molecules and for incorporation of laminin into the extracellular matrix.[4,5]

The role of the laminin proteins has been closely linked to their interactions with integrins, heterodimeric transmembrane proteins composed of associations between α and β subunits. The specifics of laminin-integrin interaction remained largely unsolved until recently, when it was shown that the glutamic acid residue at the third position from the C-terminal region of the laminin γ chain is critically involved in the recognition of laminin by integrins.[6,7] It is now also known that whereas the laminin γ chain is involved in this initial recognition, the affinity of binding between laminin and integrin is modulated by the β chain of the C terminus.[1]

In addition to its role in the assembly of the BMZ, laminins interact with cells to influence proliferation, adhesion, and migration. To fully understand the role of laminin in pathologic states, it is important to examine the critical roles of individual laminin proteins.

Laminin-332

Laminin-332 is initially synthesized, assembled, and secreted by keratinocytes in a precursor form consisting of an α3 chain, γ2 chain, and β3 chain. Each of these chains is truncated compared with most other laminins, structurally depicted in **Fig. 2**, by comparison with laminin-511, one of the other major laminins of the skin. Laminin-332 becomes even smaller after it is secreted, because it undergoes processing extracellularly at one position of its γ2 chain and at two positions of its α3 chain. The major processing enzyme is mammalian Tolloid, which is a member of the family of C-proteinases.[8] The protein BMP-1 is another enzyme of this family that is less highly expressed in keratinocytes and fibroblasts in the skin.[9] One of the processing sites, on the laminin α3 globular G3-4 domain, seems to have less specificity and non–C-proteinase enzymes, such as plasmin, and several MMPs has also been shown to cleave this domain.[8,10] Processing of laminin-332 seems to play an important role in the skin, both during wound healing[11] and carcinoma development.[12,13]

Compared with other laminins, laminin-332 has unique activity and structure. One of its unique functions is that it interacts with two major epithelial integrin receptors, α3β1 and α6β4,[14,15] and promotes the formation of two separate types of attachment structures, focal adhesions and stable anchoring contacts.[16,17] Laminin-332 localizes to focal adhesions through the α3β1 integrin, on which focal adhesions contribute to the migration and attachment of normal and malignant cells.[17–19] It also interacts with α6β4 integrin to promote the assembly of stable anchoring contacts. Whereas

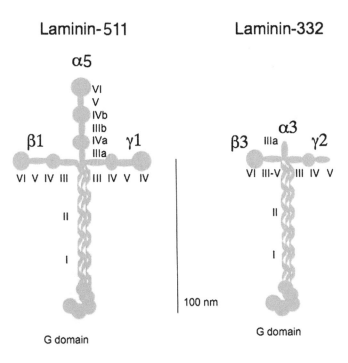

Fig. 2. Domain structure of two major laminins of the dermal-epidermal basement membrane. To the right is a schematic depiction of the laminin-511 molecule with its extended domain structure contained in its three short arms. To the left is laminin-332 showing a more compact structure of its short arms, containing fewer domains.

focal adhesions provide short-term adhesion through reversible association of integrins, stable anchoring contacts–derived stable adhesion in epidermal cells provides increased resistance to disruptive forces. It is generally believed that focal adhesions evolve into stable anchoring contacts over time within the same area of deposited laminin-332.[20,21] Structurally, laminin-332 presents unique truncations in its N-terminal regions (short arms) compared with other members of the laminin family. Despite their relatively small size, certain N-terminal domains of the short arm are important because of their ability to interact with other BMZ proteins.[13] For example, it is known that the laminin β3 short arm domain V-III binds directly to the type VII collagen NC1 domain.[22–24] It is also believed the short arm of the laminin β3 also enhances the matrix assembly of another BMZ laminin, laminin-511.[15]

Laminin-332 is involved in various blistering diseases and skin wounds. It has been shown that during re-epithelialization after skin wounding, laminin-332 is deposited over the provisional matrix during the migration and hyperproliferation of keratinocytes. Studies using K14-Cre mice lacking the α3 subunit in the basal layer of the epidermis have shown that integrin α3β1 binds to laminin-332 that is newly deposited on the wound bed, thereby delaying keratinocyte directional migration and wound re-epithelizalization in the skin.[14]

The crucial role of laminin-332 in epidermal adhesion was highlighted by the demonstration of its absence in the severe and lethal blistering Herlitz disease, junctional epidermolysis bullosa

(JEB),[25–27] a result of underlying laminin-332 gene mutations.[25,28,29] JEB is just one of the many forms of epidermolysis bullosa (EB) and is characterized by intralaminar lucida blistering as depicted in **Fig. 3.** JEB has largely been accepted as an untreatable genodermatosis. Recent studies have cast more light on potential therapeutic measures. Igoucheva and colleagues[28] have demonstrated the applicability of using recombinant protein therapy for JEB by developing a protocol for production and purification of the active recombinant β3 chain that was incorporated into human keratinocytes that lack the β3 subunit. An animal model has also now been established, demonstrating the sustained phenotypic reversion of JEB in dog keratinocytes.[25]

Most exciting are the recent results of a clinical trial of gene therapy of a non-Herlitz JEB patient.[30] In these studies, corrective expression of laminin-332 β3 chain cDNA delivered by a retrovirus to the patient's cells ex vivo resulted in maintenance of expression of laminin-332 and a reduction in the blistering phenotype of the localized corrected skin cell grafts even as long as 1 year after treatment. Although only performed with a single patient, these landmark studies represent the first demonstration of corrective BMZ therapy in genetic skin disease and pave the way toward future studies in this area.

Laminin-511

Laminin-511 (previously known as laminin 10) is a protein that is expressed abundantly in the

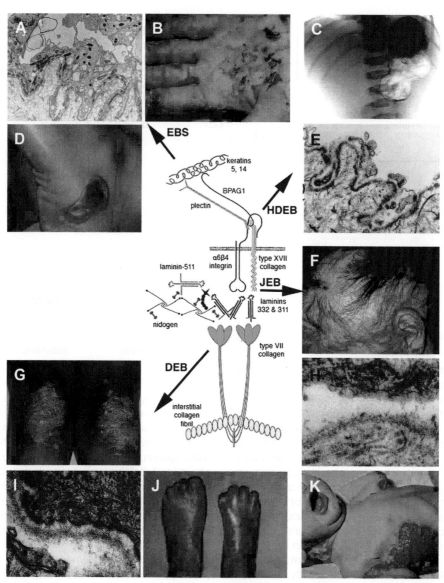

Fig. 3. Correlation of basement membrane assembly, ultrastructural abnormalities, and clinical features in various types of epidermolysis bullosa. (*A*) Electron micrograph showing intraepidermal separation of epidermolysis bullosa simplex (EBS) (original magnification × 7800). (*B*) Severe blistering and hyperkeratosis seen in EBS of Koebner. (*C*) Radiologic findings associated with epidermolysis bullosa with pyloric atresia (EB-PA). (*D*) Blistering seen in milder Weber-Cockayne variant of EBS. (*E*) Electron micrograph showing level of blistering associated with EB-PA termed hemidesmosomal EB, and showing separation just above the plasma membrane (original magnification × 12,500). (*F*) Nonscarring diffuse alopecia in patient with the nonlethal junctional epidermolysis bullosa (JEB) variant generalized atrophic benign epidermolysis bullosa. (*G*) Dystrophic scarring in dominant dystrophic epidermolysis bullosa (DEB). (*H*) Electron micrograph showing intralamina lucida level of separation in JEB. (*I*) Electron micrograph showing sublamina densa level of separation in DEB (original magnification × 15,500). (*J*) Clinical feature of pseudosyndactyly (a scar-induced fusion of skin around the digits) in recessive DEB. (*K*) Extensive blistering associated with loss of laminin-332 in the severe Herlitz's variant of JEB (original magnification × 15,500).

BMZ underlying the interfollicular epidermis and the blood vessels in the dermis.[31] It was first identified with the molecular cloning of the laminin α5 chain.[32] In the first years following the initial characterization of the protein, laminin-511 remained somewhat of an enigmatic protein.

In recent years, however, advances in molecular techniques have allowed for better characterization of the structure of laminin-511 and its role in development and various skin and systemic diseases. Laminin-511 consists of three chains associated with α5, γ1, and β1 chains.[33,34] It has been shown to interact with $\alpha3\beta1$ integrin[35–37] and with α-dystroglycan.[38] The G domain of the α 5-chain is responsible for laminin-511's interactions with both dystroglycan and $\alpha3\beta1$ integrin.[38,39] Attempts have been made to investigate further the specific epitope of the G domain that is responsible for recognition of $\alpha3\beta1$ integrin by using a function-blocking monoclonal antibody, 4C7. The integrin binding activity did not parallel the 4C7 reactivity, however, suggesting that binding may require a strictly defined conformation of the LG domain–like 1 module, which can only be attained within an array of the LG 1 to 3 modules.[40] Future studies need to be conducted to elucidate fully the specifics behind the interaction between laminin-511 and $\alpha3\beta1$ integrin. It is most likely that $\beta1$ integrin and α-dystroglycan binding sites are localized to different LG modules within the laminin $\alpha5$ chain G domain.[38]

Like laminin-332, laminin-511 is involved in important skin functions. Laminin-511 is produced by human dermal microvascular endothelial cells, and highly expressed in blood vessels skin wounds. It is thought that the interaction between laminin-511 and its corresponding integrin mediates the interactions between cells and the extracellular matrix during wound angiogenesis.[41] It has also been implicated to be an alternative adhesive ligand for promoting the proliferation and migration of epidermal keratinocytes during wound healing.[31]

Laminin-311

Laminin-311 (previously known as laminin 6) contains the $\alpha3$, $\beta1$, and γ 1 chains.[42] It has been hypothesized that one of the unpaired cysteine residues in the laminin-311 $\alpha3$ chain domain 3 EGF1 region binds to an unpaired cysteine residue in the $\beta3$ domain 6 region of laminin-332.[43] The $\alpha3$ and $\gamma2$ chains of laminin-332 are completely processed when laminin-332 is complexed with laminin-311, and these processing steps are probably necessary in the covalent association of the two laminins. Because laminins-311 and -332 share the common integrin-binding domain in the laminin $\alpha3$ chain, the two have been thought to cooperatively regulate cellular functions.[44] The mechanism of such cellular regulation is different, however, between the two proteins; laminin-311 is activated by proteolytic processing and regulates cellular adhesion and migration differently from laminin-332.[44]

Laminins as Facilitators of Signal Transduction

The role of BMZ laminin proteins as cell-migration–promoting adhesion molecules has been widely studied and undisputed. To appreciate fully the role of laminins in the BMZ, however, it is important to appreciate the role of laminin proteins not only as facilitators of cell adhesion, but also as facilitators of critical signal transduction pathways.

It has been shown that when the $\gamma2$ chain of laminin-332's short arm is processed by proteolysis, laminin is converted from an adhesion type to a motility type. This mobilized laminin-332 was shown to bind to syndecan-1. Such binding triggers intracellular signaling events, which negatively regulates $\beta4$ integrin, and leads to the regulation of keratinocyte adhesion and motility.[45,46] In 2005, Jones and colleagues[47] suggested that laminin-311 assembles into multimolecular fibrillar complexes with perlecan and participates in mechanical-signal transduction by a dystroglycan-dependent, integrin-dependent mechanism. These results provide new insight into the role of laminin-311 in dictating the response of epithelial cells to mechanical stimulation, carrying broad implications for the usage of mechanical ventilators in lung injury.

Finally, the dual role of laminin in promoting both cellular adhesion and signal transduction was demonstrated by the role of laminin-511 in T-cell recruitment across blood-brain barrier. In an experiment studying autoimmune encephalomyelitis, Sixt and colleagues[48] suggested two possible roles for laminin in the endothelial BMZ: one at the level of endothelial cells resulting in reduced adhesion, and secondly at the level of T cells providing direct signals to the transmigrating cells.

INTEGRINS OF THE DERMAL-EPIDERMAL BMZ

Integrins are a large family of heterodimeric receptor molecules comprised of transmembrane α and β subunits that are receptors for cell adhesion to the extracellular matrix or to other cells.[49,50] Integrin expression is normally restricted to the basal, proliferative cell layers of the epidermis and keratinocytes.

The two main integrins of the dermal-epidermal BMZ are $\alpha6\beta4$ and $\alpha3\beta1$. These integrins are abundant in keratinocytes and function as cell adhesion receptors for laminin-332. Both $\alpha6\beta4$ and $\alpha3\beta1$ are important for maintaining the integrity of the epidermis. Ablation in mice of either of the two integrins through null mutations resulted in epidermal blistering of varying intensity. Even in the absence of $\alpha6\beta4$ and $\alpha3\beta1$, however, the keratinocytes retained their capacity to proliferate in the epidermis, and epidermal stratification and differentiation was normal before blister formation. These results suggested that the integrins are not essential for epidermal morphogenesis during skin development.[51]

Despite their shared functions as receptors for laminin-332, α6β4 and α3β1 integrins are recruited to different cell adhesion structures. It is important to address the functions of the two integrins separately.

α6β4 Integrin

α6β4 Integrin is an essential component of the hemidesmosome,[52] multiprotein adhesion complexes that promote cell-substrate adhesion in stratified and complex epithelia. It has been shown to be important in assembly of hemidesmosomes; mutating the phosphorylation of the β4 integrin, S(1424), resulted in a gradual disassembly of the hemidesmosomes.[52] The extracellular domains of the α6β4 subunits combine together to form a ligand-binding site, whereas the intracellular domains interact with other hemidesmosomal components. The β4 integrin is only known to combine with the α6 subunit, whereas the α6 subunit can combine with either β4 or β1 subunits.[53] As a receptor for laminin-332, α6β4 links laminin-332 anchoring filaments outside the cell with the keratin filament inside the cell. Such laminin-332 linking abilities of α6β4 integrin allow it to determine the organization of laminin-332, thereby to regulate keratinocyte adhesion, motility, and proliferation.[21,54] One possible mechanism by which this happens is through β4 signaling that results in laminin-332–dependent nuclear entry of mitogen-activated protein kinases and NF-kappaB.[55]

Deficiency or defects in α6β4 leads to epidermal diseases. Patients with mutations in the hemidesmosomal genes ITGA6 and ITGB4, which encode the α6 and β4 polypeptides, respectively, present with EB with pyloric atresia (EB-PA).[56] The level of separation in this disease is often just above the plasma membrane, with characteristic small fragments of the basal keratinocyte plasma membrane remaining attached to the dermal side of the separation. This level of split, termed "hemidesmosomal" EB[57] (see **Fig. 3**), is not one of the three recognized major levels of separation listed in a recent EB consensus.[58] Nonetheless, it can be a useful feature to appreciate in making the ultrastructural diagnosis of EB. EB-PA is an autosomal-recessive disorder characterized clinically by mucocutaneous fragility and gastrointestinal atresia, which affects the pylorus. Additional complications include involvement of the urogenital tract, aplasia cutis, and failure to thrive. Prognosis of patients varies, although most affected patients die in infancy.[56,59] Recent immunofluorescence analysis of villous trophoblasts reported seven previously unreported mutations in the α6β4 integrin genes in 19 pregnancy cases of PA-JEB, suggesting potential mechanisms for prenatal screening of this deadly disease.[60]

α3β1 Integrin

In contrast to α6β4 integrin, α3β1 integrin is recruited to focal contacts in keratinocytes and other cells in culture. It thereby links the extracellular matrix to components of actin cytoskeleton.[61] Similar to α6β4 integrin, α3β1 activates distinct signal transduction pathways, resulting in tyrosine phosphorylation of various cellular proteins, and activation of Rac 1.[62] One unique characteristic of α3β1 is that only α3β1-dependent adhesion of laminin-332 is dependent on Rap1. This result provides evidence for a functional of camp-Epac-Rap1 pathway in cell adhesion and spreading.[63]

α3β1 Integrin may also play a role in certain disease states. Recently, it was shown that epithelial cell α3β1 integrin links β-catenin and Smad signaling, which contribute to myofibroblast formation, and ultimately pulmonary fibrosis.[64] It is also involved in metastasis of cancer and human development (discussed later).

KERATIN LINKERS OF THE DERMAL-EPIDERMAL BMZ
Bullous Pemphigoid Antigen 1 (BPAG1/BP230)

Bullous pemphigoid antigen I (BPAG1) is a component of hemidesmosomes, multiprotein adhesion complexes that promote cell-substrate adhesion in stratified and complex epithelia. Molecular biologic studies indicated that the epidermal isoform of BPAG1 (BPAG1-e), a 230-kd protein, has cytoskeletal linker properties.[65,66] The amino (N) terminal head domain is homologous to that of other plakin family members (hence called the "plakin domain"), and the carboxy (C) terminus consists of two homologous repeats and has been proposed to be an intermediate filament-binding domain.[67–70] BPAG1 localizes to the inner plate on the cytoplasmic surface of the hemidesmosome and functions in the connection between hemidesmosomes and intermediate filaments. In 2000, a yeast two-hybrid screen was performed to identify the specific proteins that interact with the N terminus of human BPAG1-e. This yeast hybrid screen uncovered a protein belonging to the LAP/LERP protein family with 16 N-terminal leucine-rich repeats and a C-terminal PDZ domain. This protein, ERBIN, was shown to interact with not only BPAG1-e, but also with the

C-terminus of the cytoplasmic domain of integrin β4 subunit. ERBIN was subsequently shown to be expressed in keratinocytes.[71]

In a study by Guo and colleagues,[72] it was shown that in BPAG1 negative transgenic mice that lacked the connection between hemidesmosomes and intermediate filaments, neither hemidesmosome stability nor cell substratum adhesion was weakened. BPAG1-e does not seem vital for hemidesmosome or BMZ assembly. Nonetheless, BPAG1-e has been shown to be involved in various diseases. It is a major protein targeted by autoantigens in patients with bullous pemphigoid, a subepidermal blistering disease first described by Lever in 1953.[52,73,74] It has also been reported as an autoantigen in patients with paraneoplastic pemphigus, an autoimmune bullous skin disease induced by underlying malignant or benign neoplasias. Clinical symptoms of paraneoplastic pemphigus are variable, ranging from polymorphous blistering skin eruptions to severe, painful mucocutaneous ulcerations.[75] There have been recent reports that BPAG1-e expression may be decreased in patients with dermatitis herpetiformis vulnerable to blistering, but further investigation is necessary to characterize the nature of this deficit.[76]

Plectin

Plectin is a 450- to 500-kd cytoskeletal linker protein of 200 nm in length. It is widely distributed in a variety of stratified epithelia, muscle, and brain.[76,77] In many tissues, plectin interacts with various cytoskeletal structures including actin microfilaments; intermediate filaments (keratin, desmin, vimentin); or microtubules.[78] In skin, plectin links kertain intermediate filaments to the transmembrane collagen XVII[79] and α6β4 integrin in the hemidesmosomes.[80,81] More specifically, its interaction with integrin α6β4 is essential for the assembly and stability of hemidesmosomes. Recent investigations in the resolution of the primary α6β4-plectin complex showed that a major rearrangement of the β4 moiety follows the binding of the integrin with plectin, promoting stable adhesion or cell migration and an allosteric control of the integrin.[82]

Patients with genetic defects in the epidermal expression of plectin form the basis of at least three disease subtypes: (1) a rare, mild form of dominant EB simplex (EBS) with mottled pigmentation[83,84]; (2) a severe recessive form of EB associated with PA and loss of skin[56]; and (3) a recessive form of EBS associated with muscular dystrophy.[60,85,86] Of these diseases, the EBS associated with muscular dystrophy is the major one caused by plectin deficiency. In EBS associated with muscular dystrophy, plectin defects have been implicated to affect plasma membrane-cytoskeletal interactions in skin and muscle, thereby leading to epidermal blistering and muscle weakness.[60,85] Even though classified as EBS, plectin deficiency usually produces a hemidesmosomal level of skin separation similar to that seen in the JEB subtype EP-PA described previously.[57] When mutational analysis and immunohistochemistry were performed on EBS associated with muscular dystrophy and control skeletal muscle, a novel homozygous plectin-exon32 rod domain mutation (R2465X) was revealed.[85]

COLLAGENS OF THE DERMAL-EPIDERMAL BMZ
Type XVII Collagen (BPAG2/BP180)

Type XVII collagen (BPAG2 or BP180) is a 180-kd, transmembrane component of the dermal-epidermal anchoring complex, which projects beneath hemidesmosomes to mediate the adhesion of epidermal keratinocytes and other epithelial cells to the underlying BMZs.[87] Recent molecular studies indicated that BPAG2 consists of 1532 amino acids, of which 1000 residues form a large extracellular carboxy-terminus extracellular domain, containing 15 collagenous domains.[88,89] The extracellular portion of BPAG2 is constitutively shed from cell surface by ADAMs (proteinases that contain adhesive and metalloprotease domains).[90,91]

BPAG2 is involved in various human diseases of the dermal-epidermal junction, in which it is either generally defective or absent. Absence of type XVII collagen has been demonstrated[92] in a form of nonlethal JEB termed "generalized atrophic benign EB."[93,94] These patients exhibit a nonscarring alopecia (see **Fig. 3**) and extensive cutaneous blistering; however, mucosal blistering is not as pronounced as it is in the more severe JEB subtypes. Interestingly, revertant mosaicism of the COL17A1 gene occurs in some generalized atrophic benign EB patients.[95,96] Autoantibodies against BPAG2 are seen in bullous pemphigoid, pemphigoid gestations mucous membrane pemphigoid, linear IgA disease, lichen planus pemphigoides, and pemphigoid nodularis.[73,87,97–103]

Type VII Collagen

Type VII collagen is a large protein 426 nm in length,[104] and is the main constituent of anchoring fibrils that are observed beneath the lamina densa.[105,106] Like all collagens, type VII collagen assembles into a triple helix, and requires sufficient ascorbic acid as a cofactor for the enzyme prolyl hydroxylase to properly convert certain prolines to hydroxyproline, which is necessary for collagen molecular stability.[107] Analysis of the deduced amino acid sequence of type VII collagen[108] revealed the presence of a long central collagenous region characterized by repeating Gly-X-Y sequences that contain a number of non-collagenous interruptions, including a 39 amino acid noncollagenous segment in the center of the helix.[109] Although it is initially secreted as a single triple helical molecule consisting of three chains, type VII collagen mostly exists as an antiparallel dimer, consisting of two triple helices joined by tail-to-tail carboxy-terminal overlap at the NC2 domains. The dimers then aggregate to form the anchoring fibril of 785 nm in length.[104,106] The group of C-proteinases including BMP-1 and mammalian Tolloid, discussed in conjunction with laminin processing previously, also process type VII collagen in the NC2 region,[110] which seems to facilitate antiparallel dimer formation. Type VII collagen is critical for the integrity of the epidermal-dermal junction through its ability to bind laminin-332, as discussed previously. Type VII collagen has the ability to intertwine between interstitial collagen fibrils, and to act as a purse-string to attach the lamina densa to the papillary dermis. In vitro binding studies demonstrated that a von Willebrand factor–like motif is essential for binding of type VII collagen to collagen fibrils.[111]

The importance of type VII collagen in maintaining the cohesion of the dermal-epidermal BMZ is demonstrated by its absence or by its functional defects because of underlying gene mutations in inherited blistering diseases collectively known as "dystrophic" EB (DEB), which is characterized by a sublamina densa level of skin separation (see **Fig. 3**). Type VII collagen defects have been shown to cause both dominant and recessive DEB, and hundreds of mutations have been identified and reported.[112] These distinct, dystrophic forms of DEB show considerable phenotypic variability. Recently, a mutation analysis on approximately 1000 families with different forms of EB suggested a possible phenotype-genotype correlation in the dystrophic subtypes, providing the basis for more accurate genetic counseling and prenatal diagnosis for at-risk families.[112] Additional future studies will cast more light on the use of phenotype-genotype correlations in DEB.

Many studies are being conducted not only to characterize type VII collagen defects in DEB, but also to investigate possible therapies for DEB patients. Protein-based therapies have been a topic of much investigation. There is some evidence that intradermal injection of recombinant human type VII collagen can restore collagen function in murine models.[113,114] Mice receiving protein therapy showed decreased skin fragility, reduced new blister formation, and markedly prolonged survival. These promising results carry implications for the future of DEB treatment strategies. As a therapy with a more long-term corrective potential, type VII collagen gene delivery either to keratinocytes or fibroblasts has proved successful in reducing the blistering phenotype in a number of preclinical studies.[115–118]

One interesting fact about patients with recessive DEB is that they often have epidermal cancers. Such predisposition arises from the fact that type VII collagen defects also lead to epidermal carcinogenesis. The relationship between type VII collagen defects and cancer is discussed later.

UBIQUITOUS COMPONENTS OF THE DERMAL-EPIDERMAL BMZ

All dermal-epidermal BMZs contain some type of laminin, collagen IV, nidogen, and perlecan, a large heparin sulfate proteoglycan.[119] These ubiquitous components of the BMZ are important players in the assembly and stability of the BMZ. It further seems that these molecules are intricately linked to determine each other's role in the BMZ, thereby challenging some of the classical views of BMZ assembly. For example, nidogens have been touted for a long time as key contributors to BMZ formation. Recent findings suggest, however, that even in the absence of nidogens, the deposition of laminin, collagen IV, and perlecan occurs, allowing for the formation of the BMZ. For example, it was shown to be the skin composition of laminin that determines whether nidogens are required for BMZ assembly and stabilization.[120] Similarly, in a recent drosophila study, it was shown that preinvasive polar cells undergo an asymmetric apical capping consisting of two collagen IV α chains, laminin A and perlecan. Such synergistic capping allowed for the transcytosis mechanism of the polar cells.[121] Interestingly, it is now also believed that although perlecan is necessary for organization and stratification of the epidermis, it is not required for the lining and deposition of major BMZ components or the distribution of integrin subunits.[122]

Recent evidence on these ubiquitous components suggests that these players act in concert, to establish and maintain the integrity of the dermal-epidermal BMZ. With improvements in molecular techniques, pre-existing dogma on the BMZ molecules is being challenged and will continue to be challenged. Nonetheless, it is worthwhile to appreciate the intricate interplay between the BMZ components, and to realize that disease states arise not from absence of one particular molecule, but rather from an interruption of the balance of many key players.

BMZ IN CANCER

The importance and ubiquity of BMZ can be appreciated by acknowledging its contribution to various human diseases. This section seeks to address a few of the ways by which BMZ constituents play into pathophysiology of cancer.

The BMZ laminin proteins are important regulators of cancer progression. Many studies have examined the role of laminin-332 as a regulator of cancer invasion. Laminin-332 was shown to be highly expressed in various squamous and other epithelial tumors, including cutaneous, oral, esophageal, laryngeal, tracheal, cervical, and colon carcinomas. In these tumors, laminin-332 often is noted to accumulate at the interface of the tumor with the surrounding stroma. Laminin-332 expression has been shown to correlate well with tumor invasiveness, and poor patient prognosis in various squamous cell carcinoma (SCC) subtypes.[13,123–134] Such a role of laminin-332 in various human cancers is a topic of great investigation. In recent studies targeting a tumor-specific, laminin-332 domain has shown induction of SCC tumor apoptosis, decreased SCC tumor proliferation, and markedly impaired SCC tumorigenesis in vivo.[135] It has further been shown that N-glycosylation of laminin-332 may regulate the protein's biologic function, implicating potential therapeutic strategies for various types of cancer.[136] Although laminin-332 has been the more widely studied laminin in cancer, recent evidence supports a tumor-derived laminin-511 in metastatic progression of breast cancer.[137] It has been shown that laminin-511 provides a proliferative signal for neonatal foreskin keratinocytes, adult breast skin keratinocytes, and a human papillomavirus type-18 transformed tumorigenic keratinocyte cell line in vitro, suggesting that such proliferation may be the mechanism by which laminin-511 contributes to cancer metastasis.[31]

Intricately associated with the expression of laminins-332 and -511 are the expression of their integrins. The expression of the $\alpha6\beta4$ integrin is associated with poor patient prognosis and reduced survival in a variety of human cancers including carcinomas and breast cancer.[138] It has been shown that $\alpha6\beta4$ promotes carcinoma progression by contributing to the evasion of apoptosis, invasion, and metastasis of cancer cells. One proposed mechanism for such a role is through the expression of specific, cancer-promoting genes. Thus far, 538 genes have been identified whose expression is controlled by $\alpha6\beta4$, and of these genes, 36 have been directly linked to pathways implicated in cell motility and metastasis. One such gene is the S100A4/metastasin, whose expression is well correlated with integrin $\alpha6\beta4$ expression.[139] One proposed mechanism by which the integrin participates in such pathways is by Y1494, a tyrosine residue in the $\beta4$ subunit of the cytoplasmic domain.[138] To transduce intracellular signals, however, coexpression of other factors, such as neuroepithelioma transforming gene 1 (Net1), has been shown to be important.[140] Future studies on the morphologic and functional properties of $\alpha6\beta4$ integrin will provide more evidence to elucidate the role of $\alpha6\beta4$ and its ligand laminin-332 in cancer progression, and potential therapeutic interventions.

Although $\alpha6\beta4$ is certainly the more widely studied integrin in cancer, various studies have characterized the role of $\alpha3\beta1$ integrin in contributing to tumor metastasis. Recent work done by Kremser and colleagues[141] suggests that the $\alpha3\beta1$ integrin possessed heavily sialylated and fucosylated glycans, which may contribute to migration of melanoma.

Efforts to study carcinogenic roles of type VII collagen stemmed from the observation that recessive DEB, a blistering skin disorder that arises from defects in type VII collagen, is often accompanied by SCCs. Type VII collagen seems to act on tumorigenesis by its amino-terminal non-collagenous domain, NC1. Using a well-characterized in vivo model of human SCC tumorigenesis, forced NC1 expression was able to restore tumorigenicity to type VII collagen-null epidermis, and fibronectin-like sequences within NC1 promoted tumor cell invasion in laminin-332–dependent manner.[142] Hence, it was shown that retention of NC1 sequences in a subset of recessive DEB patients may contribute to their increased susceptibility to SCC.

Deletion of the type VII collagen NC1 binding site on laminin-332's $\beta3$ chain, in the region of domain V-III, also led to a lack of human SCC tumorigenesis in vivo.[124] These studies suggest that type VII collagen NC1 domain contributions to SCC tumorigenesis take place through its interaction with laminin-332. Inhibition of normal and EB keratinocyte derived SCC tumors in vivo by laminin-332[135,143] or type VII collagen[142] antibodies further illustrates the role these molecules seem to play in human SCC.

Although these mechanisms certainly seem applicable to many SCCs, it should be noted that mutational activation of genes upstream from extracellular matrix–induced signaling has the potential to modify a given tumor's extracellular matrix requirements. For example, overexpression of an activated mutant catalytic subunit of phosphatidyl-3 kinase restored SCC tumorigenesis from RDEB cells lacking type VII collagen and from JEB cells lacking the type VII collagen-binding domain on laminin-332.[124]

This could help explain the observation that although approximately three quarters of SCCs show moderate to high level of laminin-332 expression, about one quarter do not.[135,144] Also, although three quarters of RDEB patients with SCC show type VII collagen NC1 expression, at least two RDEB patients with SCC lack detectable type VII collagen NC1.[145] Although BMZ inhibition as an approach to cancer therapy depends on identification of the most effective protein targets,[13] identification of the most responsive patient population for these targeted therapies is an equally important consideration.

BMZ IN SKIN DEVELOPMENT

The BMZ proteins, particularly the laminins, have been widely studied for their role in development. The structure and composition of both laminins and the BMZ seem to be critical for embryogenesis. In a targeted mutation analysis, laminin-111–deficient mouse embryos died within a day of implantation. Likewise, when composition of the BMZ was disturbed, the experimental mice were halted in their embryonic development.[146]

Not all laminins display morphogenic properties. For example, although lack of laminin-332 in Herlitz JEB results in extensive blistering, no developmental abnormalities aside from pitting of dental enamel have been described in these patients.[147] In contrast, laminin-511 mice, despite having little or no blistering, nonetheless display a myriad of developmental abnormalities including lack of neural tube formation; exencephaly; syndactyly; and kidney, lung, and heart defects.[32] These findings illustrate the divergent roles individual members of the laminin family play with respect to structure, distribution, and especially function.

Laminin-511 plays a critical role in the skin in the area of hair follicle development because transgenic mice lacking laminin-511 showed an arrest of hair development at the hair derm stage.[148] Interestingly, absence of laminin-511's main receptor, $\alpha3\beta1$ integrin, in transgenic mice produced a similar arrest of hair development.[149] Interesting, it was shown that a single application of purified laminin-511 to laminin-511 null skin was sufficient to restore hair formation.[148] Similarly, postnatal hair follicle culture studies have shown that laminin-511–rich human placental laminin enhanced hair growth.[150] Even though it is an epithelially derived product, laminin-511's main role in hair formation seems to be on dermal papilla development and function. Antibody-induced inhibition of laminin-511 or its integrin receptor in human skin xenografts caused a complete loss of appendageal structures, a hallmark of the type of permanent hair loss seen in scarring.[148] Although laminin-511 has been mainly studied for its ability to maintain the dermal papilla of skin, it is possible that its effects on mesenchymal stem cells may extend outside the skin to other organs. In addition to its role as a potential target of therapy for hair disorders, a cause of significant morbidity and emotional distress in approximately half of Americans by the age of 50,[151] its possible that laminin-511 could serve a broader role in tissue regeneration of other organs. These are important studies to address in the future.

REFERENCES

1. Taniguchi Y, Ido H, Sanzen N, et al. The carboxyl-terminal region of laminin beta chains modulates the integrin binding affinities of laminins. J Biol Chem 2009;284:7820–31.
2. Aumailley M, Bruckner-Tuderman L, Carter WG, et al. A simplified laminin nomenclature. Matrix Biol 2005;24(5):326–32.
3. Nguyen N, Senior R. Laminin isoforms and lung development: all isoforms are not equal. Dev Biol 2006;294(2):271–9.
4. Miyazaki K. Laminin-5 (laminin-332): unique biological activity and role in tumor growth and invasion. Cancer Sci 2006;97(2):91–8.
5. Colognato H, Yurchenco PD. Form and function: the laminin family of heterotrimers. Dev Dyn 2000; 218(2):213–34.
6. Ido H, Ito S, Taniguchi Y, et al. Laminin isoforms containing the gamma3 chain are unable to bind to integrins due to the absence of the glutamic acid residue conserved in the C-terminal regions of the gamma1 and gamma2 chains. J Biol Chem 2008;283(42):28149–57.
7. Ido H, Nakamura A, Kobayashi R, et al. The requirement of the glutamic acid residue at the third position from the carboxyl termini of the laminin gamma chains in integrin binding by laminins. J Biol Chem 2007;282(15):11144–54.
8. Veitch DP, Nokelainen P, McGowan KA, et al. Mammalian tolloid metalloproteinase, and not matrix metalloprotease 2 or membrane type 1 metalloprotease, processes laminin-5 in keratinocytes and skin. J Biol Chem 2003;278(18):15661–8.
9. Amano S, Scott IC, Takahara K, et al. Bone morphogenetic protein 1 is an extracellular processing

enzyme of the laminin 5 gamma 2 chain. J Biol Chem 2000;275(30):22728–35.

10. Goldfinger LE, Stack MS, Jones JC. Processing of laminin-5 and its functional consequences: role of plasmin and tissue-type plasminogen activator. J Cell Biol 1998;141(1):255–65.

11. Sigle RO, Gil SG, Bhattacharya M, et al. Globular domains 4/5 of the laminin alpha3 chain mediate deposition of precursor laminin 5. J Cell Sci 2004; 117(Pt 19):4481–94.

12. Giannelli G, Falk-Marzillier J, Schiraldi O, et al. Induction of cell migration by matrix metalloprotease-2 cleavage of laminin-5. Science 1997; 277(5323):225–8.

13. Marinkovich MP. Tumour microenvironment: laminin 332 in squamous-cell carcinoma. Nat Rev Cancer 2007;7(5):370–80.

14. Margadant C, Raymond K, Kreft M, et al. Integrin {alpha}3{beta}1 inhibits directional migration and wound re-epithelialization in the skin. J Cell Sci 2009;122(Pt 2):278–88.

15. Nakashima Y, Kariya Y, Miyazaki K. The beta3 chain short arm of laminin-332 (laminin-5) induces matrix assembly and cell adhesion activity of laminin-511 (laminin-10). J Cell Biochem 2007;100(3): 545–56.

16. Xia Y, Gil SG, Carter WG. Anchorage mediated by integrin alpha6beta4 to laminin 5 (epiligrin) regulates tyrosine phosphorylation of a membrane-associated 80-kD protein. J Cell Biol 1996;132(4): 727–40.

17. Carter WG, Kaur P, Gil SG, et al. Distinct functions for integrins alpha 3 beta 1 in focal adhesions and alpha 6 beta 4/bullous pemphigoid antigen in a new stable anchoring contact (SAC) of keratinocytes: relation to hemidesmosomes. J Cell Biol 1990;111(6 Pt 2):3141–54.

18. Tang J, Wu YM, Zhao P, et al. {beta}ig-h3 Interacts with {alpha}3{beta}1 integrin to promote adhesion and migration of human hepatoma cells. Exp Biol Med (Maywood) 2009;234(1):35–9.

19. Campbell ID. Studies of focal adhesion assembly. Biochem Soc Trans 2008;36(Pt 2):263–6.

20. Litjens S, de Pereda J, Sonnenberg A. Current insights into the formation and breakdown of hemidesmosomes. Trends Cell Biol 2006;16:376–83.

21. Geuijen CA, Sonnenberg A. Dynamics of the alpha6beta4 integrin in keratinocytes. Mol Biol Cell 2002;13(11):3845–58.

22. Rousselle P, Keene DR, Ruggiero F, et al. Laminin 5 binds the NC-1 domain of type VII collagen. J Cell Biol 1997;138(3):719–28.

23. Chen M, Marinkovich M, Veis A, et al. Interactions of the amino-terminal noncollagenous (NC1) domain of type VII collagen with extracellular matrix components: a potential role in epidermal-dermal adherence in human skin. J Biol Chem 1997; 272(23):14516–22.

24. Chen M, Marinkovich MP, Jones JC, et al. NC1 domain of type VII collagen binds to the beta3 chain of laminin 5 via a unique subdomain within the fibronectin-like repeats. J Invest Dermatol 1999;112(2):177–83.

25. Spirito F, Capt A, Del Rio M, et al. Sustained phenotypic reversion of junctional epidermolysis bullosa dog keratinocytes: establishment of an immunocompetent animal model for cutaneous gene therapy. Biochem Biophys Res Commun 2006; 339(3):769–78.

26. Marinkovich MP, Verrando P, Keene DR, et al. The basement membrane proteins kalinin and nicein are structurally and immunologically identical. Lab Invest 1993;69:295–9.

27. Meneguzzi G, Marinkovich MP, Aberdam D, et al. Kalinin is abnormally expressed in epithelial basement membranes of Herlitz's junctional epidermolysis bullosa patients. Exp Dermatol 1992;1(5): 221–9.

28. Igoucheva O, Kelly A, Uitto J, et al. Protein therapeutics for junctional epidermolysis bullosa: incorporation of recombinant beta3 chain into laminin 332 in beta3-/- keratinocytes in vitro. J Invest Dermatol 2008;128(6):1476–86.

29. Nakano A, Chao SC, Pulkkinen L, et al. Laminin 5 mutations in junctional epidermolysis bullosa: molecular basis of Herlitz vs. non-Herlitz phenotypes. Hum Genet 2002;110(1):41–51.

30. Mavilio F, Pellegrini G, Ferrari S, et al. Correction of junctional epidermolysis bullosa by transplantation of genetically modified epidermal stem cells. Nat Med 2006;12(12):1397–402.

31. Pouliot N, Saunders NA, Kaur P. Laminin 10/11: an alternative adhesive ligand for epidermal keratinocytes with a functional role in promoting proliferation and migration. Exp Dermatol 2002;11(5): 387–97.

32. Miner J, Lewis R, Sanes J. Molecular cloning of a novel laminin chain, alpha 5, and widespread expression in adult mouse tissues. J Biol Chem 1995;270(48):28523–6.

33. Makino M, Okazaki I, Kasai S, et al. Identification of cell binding sites in the laminin alpha5-chain G domain. Exp Cell Res 2002;277(1):95–106.

34. Miner JH, Patton BL, Lentz SI, et al. The laminin alpha chains: expression, developmental transitions, and chromosomal locations of alpha1-5, identification of heterotrimeric laminins 8-11, and cloning of a novel alpha3 isoform. J Cell Biol 1997;137(3):685–701.

35. Tiger CF, Champliaud MF, Pedrosa-Domellof F, et al. Presence of laminin alpha5 chain and lack of laminin alpha1 chain during human muscle

development and in muscular dystrophies. J Biol Chem 1997;272(45):28590–5.

36. Kikkawa Y, Sanzen N, Sekiguchi K. Isolation and characterization of laminin-10/11 secreted by human lung carcinoma cells. laminin-10/11 mediates cell adhesion through integrin alpha3 beta1. J Biol Chem 1998;273(25):15854–9.

37. Kikkawa Y, Sanzen N, Fujiwara H, et al. Integrin binding specificity of laminin-10/11: laminin-10/11 are recognized by alpha 3 beta 1, alpha 6 beta 1 and alpha 6 beta 4 integrins. J Cell Sci 2000; 113(Pt 5):869–76.

38. Yu H, Talts JF. Beta1 integrin and alpha-dystroglycan binding sites are localized to different laminin-G-domain-like (LG) modules within the laminin alpha5 chain G domain. Biochem J 2003;371(Pt 2):289–99.

39. Nielsen PK, Yamada Y. Identification of cell-binding sites on the laminin alpha 5 N-terminal domain by site-directed mutagenesis. J Biol Chem 2001; 276(14):10906–12.

40. Ido H, Harada K, Yagi Y, et al. Probing the integrin-binding site within the globular domain of laminin-511 with the function-blocking monoclonal antibody 4C7. Matrix Biol 2006;25(2):112–7.

41. Li J, Zhang YP, Kirsner RS. Angiogenesis in wound repair: angiogenic growth factors and the extracellular matrix. Microsc Res Tech 2003;60(1):107–14.

42. Marinkovich MP, Lundstrum GP, Keene DR, et al. The dermal-epidermal junction of human skin contains a novel laminin variant. J Cell Biol 1992; 119:695–703.

43. Champliaud MF, Lunstrum GP, Rousselle P, et al. Human amnion contains a novel laminin variant, laminin 7, which like laminin 6, covalently associates with laminin 5 to promote stable epithelial-stromal attachment. J Cell Biol 1996;132(6): 1189–98.

44. Hirosaki T, Tsubota Y, Kariya Y, et al. Laminin-6 is activated by proteolytic processing and regulates cellular adhesion and migration differently from laminin-5. J Biol Chem 2002;277(51):49287–95.

45. Ogawa T, Tsubota Y, Hashimoto J, et al. The short arm of laminin gamma2 chain of laminin-5 (laminin-332) binds syndecan-1 and regulates cellular adhesion and migration by suppressing phosphorylation of integrin beta4 chain. Mol Biol Cell 2007; 18(5):1621–33.

46. Bachy S, Letourneur F, Rousselle P. Syndecan-1 interaction with the LG4/5 domain in laminin-332 is essential for keratinocyte migration. J Cell Physiol 2007;214: 238–49.

47. Jones JC, Lane K, Hopkinson SB, et al. Laminin-6 assembles into multimolecular fibrillar complexes with perlecan and participates in mechanical-signal transduction via a dystroglycan-dependent, integrin-independent mechanism. J Cell Sci 2005; 118(Pt 12):2557–66.

48. Sixt M, Engelhardt B, Pausch F, et al. Endothelial cell laminin isoforms, laminins 8 and 10, play decisive roles in T cell recruitment across the blood-brain barrier in experimental autoimmune encephalomyelitis. J Cell Biol 2001;153(5):933–46.

49. Ziegler WH, Gingras AR, Critchley DR, et al. Integrin connections to the cytoskeleton through talin and vinculin. Biochem Soc Trans 2008;36(Pt 2): 235–9.

50. Pawar SC, Demetriou MC, Nagle RB, et al. Integrin alpha6 cleavage: a novel modification to modulate cell migration. Exp Cell Res 2007;313(6):1080–9.

51. DiPersio CM, van der Neut R, Georges-Labouesse E, et al. Alpha3beta1 and alpha6beta4 integrin receptors for laminin-5 are not essential for epidermal morphogenesis and homeostasis during skin development. J Cell Sci 2000;113(Pt 17): 3051–62.

52. Germain EC, Santos TM, Rabinovitz I. Phosphorylation of a novel site on the {beta}4 integrin at the trailing edge of migrating cells promotes hemidesmosome disassembly. Mol Biol Cell 2009;20(1): 56–67.

53. Askari JA, Buckley PA, Mould AP, et al. Linking integrin conformation to function. J Cell Sci 2009; 122(Pt 2):165–70.

54. Sehgal BU, DeBiase PJ, Matzno S, et al. Integrin beta4 regulates migratory behavior of keratinocytes by determining laminin-332 organization. J Biol Chem 2006;281(46):35487–98.

55. Nikolopoulos SN, Blaikie P, Yoshioka T, et al. Targeted deletion of the integrin beta4 signaling domain suppresses laminin-5-dependent nuclear entry of mitogen-activated protein kinases and NF-kappaB, causing defects in epidermal growth and migration. Mol Cell Biol 2005;25(14):6090–102.

56. Pfendner E, Uitto J. Plectin gene mutations can cause epidermolysis bullosa with pyloric atresia. J Invest Dermatol 2005;124(1):111–5.

57. Smith LT. Ultrastructural findings in epidermolysis bullosa. Arch Dermatol 1993;129(12):1578–84.

58. Fine JD, Eady RA, Bauer EA, et al. The classification of inherited epidermolysis bullosa (EB): report of the Third International Consensus Meeting on Diagnosis and Classification of EB. J Am Acad Dermatol 2008;58(6):931–50.

59. Ashton GH, Sorelli P, Mellerio JE, et al. Alpha6-beta4 integrin abnormalities in junctional epidermolysis bullosa with pyloric atresia. Br J Dermatol 2001;144(2):408–14.

60. D'Alessio M, Zambruno G, Charlesworth A, et al. Immunofluorescence analysis of villous trophoblasts: a tool for prenatal diagnosis of inherited epidermolysis bullosa with pyloric atresia. J Invest Dermatol 2008;128:2815–9.

61. DiPersio CM, Hodivala-Dilke KM, Jaenisch R, et al. Alpha3beta1 Integrin is required for normal

development of the epidermal basement membrane. J Cell Biol 1997;137(3):729–42.

62. Choma DP, Pumiglia K, DiPersio CM. Integrin alpha3beta1 directs the stabilization of a polarized lamellipodium in epithelial cells through activation of Rac1. J Cell Sci 2004;117(Pt 17):3947–59.

63. Enserink JM, Price LS, Methi T, et al. The cAMP-Epac-Rap1 pathway regulates cell spreading and cell adhesion to laminin-5 through the alpha3beta1 integrin but not the alpha6beta4 integrin. J Biol Chem 2004;279(43):44889–96.

64. Kim KK, Wei Y, Szekeres C, et al. Epithelial cell alpha3beta1 integrin links beta-catenin and Smad signaling to promote myofibroblast formation and pulmonary fibrosis. J Clin Invest 2009;119(1):213–24.

65. Aizu T, Tamai K, Nakano H, et al. Calcineurin/NFAT-dependent regulation of 230-kDa bullous pemphigoid antigen (BPAG1) gene expression in normal human epidermal keratinocytes. J Dermatol Sci 2008;51(1):45–51.

66. Kaneko T, Tamai K, Matsuzaki Y, et al. Interferon-gamma down-regulates expression of the 230-kDa bullous pemphigoid antigen gene (BPAG1) in epidermal keratinocytes via novel chimeric sequences of ISRE and GAS. Exp Dermatol 2006;15(4):308–14.

67. Leung CL, Zheng M, Prater SM, et al. The BPAG1 locus: alternative splicing produces multiple iso-forms with distinct cytoskeletal linker domains, including predominant isoforms in neurons and muscles. J Cell Biol 2001;154(4):691–7.

68. Tang HY, Chaffotte AF, Thacher SM. Structural analysis of the predicted coiled-coil rod domain of the cytoplasmic bullous pemphigoid antigen (BPAG1): empirical localization of the N-terminal globular domain-rod boundary. J Biol Chem 1996;271(16):9716–22.

69. Tamai K, Silos SA, Li K, et al. Tissue-specific expression of the 230-kDa bullous pemphigoid antigen gene (BPAG1): identification of a novel ker-atinocyte regulatory cis-element KRE3. J Biol Chem 1995;270(13):7609–14.

70. Sawamura DK, Li K, Chu M-L, et al. Human bullous pemphigoid antigen (BPAG1): amino acid sequence deduced from cloned cDNAs predicts biologically important peptide segments and protein domains. J Biol Chem 1991;266:17784–90.

71. Favre B, Fontao L, Koster J, et al. The hemidesmo-somal protein bullous pemphigoid antigen 1 and the integrin beta 4 subunit bind to ERBIN: molec-ular cloning of multiple alternative splice variants of ERBIN and analysis of their tissue expression. J Biol Chem 2001;276(35):32427–36.

72. Guo L, Degenstein L, Dowling J, et al. Gene target-ing of BPAG1: abnormalities in mechanical strength

and cell migration in stratified epithelia and neuro-logic degeneration. Cell 1995;81(2):233–43.

73. Iwata Y, Komura K, Kodera M, et al. Correlation of IgE autoantibody to BP180 with a severe form of bullous pemphigoid. Arch Dermatol 2008;144(1):41–8.

74. Olivry T, Chan LS, Xu L, et al. Novel feline autoim-mune blistering disease resembling bullous pem-phigoid in humans: IgG autoantibodies target the NC16A ectodomain of type XVII collagen (BP180/BPAG2). Vet Pathol 1999;36(4):328–35.

75. Preisz K, Karpati S. [Paraneoplastic pemphigus]. Orv Hetil 2007;148(21):979–83.

76. Leivo T, Kiistala U, Vesterinen M, et al. Re-epitheli-alization rate and protein expression in the suction-induced wound model: comparison between intact blisters, open wounds and calcipotriol-pretreated open wounds. Br J Dermatol 2000;142(5):991–1002.

77. Pfendner E, Rouan F, Uitto J. Progress in epider-molysis bullosa: the phenotypic spectrum of plectin mutations. Exp Dermatol 2005;14(4):241–9.

78. Wiche G. Role of plectin in cytoskeleton organiza-tion and dynamics. J Cell Sci 1998;111(Pt 17):2477–86.

79. Koster J, Geerts D, Favre B, et al. Analysis of the interactions between BP180, BP230, plectin and the integrin alpha6beta4 important for hemidesmo-some assembly. J Cell Sci 2003;116(Pt 2):387–99.

80. Litjens SH, Wilhelmsen K, de Pereda JM, et al. Modelling and experimental validation of the binary complex of the plectin actin-binding domain and the first pair of fibronectin type III (FNIII) domains of the {beta}4 Integrin. J Biol Chem 2005;280(23):22270–7.

81. Koster J, van Wilpe S, Kuikman I, et al. Role of binding of plectin to the integrin beta4 subunit in the assembly of hemidesmosomes. Mol Biol Cell 2004;15(3):1211–23.

82. de Pereda JM, Lillo MP, Sonnenberg A. Structural basis of the interaction between integrin alpha6-beta4 and plectin at the hemidesmosomes. EMBO J 2009;28:1180–90.

83. Koss-Harnes D, Hoyheim B, Anton-Lamprecht I, et al. A site-specific plectin mutation causes domi-nant epidermolysis bullosa simplex Ogna: two identical de novo mutations. J Invest Dermatol 2002;118(1):87–93.

84. Koss-Harnes D, Jahnsen FL, Wiche G, et al. Plectin abnormality in epidermolysis bullosa simplex Ogna: non-responsiveness of basal keratinocytes to some anti-rat plectin antibodies. Exp Dermatol 1997;6(1):41–8.

85. McMillan JR, Akiyama M, Rouan F, et al. Plectin defects in epidermolysis bullosa simplex with muscular dystrophy. Muscle Nerve 2007;35(1):24–35.

86. Schara U, Tucke J, Mortier W, et al. Severe mucous membrane involvement in epidermolysis bullosa simplex with muscular dystrophy due to a novel plectin gene mutation. Eur J Pediatr 2004; 163(4-5):218–22.

87. Powell A, Sakuma-Oyama Y, Oyama N, et al. Collagen XVII/BP180: a collagenous transmembrane protein and component of the dermoepidermal anchoring complex. Clin Exp Dermatol 2005; 30(6):682–7.

88. Giudice GJ, Emery DJ, Zelickson BD, et al. Bullous pemphigoid and herpes gestationis autoantibodies recognize a common non-collagenous site on the BP180 ectodomain. J Immunol 1993;151(10): 5742–50.

89. Gatalica B, Pulkkinen L, Li KH, et al. Cloning of the human type XVII collagen gene (COL17A1), and detection of novel mutations in generalized atrophic benign epidermolysis bullosa. Am J Hum Genet 1997;60(2):352–65.

90. Franzke CW, Tasanen K, Borradori L, et al. Shedding of collagen XVII/BP180: structural motifs influence cleavage from cell surface. J Biol Chem 2004; 279(23):24521–9.

91. Franzke CW, Tasanen K, Schacke H, et al. Transmembrane collagen XVII, an epithelial adhesion protein, is shed from the cell surface by ADAMs. EMBO J 2002;21(19):5026–35.

92. Jonkman MF, de Jong MC, Heeres K, et al. Generalized atrophic benign epidermolysis bullosa: either 180-kd bullous pemphigoid antigen or laminin-5 deficiency. Arch Dermatol 1996;132(2): 145–50.

93. Hintner H, Wolff K. Generalized atrophic benign epidermolysis bullosa. Arch Dermatol 1982; 118(6):375–84.

94. Hashimoto I, Schnyder UW, Anton-Lamprecht I. Epidermolysis bullosa hereditaria with junctional blistering in an adult. Dermatologica 1976;152(2): 72–86.

95. Pasmooij A, Pas H, Deviaene F, et al. Multiple correcting COL17A1 mutations in patients with revertant mosaicism of epidermolysis bullosa. Am J Hum Genet 2005;77(5):727–40.

96. Jonkman MF, Scheffer H, Stulp R, et al. Revertant mosaicism in epidermolysis bullosa caused by mitotic gene conversion. Cell 1997;88(4):543–51.

97. Song HJ, Han SH, Hong WK, et al. Paraneoplastic bullous pemphigoid: clinical disease activity correlated with enzyme-linked immunosorbent assay index for the NC16A domain of BP180. J Dermatol 2009;36(1):66–8.

98. Liu Z, Sui W, Zhao M, et al. Subepidermal blistering induced by human autoantibodies to BP180 requires innate immune players in a humanized bullous pemphigoid mouse model. J Autoimmun 2008;31(4):331–8.

99. Ishii N, Ohyama B, Yamaguchi Z, et al. IgA autoantibodies against the NC16a domain of BP180 but not 120-kDa LAD-1 detected in a patient with linear IgA disease. Br J Dermatol 2008;158(5):1151–3.

100. Desai N, Allen J, Ali I, et al. Autoantibodies to basement membrane proteins BP180 and BP230 are commonly detected in normal subjects by immunoblotting. Australas J Dermatol 2008;49(3):137–41.

101. Mulyowa G, Jaeger G, Sitaru C, et al. Scarring autoimmune bullous disease in a Ugandan patient with autoantibodies to BP180, BP230, and laminin 5. J Am Acad Dermatol 2006;54(Suppl 2):S43–6.

102. Blank M, Gisondi P, Mimouni D, et al. New insights into the autoantibody-mediated mechanisms of autoimmune bullous diseases and urticaria. Clin Exp Rheumatol 2006;24(1 Suppl 40):S20–5.

103. Zillikens D. BP180 as the common autoantigen in blistering diseases with different clinical phenotypes. Keio J Med 2002;51(1):21–8.

104. Lunstrum GP, Sakai LY, Keene DR, et al. Large complex globular domains of type VII procollagen contribute to the structure of anchoring fibrils. J Biol Chem 1986;261:9042–8.

105. Sesarman A, Mihai S, Chiriac MT, et al. Binding of avian IgY to type VII collagen does not activate complement and leucocytes and fails to induce subepidermal blistering in mice. Br J Dermatol 2008;158:463–71.

106. Sakai LY, Keene DR, Morris NP, et al. Type VII collagen is a major structural component of anchoring fibrils. J Cell Biol 1986;103(4):1577–86.

107. Olsen D, Yang C, Bodo M, et al. Recombinant collagen and gelatin for drug delivery. Adv Drug Deliv Rev 2003;55(12):1547–67.

108. Parente MG, Chung LC, Ryynanen J, et al. Human type VII collagen: cDNA cloning and chromosomal mapping of the gene (COL7A1) on chromosome 3 to dominant dystrophic epidermolysis bullosa. Am J Hum Genet 1991;24:119–35.

109. Bachinger HP, Morris NP, Lundstrum GP. The relationship of the biophysical and biochemical characteristics of type VII collagen to the function of anchoring fibrils. J Biol Chem 1990;265: 10095–101.

110. Rattenholl A, Pappano WN, Koch M, et al. Proteinases of the bone morphogenetic protein-1 family convert procollagen VII to mature anchoring fibril collagen. J Biol Chem 2002;277(29):26372–8.

111. Villone D, Fritsch A, Koch M, et al. Supramolecular interactions in the dermo-epidermal junction zone: anchoring fibril-collagen VII tightly binds to banded collagen fibrils. J Biol Chem 2008;283(36): 24506–13.

112. Varki R, Sadowski S, Uitto J, et al. Epidermolysis bullosa. II. Type VII collagen mutations and phenotype-genotype correlations in the dystrophic subtypes. J Med Genet 2007;44(3):181–92.

113. Remington J, Wang X, Hou Y, et al. Injection of recombinant human type VII collagen corrects the disease phenotype in a murine model of dystrophic epidermolysis bullosa. Mol Ther 2009;17(1):26–33.

114. Woodley DT, Keene DR, Atha T, et al. Injection of recombinant human type VII collagen restores collagen function in dystrophic epidermolysis bullosa. Nat Med 2004;10(7):693–5.

115. Woodley DT, Keene DR, Atha T, et al. Intradermal injection of lentiviral vectors corrects regenerated human dystrophic epidermolysis bullosa skin tissue in vivo. Mol Ther 2004;10(2):318–26.

116. Chen M, Kasahara N, Keene DR, et al. Restoration of type VII collagen expression and function in dystrophic epidermolysis bullosa. Nat Genet 2002;32(4):670–5.

117. Ortiz-Urda S, Thyagarajan B, Keene DR, et al. Stable nonviral genetic correction of inherited human skin disease. Nat Med 2002;8(10):1166–70.

118. Ortiz-Urda S, Lin Q, Green CL, et al. Injection of genetically engineered fibroblasts corrects regenerated human epidermolysis bullosa skin tissue. J Clin Invest 2003;111(2):251–5.

119. Sercu S, Zhang M, Oyama N, et al. Interaction of extracellular matrix protein 1 with extracellular matrix components: ECM1 is a basement membrane protein of the skin. J Invest Dermatol 2008;128:1397–408.

120. Mokkapati S, Baranowsky A, Mirancea N, et al. Basement membranes in skin are differently affected by lack of nidogen 1 and 2. J Invest Dermatol 2008;128:2259–67.

121. Medioni C, Noselli S. Dynamics of the basement membrane in invasive epithelial clusters in Drosophila. Development 2005;132(13):3069–77.

122. Sher I, Zisman-Rozen S, Eliahu L, et al. Targeting perlecan in human keratinocytes reveals novel roles for perlecan in epidermal formation. J Biol Chem 2006;281(8):5178–87.

123. Sugawara K, Tsuruta D, Ishii M, et al. Laminin-332 and -511 in skin. Exp Dermatol 2008;17(6):473–80.

124. Waterman EA, Sakai N, Nguyen NT, et al. A laminin-collagen complex drives human epidermal carcinogenesis through phosphoinositol-3-kinase activation. Cancer Res 2007;67(9):4264–70.

125. Mizushima H, Hirosaki T, Miyata S, et al. Expression of laminin-5 enhances tumorigenicity of human fibrosarcoma cells in nude mice. Jpn J Cancer Res 2002;93(6):652–9.

126. Mizushima H, Miyagi Y, Kikkawa Y, et al. Differential expression of laminin-5/ladsin subunits in human tissues and cancer cell lines and their induction by tumor promoter and growth factors. J Biochem 1996;120(6):1196–202.

127. Turck N, Gross I, Gendry P, et al. Laminin isoforms: biological roles and effects on the intracellular distribution of nuclear proteins in intestinal epithelial cells. Exp Cell Res 2005;303(2):494–503.

128. Katayama M, Sanzen N, Funakoshi A, et al. Laminin gamma2-chain fragment in the circulation: a prognostic indicator of epithelial tumor invasion. Cancer Res 2003;63(1):222–9.

129. Souza LF, Souza VF, Silva LD, et al. Expression of basement membrane laminin in oral squamous cell carcinomas. Braz J Otorhinolaryngol 2007;73(6):768–74.

130. Boulet GA, Schrauwen I, Sahebali S, et al. Correlation between laminin-5 immunohistochemistry and human papillomavirus status in squamous cervical carcinoma. J Clin Pathol 2007;60(8):896–901.

131. Yamamoto H, Itoh F, Iku S, et al. Expression of the gamma(2) chain of laminin-5 at the invasive front is associated with recurrence and poor prognosis in human esophageal squamous cell carcinoma. Clin Cancer Res 2001;7(4):896–900.

132. Kurokawa A, Nagata M, Kitamura N, et al. Diagnostic value of integrin alpha3, beta4, and beta5 gene expression levels for the clinical outcome of tongue squamous cell carcinoma. Cancer 2008;112:1272–81.

133. Nordemar S, Kronenwett U, Auer G, et al. Laminin-5 as a predictor of invasiveness in cancer in situ lesions of the larynx. Anticancer Res 2001;21(1B):509–12.

134. Giannelli G, Fransvea E, Bergamini C, et al. Laminin-5 chains are expressed differentially in metastatic and nonmetastatic hepatocellular carcinoma. Clin Cancer Res 2003;9(10 Pt 1):3684–91.

135. Tran M, Rousselle P, Nokelainen P, et al. Targeting a tumor-specific laminin domain critical for human carcinogenesis. Cancer Res 2008;68(8):2885–94.

136. Kariya Y, Kato R, Itoh S, et al. N-glycosylation of laminin-332 regulates its biological functions: a novel function of the bisecting GlcNAc. J Biol Chem 2008;283(48):33036–45.

137. Chia J, Kusuma N, Anderson R, et al. Evidence for a role of tumor-derived laminin-511 in the metastatic progression of breast cancer. Am J Pathol 2007;170(6):2135–48.

138. Dutta U, Shaw L. A key tyrosine (Y1494) in the {beta}4 integrin regulates multiple signaling pathways important for tumor development and progression. Cancer Res 2008;68(21):8779–87.

139. Chen M, Sinha M, Luxon BA, et al. Integrin alpha6-beta4 controls the expression of genes associated with cell motility, invasion, and metastasis, including S100A4/metastasin. J Biol Chem 2009;284(3):1484–94.

140. Gilcrease MZ, Kilpatrick SK, Woodward WA, et al. Coexpression of {alpha}6{beta}4 integrin and guanine nucleotide exchange factor net1 identifies node-positive breast cancer patients at high risk

for distant metastasis. Cancer Epidemiol Biomarkers Prev 2009;18(1):80–6.

141. Kremser ME, Przybylo M, Hoja-Lukowicz D, et al. Characterisation of alpha3beta1 and alpha(v)beta3 integrin N-oligosaccharides in metastatic melanoma WM9 and WM239 cell lines. Biochim Biophys Acta 2008;1780(12):1421–31.

142. Ortiz-Urda S, Garcia J, Green CL, et al. Type VII collagen is required for Ras-driven human epidermal tumorigenesis. Science 2005;307(5716):1773–6.

143. Dajee M, Lazarov M, Zhang JY, et al. NF-kappaB blockade and oncogenic Ras trigger invasive human epidermal neoplasia. Nature 2003; 421(6923):639–43.

144. Pyke C, Salo S, Ralfkiaer E, et al. Laminin-5 is a marker of invading cancer cells in some human carcinomas and is coexpressed with the receptor for urokinase plasminogen activator in budding cancer cells in colon adenocarcinomas. Cancer Res 1995;55(18):4132–9.

145. Pourreyron C, Cox G, Mao X, et al. Patients with recessive dystrophic epidermolysis bullosa develop squamous-cell carcinoma regardless of type VII collagen expression. J Invest Dermatol 2007;127(10):2438–44.

146. Miner JH, Li C, Mudd JL, et al. Compositional and structural requirements for laminin and basement membranes during mouse embryo implantation and gastrulation. Development 2004;131(10): 2247–56.

147. Tzu J, Marinkovich MP. Bridging structure with function: structural, regulatory, and developmental role of laminins. Int J Biochem Cell Biol 2008; 40(2):199–214.

148. Li J, Tzu J, Chen Y, et al. Laminin-10 is crucial for hair morphogenesis. EMBO J 2003;22(10):2400–10.

149. Conti FJ, Rudling RJ, Robson A, et al. alpha3beta1-integrin regulates hair follicle but not interfollicular morphogenesis in adult epidermis. J Cell Sci 2003;116(Pt 13):2737–47.

150. Sugawara K, Tsuruta D, Kobayashi H, et al. Spatial and temporal control of laminin-332(5) and -511 (10) expression during induction of anagen hair growth. J Histochem Cytochem 2007;55(1):43–55.

151. Gao J, DeRouen MC, Chen CH, et al. Laminin-511 is an epithelial message promoting dermal papilla development and function during early hair morphogenesis. Genes Dev 2008;22(15): 2111–24.

Mutation Mechanisms

Daniele Castiglia, PhD, Giovanna Zambruno, MD*

KEYWORDS

- Mendelian diseases • Inheritance patterns
- Mutation types • Epidermolysis bullosa

A mutation is an event that produces heritable changes in the DNA. There are many different types of mutations, including point mutations (changes that imply loss, duplication, or alterations of small DNA segments, often involving a single or a few nucleotides) and major DNA changes (loss, duplication, or rearrangements of entire genes or of gene segments). Each of these alterations is able to cause diseases.[1] Simple patterns of mutation inheritance are observed in Mendelian diseases, that is when a single mutated gene is involved. The mode of inheritance in Mendelian conditions, such as all inherited forms of epidermolysis bullosa (EB), depends on whether a clinical phenotype is observed in the heterozygous carrier of the mutation (dominant inheritance) or only in the homozygote subjects born of healthy parents, who are heterozygous carriers of the mutation (recessive inheritance). Both recessive and dominant inheritance may be seen for mutant genes mapping on X sex chromosome (X-linked inheritance) and on autosomes (ie, nonsex chromosomes [autosomal inheritance]).[2] Specifically, all genes involved in EB map on autosomes. The simplex (EBS) and dystrophic (DEB) EB types comprise variants with either dominant or recessive mode of inheritance; Kindler syndrome is a recessive condition, and junctional EB (JEB) is almost always recessively inherited.[3]

The pattern of inheritance can be deduced on the basis of the family history; a pedigree (ie, a graphical diagram illustrating how the disease segregates in family members) can be drawn. In the case of an autosomal-dominant condition, the pedigree will show the transmission of the trait from generation to generation, usually without skipping (vertical transmission) and with several affected members, while the trait will be rare in autosomal-recessive conditions, presenting in one or more siblings who have healthy parents and offspring. Recessive inheritance should be suspected in consanguineous kindreds.

In exceptional cases, a recessive condition can arise from reduction to homozygosity of a mutation carried by a single parent. This phenomenon results from uniparental disomy (UPD, ie, the paradoxic inheritance of two copies of a mutant allele from one parent only).[4] UPD is the result of events that operate to restore the correct chromosomal number in the embryo. Indeed, this number may become altered because of errors during meiosis and gamete maturation.[5] UPD has been documented as the cause of EB in several cases.[6,7]

Not all mutations are inherited. In some cases, a mutation can originate as a new event in the patient who will be a sporadic case of a dominant condition. However, a new mutation, also may involve germ cells in the gonad of a proband's parent who, therefore, is a healthy mosaic for the disease allele. In this instance, an increased recurrence risk for what appears to be a new dominant mutation may occur; two affected children demonstrate the presence of germline mosaicism in one of the parents.[2,8,9] In rare cases, specific types of new mutations also can result, when combined with a second inherited mutation, in a recessive condition. This can lead to diagnostic dilemmas in sporadic patients affected with diseases, such as DEB, which can be transmitted in either a dominant or recessive manner.[10] Finally, a spontaneous mutation may occur postnatally within a somatic cell of an affected patient. If this event takes place in an EB individual and leads to the correction of the primary defect caused by the inherited

---

This work was supported by grants from the Istituto Superiore di Sanità (numbers 526D/4 and E-Rare 1, acronym Kindlernet).

Laboratory of Molecular and Cell Biology, IDI-IRCCS, Via dei Monti di Creta 104, 00167 Rome, Italy
* Corresponding author.
E-mail address: g.zambruno@idi.it (G. Zambruno).

mutation (genetic reversion), then the patient shows revertant somatic mosaicism, which manifests clinically as small patches of healthy nonblistering skin where blistering is no longer inducible. Such phenotypic rescue is caused by the expansion of the reverted somatic cells and might explain some atypical phenotypes that are milder than expected. Somatic reversion events are not so rare and have been documented extensively in JEB.[11]

Mutations may alter inherited traits by affecting gene transcription, pre-mRNA splicing or protein translation, thus impacting on the expression or function of the protein product.[2]

This article reviews how different types of mutation may result in defective gene expression.

POINT MUTATIONS
Missense Mutations

Point mutations occur with the highest frequency in the human genome.[1] If codons are changed by a single nucleotide substitution, these point mutations are defined as missense mutations.[2] They directly involve crucial residues, such as at a catalytic site, or can alter the three-dimensional structure of the protein such that its function is compromised. Alternatively, they can perturb the correct assembly of protein subunits.[12,13] An EB subtype that has clearly been shown to be caused by many different missense mutations affecting a specific protein domain is dominant dystrophic EB (DDEB). Such mutations lead to glycine substitutions in the triple helix of type VII collagen encoded by the COL7A1 gene.[14,15] Type VII collagen is a trimer of identical chains [α1(VII) polypeptides].[16] Each chain is composed by a central large collagenous domain flanked by N- and C-terminal noncollagenous domains. The primary structure of the collagenous domain is remarkable, being formed, for the most of its length, by regular repeats of three amino acids, in which nearly every third residue is glycine (X-Y-Gly). Glycine is a key amino acid in this structure, because it occupies very little space and thereby allows the collagenous domain of three separate chains to come together and form a triple-stranded helical rod. Thus, a glycine substitution mutation in the α1(VII) polypeptide has a deleterious effect, because it becomes part of a triple-stranded structure, which will be partly unfolded, resulting in impaired collagen VII secretion into the extracellular matrix.[17] From a genetic point of view, the allele with the missense mutation is dominant over the normal allele. It should be kept in mind, however, that not all glycine substitutions in the triple helix of type VII collagen result in dominant

inheritance, as several of these missense mutations behave in a recessive manner.[17]

Nonsense Mutations

This type of point mutation affects protein translation via a nucleotide substitution that produces a premature termination codon (PTC) (**Fig. 1**). PTC formation results in truncated proteins, which are usually unstable and degraded.[2] PTC upstream of the penultimate exon, however, triggers a mechanism that leads to rapid degradation of the mutant transcript. This active process, called nonsense mediated mRNA decay (NMD), is evolutionary conserved and provides surveillance against faulty open reading frames (ORFs) by eliminating imperfect messages that contain PTCs and code for nonfunctional and potentially harmful polypeptides.[18] For these reasons, nonsense mutations result in recessive inheritance and are normally associated, when present in both alleles, with the most severe variants of recessive DEB (RDEB) and JEB, which are characterized by a complete loss of expression of the protein product in the skin.[19,20]

Frameshift Mutations

These are either deletions or insertions of one or a few nucleotides in the coding region of the gene (see **Fig. 1**).[2,14,15,20] These mutations change the triplet code for all codons that follow and thus completely alter the downstream protein sequence, often leading to PTC formation. Therefore, they are genetically and functionally similar to the nonsense mutations.

Splicing Mutations

RNA splicing is crucial to normal gene expression, because introns must be excised precisely from the pre-mRNA to produce a mature mRNA for translation into protein.[21] This process is performed by the spliceosome, a macromolecular apparatus endowed with the catalytic functions needed to join exons, and requires conserved sequence motifs at the intron–exon borders. These sequences are known as splice sites. The 5′ exon/intron junction is called the donor splice site, and the 3′ intron/exon junction is the acceptor splice site. The 5′ end of the intron almost invariably begins with nucleotides GU, and the 3′ end of the intron always bears the nucleotides AG. In the acceptor region, there are two other conserved elements upstream of the AG dinucleotide: the branchpoint sequence (BPS), which lies 18 to 40 bases upstream the AG, and the polypyrimidine (Py) tract placed downstream the BPS. The splicing process begins with a cut at the donor

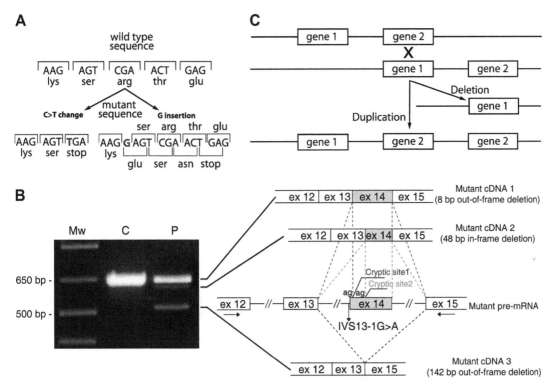

Fig. 1. Examples of different mutation types. (*A*) Point mutations. A substitution and an insertion of a single nucleotide in the coding region of a given gene are shown. Specifically, a C-to-T change involving the first nucleotide of a codon for arginine (CGA) results in a nonsense codon (TGA). The G insertion shifts the reading frame for protein translation, leading to a premature stop codon formation. (*B*) The consequences on pre-mRNA splicing of a single nucleotide substitution that involves the obligate G of an acceptor splice site are shown. Agarose gel electrophoresis reveals three polymerase chain reaction (PCR) products following amplification of the cDNA of a Kindler syndrome patient (P in the left panel), who carries the IVS13-1G→A mutation in the FERMT1 gene. A normal-sized product amplified from a healthy control (C) also is shown for comparison. Mw indicates a DNA size marker (bp, base pairs). Subsequent nucleotide sequencing of each gel-purified cDNA fragment identifies mutant mRNAs (schematically depicted on the right hand side) characterized by: the out-of-frame deletion of 8 bp due to the use of cryptic splice site 1 (*upper band*); the out-of-frame skipping of exon 14 (142 bp) (*lower band*); and the in-frame deletion of 48 bp resulting from the use of cryptic splice site 2 (*middle band*). Arrows indicate the position of the primers used to amplify the cDNA. (*C*) Major gene rearrangements. Schematic representation of a chromosome pair containing clustered high homologous genes. Mispairing during meiosis between gene 1 and 2, followed by homologous unequal crossing over (indicated by X), results in two recombined alleles bearing the deletion or the tandem duplication of gene 2.

splice site of the pre-mRNA. The excised left end of the intron becomes linked by a 5′–2′ bond to an adenosine of the BPS (branch site) forming a lariat. Then, a second cutting at the 3′ splice site releases the lariat intron, and the downstream exon is joined to the upstream exon. Other sequence motifs involved in exon definition and activation of splice site selection by stimulation of spliceosome assembly are known as exonic splicing enhancers (ESE), as they usually lie within exons. Conversely, sequences that act by blocking the spliceosome assembly are called exonic splicing silencers (ESS).[21] If a single nucleotide substitution or an insertion/deletion of a few nucleotides alters one of the previously mentioned conserved splice site sequences as well as an ESE or ESS element, this will produce aberrant splicing of the pre-mRNA, leading to deleterious effects on protein product.[22,23] For example, mutations that alter either the AG or the GU splice sites always lead to complete absence of normal splicing (see **Fig. 1**). Indeed, the spliceosome is no more able to recognize the exon and may neglect it, leading to exon skipping, or may use potential splice sites that are not normally selected, termed cryptic splice sites. These can be present in other positions within either the same exon or the flanking introns. Exon skipping and the use of cryptic splice sites are harmful, because they alter the normal ORF of the mRNA by adding pieces of intronic sequences or deleting either the entire exon or a segment of it. The resulting mutant mRNA can be: out-of-frame, thus leading to PTC formation, which is predicted to result in the translation of a truncated unstable polypeptide or NMD activation, or in-frame, and thereby compatible with the synthesis of a protein with internal amino acid deletion or insertion. When a mutation affects the splice site consensus sequence in positions other than the strictly conserved AG/GU dinucleotides, or disrupts the BPS, which is not as well-conserved in people as in yeast, its effects can be leaky or compensated by an alternative element in the vicinity, thus producing only moderately reduced splicing efficiency.[22–24] The presence of mutant in-frame transcripts or the maintenance of a minimal rate of normal splicing is compatible with the translation of a certain amount of either normal or partially functional protein products. Reduced amounts of a given protein or no protein at all often make the difference between severe and mild/moderate phenotypes of various EB subtypes, as in the case of laminin chain subunits in Herlitz JEB versus non-Herlitz JEB or type VII collagen in severe generalized RDEB versus milder generalized or localized RDEB variants.[15,25,26]

Another manner through which a point mutation can affect splicing is the creation of new splice sites. These mutations are single nucleotide substitutions occurring in introns, usually in the vicinity of canonical splice sites, or within exons. When located in an exon, they often may appear as nonpathogenic sequence variants, because they do not change the amino acid (silent mutation), or may be wrongly classified as nonsense, missense or frameshift mutations.[22,23] Thus, the consequences of a point mutation on splicing should be verified by amplification of the cDNA (the complementary copy of the mRNA) whenever a source of mRNA, such as a skin biopsy or cultured fibroblasts and keratinocytes, is available. This is strongly recommended in particular when a mutation in an ESE or the creation of a new splice site by an apparently harmless nucleotide substitution is suspected. Computational tools for the analysis of the information content and effect prediction of splice site sequence changes are now available, however. Information content splice site analysis can be freely performed via the Web interface at www.fruitfly.org/seq_tools/splice.html or www.cbs.dtu.dk/services/NetPGene/ for splice site prediction, and http://rulai.cshl.edu/cgi-bin/tools/ESE3/esefinder.cgi for ESE prediction.

Splicing mutations are believed to account up to 50% of all mutations in a given gene,[27] and most of those identified in EB patients behave in a recessive manner.[14,25] However, a few splicing mutations that affect the triple-helix domain of type VII collagen and result in in-frame deletion of X-Y-Gly repeats have a dominant pattern of inheritance and cause DDEB.[14,28]

Transcription Mutations

All point mutation types described previously fall in the coding region and result in a mutant protein with altered function. Point mutations, however, also may occur 5′ to the start codon or in residues at the 3′ end, in DNA sequences that are critical for regulating transcription. The consequence of these mutations is a decrease or an increase of the amount of a given protein, leading to a loss of normal function (common in recessive diseases) or, more rarely, gain of new biologic function (typical in some autosomal dominant traits), respectively.[2] A single regulatory mutation in the 5′ promoter region that abolishes transcription of a COL7A1 allele has been shown to cause RDEB.[29]

MAJOR GENE REARRANGEMENTS
Deletions

Gene deletions are uncommon causes of mutations. Alpha-thalassemia is the best example. It is caused by deletion of the α-globin gene cluster, which comprises two pairs (α1 and α2) of highly related sequences in close proximity to each other. Because of the sequence similarity of the genes, mispairing of chromosomes may occur during meiosis (see **Fig. 1**).[2] Following homologous unequal crossing over, one product will contain an interstitial deletion of the genetic material encompassing functional α-globin genes. Moreover, the sequence homology needed to mediate mispairing can be provided by specific sequence units of the human genome, known as Alu elements.[30] Alu sequences are a family of short interspersed repeated elements (SINE) with a consensus sequence of approximately 300 nucleotides, present in at least 500,000 copies in the human genome.[31] In some genes, they can be found at high frequency in intronic regions, where they can drive mispairing events followed by unequal recombination, either between homologous chromosomes or between sister chromatids of the same chromosome.[32] If this occurs, the net effect is a recombined allele that has lost part of its coding DNA. In addition to homologous unequal crossing over between gene sequences or repetitive sequence elements, recombination may occur between DNA regions with little or no homology. This mechanism is known as nonhomologous (illegitimate) recombination.[33] Gene rearrangements have been shown to involve the COL7A1 and

FERMT1 genes of patients affected with RDEB and Kindler syndromes, respectively.[34,35]

Duplications

Duplications of DNA sequences may be caused by mispairing between DNA sequences in close proximity, essentially with the same modalities described for deletions.[2] Most of the recombination events that follow mispairing lead to tandem duplications of genetic material that belongs to the same gene, with the consequent alteration of the reading frame. A complex intragenic duplication has been described for the LAMC2 gene and caused Herlitz JEB.[25]

Insertions

These are rare causes of mutations in people. Insertions are caused by the transposition of DNA sequences, an event that is relatively common in the human genome but normally not targeting coding regions. Sequence elements able to transpose are SINE (Alu sequences) and long interspersed repetitive sequences (LINE). If a transposition/insertion of these units involves the coding region, this can disrupt the gene function by altering the reading frame or splicing.[36] This mutation type has never been described as causing EB.

RECURRENT MUTATIONS

The spectrum of mutations affecting a given gene may be at least in part specific of a certain population with some mutations occurring at high frequency. Mutation recurrence may be caused by a founder effect, which means that an ancestral mutant allele carried by a few ancestors has spread in the population because of limited gene pool, genetic drift, and healthy carrier migration. Founder mutations usually show a restricted geographic distribution within a given country. Ethnic-specific recurrent mutations in laminin-332 and COL7A1 genes have been described in several ethnic groups.[20,37] Identical mutations, however, also may occur in more than one population. This finding can be ascribed to two mechanisms:

1. Mutations have arisen before ethnic divergence and thus are observed in different ethnic groups.
2. Mutations have arisen as independent events in distinct population groups because of the vulnerability of certain sequences.

This is the case of CpG dinucleotides, which are particularly prone (hotspot) to C-to-T single nucleotide transitions that result in nonsense and missense codons.[19] Examples of recurrent mutations with no ethnic specificity are the hotspot c.1903C-to-T substitution in the LAMB3 gene, leading to the nonsense codon p.R635X, and the c.425A-to-G splice site mutation in the COL7A1 gene, both frequently found in European patients with Herlitz JEB and RDEB, respectively.[37–39]

REFERENCES

1. Stenson PD, Mort M, Ball EV, et al. The human gene mutation database: 2008 update. Genome Med 2009;1(1):13.
2. Strachan T, Read A. Human molecular genetics. 3rd edition. London: Garland Publishing; 2004.
3. Fine JD, Eady RA, Bauer EA, et al. The classification of inherited epidermolysis bullosa (EB): report of the Third International Consensus Meeting on Diagnosis and Classification of EB. J Am Acad Dermatol 2008; 58(6):931–50.
4. Engel E. A new genetic concept: uniparental disomy and its potential effect, isodisomy. Am J Med Genet 1980;6(2):137–43.
5. Engel E. A fascination with chromosome rescue in uniparental disomy: Mendelian recessive outlaws and imprinting copyrights infringements. Eur J Hum Genet 2006;14(11):1158–69.
6. Fassihi H, Wessagowit V, Ashton GH, et al. Complete paternal uniparental isodisomy of chromosome 1 resulting in Herlitz junctional epidermolysis bullosa. Clin Exp Dermatol 2005;30(1):71–4.
7. Fassihi H, Lu L, Wessagowit V, et al. Complete maternal isodisomy of chromosome 3 in a child with recessive dystrophic epidermolysis bullosa but no other phenotypic abnormalities. J Invest Dermatol 2006;126(9):2039–43.
8. Nagao-Watanabe M, Fukao T, Matsui E, et al. Identification of somatic and germline mosaicism for a keratin 5 mutation in epidermolysis bullosa simplex in a family of which the proband was previously regarded as a sporadic case. Clin Genet 2004;66(3):236–8.
9. Cserhalmi-Friedman PB, Garzon MC, Guzman E, et al. Maternal germline mosaicism in dominant dystrophic epidermolysis bullosa. J Invest Dermatol 2001;117(5):1327–8.
10. Mallipeddi R, Bleck O, Mellerio JE, et al. Dilemmas in distinguishing between dominant and recessive forms of dystrophic epidermolysis bullosa. Br J Dermatol 2003;149(4):810–8.
11. Frank J, Happle R. Cutaneous mosaicism: right before our eyes. J Clin Invest 2007;117(5):1216–9.
12. Daniele A, Scala I, Cardillo G, et al. Functional and structural characterization of novel mutations and genotype-phenotype correlation in 51 phenylalanine hydroxylase deficient families from Southern Italy. FEBS J 2009;276(7):2048–59.
13. Turk D, Janjić V, Stern I, et al. Structure of human dipeptidyl peptidase I (cathepsin C): exclusion domain added to an endopeptidase framework

creates the machine for activation of granular serine proteases. EMBO J 2001;20(23):6570–82.

14. Dang N, Murrell DF. Mutation analysis and characterization of COL7A1 mutations in dystrophic epidermolysis bullosa. Exp Dermatol 2008;17(7):553–68.

15. Varki R, Sadowski S, Uitto J, et al. Epidermolysis bullosa. II. Type VII collagen mutations and phenotype-genotype correlations in the dystrophic subtypes. J Med Genet 2007;44(3):181–92.

16. Christiano AM, Greenspan DS, Lee S, et al. Cloning of human type VII collagen. Complete primary sequence of the alpha 1(VII) chain and identification of intragenic polymorphisms. J Biol Chem 1994; 269(32):20256–62.

17. Hammami-Hauasli N, Schumann H, Raghunath M, et al. Some, but not all, glycine substitution mutations in COL7A1 result in intracellular accumulation of collagen VII, loss of anchoring fibrils, and skin blistering. J Biol Chem 1998;273(30):19228–34.

18. Neu-Yilik G, Kulozik AE. NMD: multitasking between mRNA surveillance and modulation of gene expression. Adv Genet 2008;62:185–243.

19. Hovnanian A, Hilal L, Blanchet-Bardon C, et al. Recurrent nonsense mutations within the type VII collagen gene in patients with severe recessive dystrophic epidermolysis bullosa. Am J Hum Genet 1994;55(2):289–96.

20. Castori M, Floriddia G, De Luca N, et al. Herlitz junctional epidermolysis bullosa: laminin-5 mutational profile and carrier frequency in the Italian population. Br J Dermatol 2008;158:38–44.

21. Wang Z, Burge CB. Splicing regulation: from a parts list of regulatory elements to an integrated splicing code. RNA 2008;14(5):802–13.

22. Wessagowit V, Nalla VK, Rogan PK, et al. Normal and abnormal mechanisms of gene splicing and relevance to inherited skin diseases. J Dermatol Sci 2005;40(2):73–84.

23. Krawczak M, Thomas NS, Hundrieser B, et al. Single base pair substitutions in exon–intron junctions of human genes: nature, distribution, and consequences for mRNA splicing. Hum Mutat 2007;28(2):150–8.

24. Královicová J, Lei H, Vorechovský I. Phenotypic consequences of branch point substitutions. Hum Mutat 2006;27(8):803–13.

25. Posteraro P, De Luca N, Meneguzzi G, et al. Laminin-5 mutational analysis in an Italian cohort of patients with junctional epidermolysis bullosa. J Invest Dermatol 2004;123(4):639–48.

26. Gardella R, Belletti L, Zoppi N, et al. Identification of two splicing mutations in the collagen type VII gene (COL7A1) of a patient affected by the localisata variant of recessive dystrophic epidermolysis bullosa. Am J Hum Genet 1996;59(2):292–300.

27. López-Bigas N, Audit B, Ouzounis C, et al. Are splicing mutations the most frequent cause of hereditary disease? FEBS Lett 2005;579(9):1900–3.

28. Sakuntabhai A, Hammami-Hauasli N, Bodemer C, et al. Deletions within COL7A1 exons distant from consensus splice sites alter splicing and produce shortened polypeptides in dominant dystrophic epidermolysis bullosa. Am J Hum Genet 1998; 63(3):737–48.

29. Gardella R, Barlati S, Zoppi N, et al. A -96C→T mutation in the promoter of the collagen type VII gene (COL7A1) abolishing transcription in a patient affected by recessive dystrophic epidermolysis bullosa. Hum Mutat 2000;16(3):275.

30. Nicholls RD, Fischel-Ghodsian N, Higgs DR. Recombination at the human alpha-globin gene cluster: sequence features and topological constraints. Cell 1987;49(3):369–78.

31. Batzer MA, Deininger PL. Alu repeats and human genomic diversity. Nat Rev Genet 2002;3(5): 370–9.

32. Ringpfeil F, Nakano A, Uitto J, et al. Compound heterozygosity for a recurrent 16.5-kb Alu-mediated deletion mutation and single-base-pair substitutions in the ABCC6 gene results in pseudoxanthoma elasticum. Am J Hum Genet 2001; 68(3):642–52.

33. van Rijk A, Bloemendal H. Molecular mechanisms of exon shuffling: illegitimate recombination. Genetica 2003;118(2–3):245–9.

34. Has C, Wessagowit V, Pascucci M, et al. Molecular basis of Kindler syndrome in Italy: novel and recurrent Alu/Alu recombination, splice site, nonsense, and frameshift mutations in the KIND1 gene. J Invest Dermatol 2006;126(8):1776–83.

35. Titeux M, Mejía JE, Mejlumian L, et al. Recessive dystrophic epidermolysis bullosa caused by COL7A1 hemizygosity and a missense mutation with complex effects on splicing. Hum Mutat 2006; 27(3):291–2.

36. Deininger PL, Moran JV, Batzer MA, et al. Mobile elements and mammalian genome evolution. Curr Opin Genet Dev 2003;13(6):651–8.

37. Murata T, Masunaga T, Ishiko A, et al. Differences in recurrent COL7A1 mutations in dystrophic epidermolysis bullosa: ethnic-specific and worldwide recurrent mutations. Arch Dermatol Res 2004; 295(10):442–7.

38. Pulkkinen L, Meneguzzi G, McGrath JA, et al. Predominance of the recurrent mutation R635X in the LAMB3 gene in European patients with Herlitz junctional epidermolysis bullosa has implications for mutation detection strategy. J Invest Dermatol 1997;109(2):232–7.

39. Csikós M, Szocs HI, Lászik A, et al. High frequency of the 425A→G splice-site mutation and novel mutations of the COL7A1 gene in central Europe: significance for future mutation detection strategies in dystrophic epidermolysis bullosa. Br J Dermatol 2005;152(5):879–86.

Epidermolysis Bullosa Simplex

Eli Sprecher, MD, PhD

KEYWORDS

- Epidermolysis bullosa • Keratin • Blisters • Epidermis
- Intermediate filaments • Mutation

HISTORY

Although the first description of a congenital blistering disease is attributed to von Hebra in 1870, it is Hallopeau who highlighted the peculiar features of epidermolysis bullosa simplex (EBS) in 1898.[1] For almost a century, the pathomechanisms underlying EBS remained poorly understood. Various theories were advanced, many of which revolved around a possible role for excessive release of deleterious proteases.[2] Using electron microscopy, Anton-Lamprecht and Schnyder were the first to postulate that defective keratin function may be responsible for disease manifestations in EBS.[3] These observations and seminal studies by Ishida-Yamamoto and colleagues[4] ultimately led two groups of investigators to the discovery of pathogenic mutations in the genes encoding KRT5 and KRT14 in several families affected with EBS.[5,6] EBS is the first keratin disorder whose genetic basis has been elucidated in humans.[7]

EPIDEMIOLOGY

The prevalence of EBS is estimated to be approximately 6 to 30 per 1 million live births,[8–10] although it is evident that many cases remain undiagnosed, suggesting that the actual prevalence of the disease may be higher than that measured in clinical surveys. The percentage of EBS cases relative to the total number of epidermolysis bullosa (EB) cases depends on the populations studied. For example, although in Western countries, EBS accounts for 75% to 85% of all EB cases, in Middle Eastern countries, a significantly higher percentage of dystrophic and junctional EB cases are observed, with EBS accounting for only approximately half of all EB cases.[11]

CLASSIFICATION AND COMMON CLINICAL FEATURES

All forms of EBS manifest with blistering of the skin, usually induced by exposure to mechanical friction or trauma (**Fig. 1**A, B, and C). Palmoplantar keratoderma (thickening of the palmar and plantar skin) (see **Fig. 1**E), nail dystrophy and nail shedding, alopecia, and mucosal tissue involvement are observed in rare (and often more severe) cases. Erosions and blisters heal without scarring but can leave widespread hyperpigmentation. EB nevi have been reported in all major forms of EB and may simulate clinically and dermoscopically melanoma (although no malignant transformation of these lesions has been reported and they often disappear spontaneously).[12,13] Aplasia cutis congenita has also been reported in EBS.[14]

EBS age of onset is variable, with the most severe cases manifesting at birth and less severe cases first appearing during the second or third decade of life only.[14] Progressive improvement with age is common. High ambient temperatures and sweating are often aggravating factors.[15]

EBS classification has undergone many revisions over the past 2 decades.[9,16,17] The most recent classification refers to EBS as a group of inherited disorders caused by blister formation within the epidermis. As such, EBS encompasses the classical type of EBS, resulting from blister formation throughout the basal cell layer (EBS, basal type, referred to in this article as EBS), and rarer disorders associated with suprabasal blister formation (EBS, suprabasal type, referred to in this article as EBS-SB).[16]

EBS can be classified according to its mode of inheritance. Although the overwhelming number of EBS cases in the Western world are inherited

Department of Dermatology, Tel Aviv Sourasky Medical Center, 6, Weizmann Street, Tel Aviv 64239, Israel
E-mail address: elisp@tasmc.health.gov.il

Dermatol Clin 28 (2010) 23–32
doi:10.1016/j.det.2009.10.003

derm.theclinics.com

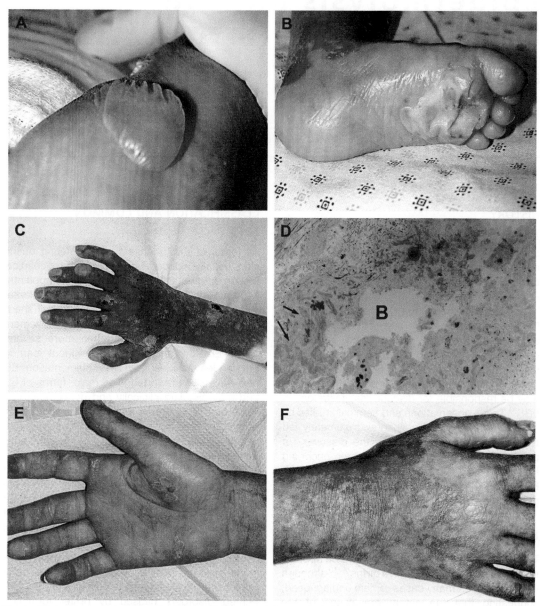

Fig. 1. Clinical features in EBS. Subepidermal blistering (*A*) over the left thigh of a young child with EBS, Dowling-Meara subtype, (*B*) on the plantar surface of an EBS patient, and (*C*) on the dorsum of an adult with EBS, Koebner subtype; (*D*) electron micrograph demonstrating blister formation through the basal cell layer (*B*) and keratin filament clumping in the basal cell cytoplasm (*arrows*); (*E*) palmar hyperkeratosis in a patient with EBS, Dowling-Meara subtype; (*F*) mottled hyperpigmentation in EBS with mottled pigmentation.

in an autosomal dominant fashion, in the Middle East, approximately 30% of the cases are caused by bilallelic recessive mutations.[11,18] Another way to classify EBS is according to the anatomic distribution of the lesions. The Weber-Cockayne subtype of EBS, (designated EBS, localized) is characterized by regional involvement of the palms and soles. The Dowling-Meara subtype of EBS is at the other end of the spectrum of severity of EBS. It is characterized by a peculiar herpetiform distribution of the blisters and is often accompanied by mucosal and nail manifestations. In contrast with other forms of EBS, EBS, Dowling-Meara subtype, is associated with atrophic scarring and milia formation. A widespread but less severe form of the disease, previously termed EBS, Koebner subtype, is today classified as EBS, other generalized.[16]

COMPLICATIONS

Severe skin blistering is associated with marked morbidity. Patients with EBS were found in one survey to experience a greater impairment in quality of life than individuals affected with dystrophic EB.[19] The birth of a child with EBS can carry serious implications for interfamilial relationships.[20] Patients report pain that can be excruciating and requires intensive treatment.[21,22] Severe infections are the most common cause of mortality in EBS patients.[23] Protein loss and involvement of the mucosae can lead to malnutrition and anemia and fluid and electrolyte imbalance.[24] Bone mineralization defects, however, may be less common in EBS than in other forms of EB.[25] Severe forms of EBS are associated with an increased risk for skin cancer[26] and death by age 1.[23]

PATHOGENESIS

EBS is usually caused by missense mutations in KRT5 and KRT14, encoding keratins mostly expressed in the epidermal basal layer.[27] Most KRT5 and KRT14 mutations have been shown to disrupt the central alpha-helical segment of these keratin molecules, thereby compromising the structure and function of the cell cytoskeleton, which becomes unable to accommodate even small amounts of mechanical stress. As a consequence of keratin cytoskeleton dysfunction, the basal cell layer is prone to fracture when exposed to friction forces. At the ultrastructural level, keratin abnormal function translates into cell vacuolization, keratin filament clumping, and blister formation, typically.[7] Phenotype-genotype analysis revealed that mutations affecting conserved areas at the beginning and end of the central rod segment are usually associated with a more severe phenotype than mutations affecting less conserved areas of the keratin molecules,[15,28,29] although many exceptions to this rule have been reported.[11,18] In addition, not only the location but also the nature of the mutation can influence the severity of the disease.[30]

The mechanisms leading to cell disintegration in EBS are still poorly understood. Although decreased mechanical resistance to cell deformation undeniably plays a major role in the development of cell fragility in EBS,[31] recent data also implicate excessive apoptotic activity, possibly induced by keratin clumps, and up-regulation of the inflammatory response in the pathogenesis of the disease.[32,33] In addition, some keratin mutations may affect the cytoskeletal dynamics or interfere with normal keratin post-translational modification.[34,35]

Most EBS-causing mutations exert a dominant negative effect, namely, the mutant molecules interfere with the function of the normal keratins encoded by the wild-type allele. This situation has direct implications for the design of genetic therapies for EBS: introduction of a wild-type allele is unlikely to benefit EBS patients; instead, effective therapies for EBS should be aimed at eliminating the deleterious keratin molecules encoded by the mutant allele (discussed later).

EBS phenotype usually evolves over time and generally shows improvement as affected individuals get older. Down-regulation of expression of mutant keratin genes and compensatory overexpression of keratins, usually weakly expressed in the basal cell layers, such as KRT15,[36] have been invoked to explain this phenomenon. Somatic genetic events may also modify the course of the disease. Revertant mosaicism refers to a situation where a second mutation attenuates or abolishes the deleterious effect of the original mutation in certain areas of the skin. This phenomenon has been reported in several patients with EBS and may be more common than previously suspected.[37,38] The phenotypic manifestations of EBS-causing keratin mutations can also be influenced by apparently silent sequence alterations.[39] Finally, genetic background is also important as exemplified by the facts that phenotype-genotype correlations differ across populations and families[11] and that keratin mutations are phenotypically expressed in a strain-dependent fashion in mice.[40]

It seems that epidermal fragility is almost exclusively associated with defective function of the conserved central regions of keratin molecules because skin blistering is unusual in disorders resulting from mutations affecting the head or tail domain of keratins (Fig. 2). For example, in Dowling-Degos disease (MIM179850), resulting from mutations in the KRT5 gene region encoding the protein head domain,[41] blistering is not observed; in contrast, melanosome transport and epithelial growth are abnormal, resulting in reticulate hyperpigmentation of the flexures, comedo-like lesions on the neck, and pitted perioral acneiform scars.[42] In Naegeli-Franceschetti-Jadassohn syndrome (MIM161000) and dermatopathia pigmentosa reticularis (MIM125595), which are caused by mutations affecting the head domain of KRT14,[43] blisters are unusual; instead, patients display reticulate hyperpigmentation and lack dermatoglyphics[44] due to deranged regulation of apoptotic activity in the basal cell layer.[45] Despite that mutations affecting the tail domain of another keratin, KRT1, are shown to affect the process of cornification but not cell resilience,[46] mutations

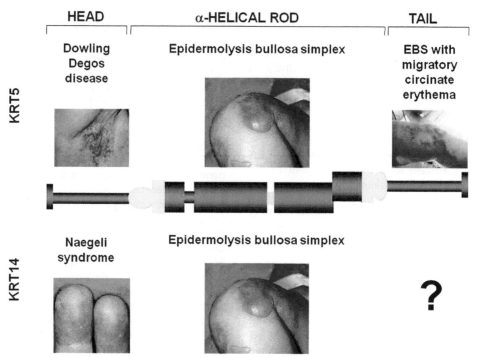

Fig. 2. Genotype-phenotype correlations. Three major domains are depicted along a scheme of a prototypic keratin with all five major KRT5- and KRT14-associated clinical phenotypes.

affecting the KRT5 tail domain are shown to cause a dominant form of EBS, in one case indistinguishable clinically from EBS associated with mutations located in the rod-segment encoding gene region.[47,48] Here, the mutation has been suggested as possibly resulting in abnormal protein folding or triggering the formation of deleterious small intracellular aggregates.[47]

UNUSUAL VARIANTS

Several unusual basal EBS variants deserve mention. Recessive EBS (MIM601001) can be caused by missense[49] or nonsense mutations,[18,36,50–54] resulting in loss of function rather than a dominant negative effect.[11] EBS with mottled pigmentation (MIM131960) is characterized by skin blistering, reticulate skin pigmentation, keratoderma, and nail dystrophy (see **Fig. 1F**). This subtype of EBS has been found to be strongly associated with a missense mutation (p.P25L) affecting the KRT5 head domain.[55] p.P25L has been suggested as impairing melanin granule aggregation and keratin filament function by interfering with post-translational processing. More recent data, however, suggest that the same phenotype may also result from other mutations in KRT5 and KRT14[56,57] or from mutations in unrelated genes.[58] EBS with migratory circinate erythema (MIM609352) is characterized by the occurrence of vesicles on the background of a migratory circinate erythema. The lesions often heal with brown pigmentation but no scarring. The disease seems to be specifically caused by a recurrent frameshift mutation affecting the structure of KRT5 tail domain.[59] The reason for this peculiar association is elusive.

Several subtypes of basal EBS are not caused by mutations in keratins per se. For example, mutations in PLEC1, encoding plectin, a large molecule that is part of the hemidesmosome and is known to interact with basal keratins, were found to cause a variety of EBS subtypes, including EBS with muscular dystrophy (MIM226677)[60]; EBS, Ogna type (MIM131950), characterized by hemorrhagic blistering[61]; lethal EBS[62]; and EBS with pyloric atresia, (MIM612138),[63] which is also caused by mutations affecting the α6β4 integrin receptor.[7] Mutations affecting other components of the hemidesmosomal plaque have similarly been found to cause EBS,[64,65] underscoring the interdependency between hemidesmosomal junctions and epidermal cell cytoskeleton functions.

Apart from these forms of EBS associated with blister formation at the level of the basal cell layer, several relatively rare forms of EBS associated with suprabasal blistering are now recognized (EBS-SB). Ectodermal dysplasia with skin fragility (MIM604536) is an autosomal recessive disorder characterized by skin fragility, nail dystrophy, palmoplantar keratoderma, and alopecia. The disease is caused by mutations in *PKF1*, encoding plakophilin 1, a component of the desmosomal plaque.[66-68] Keratin intermediate filaments binding to the desmosomal plaque, at least in lower suprabasal epidermal cells, is critically dependent on normal PKF1 function,[69] which may explain the common occurrence of blistering in EBS and in EDSF.

Lethal acantholytic EB is a new phenotype, lethal in the neonatal period, characterized by skin fragility, complete disruption of the epidermal barrier, universal alopecia, neonatal teeth, and nail loss.[70] Histology shows suprabasal clefting and acantholysis throughout the spinous layer, mimicking pemphigus. The disease was found to result from truncation of the tail domain of desmoplakin.[70]

EBS superficialis refers to a disease rarely reported and characterized by superficial erosions with scarring and milia formation.[71] In one case, the disease was found to result from mutations in *COL7A1*, suggesting that EBS superficialis represents a subset of dystrophic EB (**Table 1**).[72]

DIAGNOSIS

The laboratory tools usually used to establish a diagnosis of EBS include regular histology, electron microscopy, antigen epitope mapping, immunohistochemistry, and molecular testing. Light microscopy demonstrates intraepidermal blister formation and vacuolar changes within the epidermal basal cell layer. Electron microscopy reveals blister formation throughout the basal cell layer and keratin filament clumping in Dowling-Meara cases (see **Fig.** 1D).[15,28] Eosinophilic inclusions are the histopathologic correlate of ultrastructural filament clumping.[73] Antigen epitope mapping consists of staining frozen or paraffin-embedded sections with antibodies detecting proteins demarcating the level of epidermal-dermal separation, thereby determining the EB type.[16,74] Antigen epitope mapping is inexpensive and, in contrast with electron microscopy, readily available at most medical institutions. Comparative studies suggest that it may perform as well as electron microscopy.[75,76] Regular immunohistochemistry can be used in recessive cases to demonstrate absence of keratin intermediate filaments.[18,77]

Molecular diagnosis is generally conducted in a stepwise fashion, with screening beginning by mutation analysis of *KRT5* and *KRT14* conserved regions; data collected in Western populations have shown that more than 40% of EBS cases are caused by a mutation affecting the *KRT14* R125 residue.[78,79] The existence of KRT14 pseudogenes requires the use of special techniques to avoid amplification of nonrelevant sequences.[80] If no mutation is identified in the conserved regions of the two genes, sequence alterations are looked

Table 1
Epidermolysis bullosa simplex–associated genes and phenotypes.

Gene	Protein	Disease	OMIM
KRT5	Keratin 5	EBS, Dowling-Meara subtype	131760
		EBS, Koebner subtype	131900
		EBS, Weber-Cockayne subtype	131800
		EBS with mottled pigmentation	131960
		EBS with migratory circinate erythema	609352
		Dowling-Degos disease	179850
K14	Keratin 14	EBS, Dowling-Meara subtype	131760
		EBS, Koebner subtype	131900
		EBS, Weber-Cockayne subtype	131800
		Autosomal recessive EBS	601001
		Dermatopathia pigmentosa reticularis	125595
		Naegeli-Franceschetti-Jadassohn syndrome	161000
PLEC1	Plectin	EBS with muscular dystrophy	226670
		EBS, Ogna type	131950
		Lethal EBS	
		EBS with pyloric atresia	612138
ITGB4	Integrin beta 4	Junctional EB associated with pyloric atresia	226730
		EBS, Weber-Cockayne subtype	131800
COL17A1	Collagen type XVII	EBS, Koebner subtype	131900
DSP	Desmoplakin	EB, lethal acantholytic	609638

for in regions of the genes less often found to contain deleterious alterations. Finally, if no mutations are found in the coding regions of KRT5 and KRT14, noncoding[81,82] and nonkeratin genes,[64,65,83] such as PLEC1, ITGB4, or COL17A1, are then scrutinized. Despite intensive mutation screening, in approximately 10% to 30% of EBS cases, no mutations are found.[84]

DIFFERENTIAL DIAGNOSIS

The differential diagnosis of EBS encompasses a large spectrum of inherited blistering conditions, including non-EBS EB types; epidermolytic hyperkeratosis (MIM113800); Kindler syndrome (MIM173650), caused by mutations in kindlin, typically accompanied by pigmentary and atrophic changes affecting sun-exposed skin; EBS-SB (discussed previously); and incontinentia pigmenti (MIM318310), characterized by congenital blisters distributed along the lines of Blaschko.

EBS should also be distinguished from congenital blistering resulting from nongenetic causes, including infectious (herpetic and candida), autoimmune (pemphigus and bullous pemphigoid), neoplastic (mastocytosis), and idiopathic (congenital erosions and vesicles healing with reticulate scarring) diseases.

PREVENTION

Major advances in understanding the molecular basis of EBS and other keratin disorders have led to the development of DNA-based prenatal testing, usually performed during the first trimester. Prenatal diagnosis is provided based on previous knowledge of mutations in a family, sequencing of the fetal and parental DNA, and confirmation of the mutation using ancillary tests, such as allele-specific polymerase chain reaction.[85] As with other dominant disorders, genetic counseling can be complicated by the presence of germline mosaicism.[86]

A particular problem arises when prenatal diagnosis is requested with no prior knowledge of the mutation. Microscopic examination of fetal skin biopsy, which entails significant risks and is performed late in pregnancy, has rarely been used in such cases.[87]

Finally, for those families for whom pregnancy interruption is not an option, preimplantation diagnosis is available, although this approach is associated with maternal complications and a lower diagnostic accuracy when compared with molecular diagnosis performed on chorionic villus sampling or amniocentesis samples.[88,89]

TREATMENT

Patient care involves wound care, including lancing of blisters to prevent their spread and sterile dressings.[90–92] Nutritional support plays a critical role in promoting wound healing.[24,93] Topical antibiotics should be used for short periods of time because of problems of resistance to antibiotics and sensitization.[90] Novel therapeutic approaches include the use of biologic dressings or skin equivalents.[91,94–96]

Because heat and excessive sweating are known aggravating factors in EBS, aluminium chloride has been used in an attempt to prevent sweating with mixed results.[97,98] Recently, botulinum toxin has been used to prevent plantar blistering in EBS with some degree of success.[99]

EBS patients, in contrast with patients affected with other forms of EB, are seldom in need of surgical procedures, such as hand surgery or surgical removal of skin cancer.[100] Dental caries due to enamel hypoplasia are apparently common in EBS, however, and may require intervention.[101]

Medical options have been tried in EBS. Tetracyclines have been shown in several small studies to be of benefit to EBS patients, although results from properly conducted controlled trials are not yet available.[102–106] Other drugs of potential benefit in EBS may include sulforaphane, which, through Nrf2 induction, up-regulates the expression of KRT17, which was shown to be able to compensate for the absence of KRT14 in a mouse model.[107]

Therapeutic approaches specifically targeting the genetic defects underlying EBS are emerging. As discussed previously, given the deleterious effects of the abnormal keratin molecules generated by the mutant allele in EBS, genetic therapies are aimed in keratin disorders at eliminating the malfunctioning keratin proteins. Although such a strategy has not yet been applied to the treatment of EBS, a recent trial using local injection of a small interfering RNA specifically recognizing a mutant KRT6a keratin in pachyonychia congenita has been completed, with encouraging results.[108,109]

REFERENCES

1. Priestley GC. A bibliography of epidermolysis bullosa. Acta Derm Venereol Suppl 1987;133:1–38.
2. Winberg JO, Gedde-Dahl T. Gelatinase expression in generalized epidermolysis bullosa simplex fibroblasts. J Invest Dermatol 1986;87(3):326–9.
3. Anton-Lamprecht I, Schnyder UW. Epidermolysis bullosa herpetiformis Dowling-Meara. Report of a case and pathomorphogenesis. Dermatologica 1982;164(4):221–35.

4. Ishida-Yamamoto A, McGrath JA, Chapman SJ, et al. Epidermolysis bullosa simplex (Dowling-Meara type) is a genetic disease characterized by an abnormal keratin-filament network involving keratins K5 and K14. J Invest Dermatol 1991; 97(6):959–68.

5. Bonifas JM, Rothman AL, Epstein EH Jr. Epidermolysis bullosa simplex: evidence in two families for keratin gene abnormalities. Science 1991; 254(5035):1202–5.

6. Coulombe PA, Hutton ME, Letai A, et al. Point mutations in human keratin 14 genes of epidermolysis bullosa simplex patients: genetic and functional analyses. Cell 1991;66(6):1301–11.

7. Uitto J, Richard G, McGrath JA. Diseases of epidermal keratins and their linker proteins. Exp Cell Res 2007;313(10):1995–2009.

8. Horn HM, Priestley GC, Eady RA, et al. The prevalence of epidermolysis bullosa in Scotland. Br J Dermatol 1997;136(4):560–4.

9. Fine JD, Bauer EA, Briggaman RA, et al. Revised clinical and laboratory criteria for subtypes of inherited epidermolysis bullosa. A consensus report by the Subcommittee on diagnosis and classification of the National Epidermolysis Bullosa Registry. J Am Acad Dermatol 1991;24(1):119–35.

10. McKenna KE, Walsh MY, Bingham EA. Epidermolysis bullosa in Northern Ireland. Br J Dermatol 1992; 127(4):318–21.

11. Abu Sa'd J, Indelman M, Pfendner E, et al. Molecular epidemiology of hereditary epidermolysis bullosa in a Middle Eastern population. J Invest Dermatol 2006;126(4):777–81.

12. Lanschuetzer CM, Emberger M, Laimer M, et al. Epidermolysis bullosa naevi reveal a distinctive dermoscopic pattern. Br J Dermatol 2005;153(1): 97–102.

13. Bauer JW, Schaeppi H, Kaserer C, et al. Large melanocytic nevi in hereditary epidermolysis bullosa. J Am Acad Dermatol 2001;44(4):577–84.

14. Horn HM, Tidman MJ. The clinical spectrum of dystrophic epidermolysis bullosa. Br J Dermatol 2002;146(2):267–74.

15. Uitto J, Richard G. Progress in epidermolysis bullosa: from eponyms to molecular genetic classification. Clin Dermatol 2005;23(1):33–40.

16. Fine JD, Eady RA, Bauer EA, et al. The classification of inherited epidermolysis bullosa (EB): report of the Third International Consensus Meeting on Diagnosis and Classification of EB. J Am Acad Dermatol 2008;58(6):931–50.

17. Fine JD, Eady RA, Bauer EA, et al. Revised classification system for inherited epidermolysis bullosa: report of the Second International Consensus Meeting on diagnosis and classification of epidermolysis bullosa. J Am Acad Dermatol 2000;42(6): 1051–66.

18. Ciubotaru D, Bergman R, Baty D, et al. Epidermolysis bullosa simplex in Israel: clinical and genetic features. Arch Dermatol 2003;139(4):498–505.

19. Horn HM, Tidman MJ. Quality of life in epidermolysis bullosa. Clin Exp Dermatol 2002;27(8): 707–10.

20. Fine JD, Johnson LB, Weiner M, et al. Impact of inherited epidermolysis bullosa on parental interpersonal relationships, marital status and family size. Br J Dermatol. 2005;152(5):1009–14.

21. Weiner MS. Pain management in epidermolysis bullosa: an intractable problem. Ostomy Wound Manage 2004;50(8):13–4.

22. Fine JD, Johnson LB, Weiner M, et al. Assessment of mobility, activities and pain in different subtypes of epidermolysis bullosa. Clin Exp Dermatol 2004; 29(2):122–7.

23. Fine JD, Johnson LB, Weiner M, et al. Cause-specific risks of childhood death in inherited epidermolysis bullosa. J Pediatr 2008;152(2):276–80.

24. Haynes L. Nutritional support for children with epidermolysis bullosa. Br J Nurs 2006;15(20): 1097–101.

25. Fewtrell MS, Allgrove J, Gordon I, et al. Bone mineralization in children with epidermolysis bullosa. Br J Dermatol 2006;154(5):959–62.

26. Fine JD, Johnson LB, Weiner M, et al. Epidermolysis bullosa and the risk of life-threatening cancers: the National EB Registry experience, 1986–2006. J Am Acad Dermatol. 2009;60(2):203–11.

27. Lane EB, McLean WH. Keratins and skin disorders. J Pathol 2004;204(4):355–66.

28. Uitto J, Richard G. Progress in epidermolysis bullosa: genetic classification and clinical implications. Am J Med Genet C Semin Med Genet 2004;131C(1):61–74.

29. Liovic M, Stojan J, Bowden PE, et al. A novel keratin 5 mutation (K5V186L) in a family with EBS-K: a conservative substitution can lead to development of different disease phenotypes. J Invest Dermatol 2001;116(6):964–9.

30. Sorensen CB, Ladekjaer-Mikkelsen AS, Andresen BS, et al. Identification of novel and known mutations in the genes for keratin 5 and 14 in Danish patients with epidermolysis bullosa simplex: correlation between genotype and phenotype. J Invest Dermatol 1999;112(2):184–90.

31. Ma L, Yamada S, Wirtz D, et al. A 'hot-spot' mutation alters the mechanical properties of keratin filament networks. Nat Cell Biol 2001;3(5):503–6.

32. Yoneda K, Furukawa T, Zheng YJ, et al. An autocrine/paracrine loop linking keratin 14 aggregates to tumor necrosis factor alpha-mediated cytotoxicity in a keratinocyte model of epidermolysis bullosa simplex. J Biol Chem 2004;279(8):7296–303.

33. Lu H, Chen J, Planko L, et al. Induction of inflammatory cytokines by a keratin mutation and their

repression by a small molecule in a mouse model for EBS. J Invest Dermatol 2007;127(12):2781–9.

34. Werner NS, Windoffer R, Strnad P, et al. Epidermolysis bullosa simplex-type mutations alter the dynamics of the keratin cytoskeleton and reveal a contribution of actin to the transport of keratin subunits. Mol Biol Cell 2004;15(3):990–1002.

35. Coulombe PA, Omary MB. 'Hard' and 'soft' principles defining the structure, function and regulation of keratin intermediate filaments. Curr Opin Cell Biol 2002;14(1):110–22.

36. Jonkman MF, Heeres K, Pas HH, et al. Effects of keratin 14 ablation on the clinical and cellular phenotype in a kindred with recessive epidermolysis bullosa simplex. J Invest Dermatol 1996;107(5):764–9.

37. Schuilenga-Hut PH, Scheffer H, Pas HH, et al. Partial revertant mosaicism of keratin 14 in a patient with recessive epidermolysis bullosa simplex. J Invest Dermatol 2002;118(4):626–30.

38. Smith FJ, Morley SM, McLean WH. Novel mechanism of revertant mosaicism in Dowling-Meara epidermolysis bullosa simplex. J Invest Dermatol 2004;122(1):73–7.

39. Yasukawa K, Sawamura D, McMillan JR, et al. Dominant and recessive compound heterozygous mutations in epidermolysis bullosa simplex demonstrate the role of the stutter region in keratin intermediate filament assembly. J Biol Chem 2002; 277(26):23670–4.

40. McGowan KM, Tong X, Colucci-Guyon E, et al. Keratin 17 null mice exhibit age- and strain-dependent alopecia. Genes Dev 2002;16(11):1412–22.

41. Betz RC, Planko L, Eigelshoven S, et al. Loss-of-function mutations in the keratin 5 gene lead to Dowling-Degos disease. Am J Hum Genet 2006; 78(3):510–9.

42. Jones EW, Grice K. Reticulate pigmented anomaly of the flexures. Dowing Degos disease, a new genodermatosis. Arch Dermatol. 1978;114(8):1150–7.

43. Lugassy J, Itin P, Ishida-Yamamoto A, et al. Naegeli-Franceschetti-Jadassohn syndrome and dermatopathia pigmentosa reticularis: two allelic ectodermal dysplasias caused by dominant mutations in KRT14. Am J Hum Genet 2006;79(4): 724–30.

44. Itin PH, Lautenschlager S. Genodermatosis with reticulate, patchy and mottled pigmentation of the neck–a clue to rare dermatologic disorders. Dermatology 1998;197(3):281–90.

45. Lugassy J, McGrath JA, Itin P, et al. KRT14 haploinsufficiency results in increased susceptibility of keratinocytes to TNF-alpha-induced apoptosis and causes Naegeli-Franceschetti-Jadassohn syndrome. J Invest Dermatol 2008;128(6): 1517–24.

46. Sprecher E, Ishida-Yamamoto A, Becker OM, et al. Evidence for novel functions of the keratin tail emerging from a mutation causing ichthyosis hystrix. J Invest Dermatol 2001;116(4):511–9.

47. Gu LH, Coulombe PA. Defining the properties of the nonhelical tail domain in type II keratin 5: insight from a bullous disease-causing mutation. Mol Biol Cell 2005;16(3):1427–38.

48. Sprecher E, Yosipovitch G, Bergman R, et al. Epidermolytic hyperkeratosis and epidermolysis bullosa simplex caused by frameshift mutations altering the v2 tail domains of keratin 1 and keratin 5. J Invest Dermatol 2003;120(4):623–6.

49. Hovnanian A, Pollack E, Hilal L, et al. A missense mutation in the rod domain of keratin 14 associated with recessive epidermolysis bullosa simplex. Nat Genet 1993;3(4):327–32.

50. Has C, Chang YR, Volz A, et al. Novel keratin 14 mutations in patients with severe recessive epidermolysis bullosa simplex. J Invest Dermatol 2006; 126(8):1912–4.

51. Indelman M, Bergman R, Sprecher E. A novel recessive missense mutation in KRT14 reveals striking phenotypic heterogeneity in epidermolysis bullosa simplex. J Invest Dermatol 2005;124(1): 272–4.

52. Lanschuetzer CM, Klausegger A, Pohla-Gubo G, et al. A novel homozygous nonsense deletion/insertion mutation in the keratin 14 gene (Y248X; 744delC/insAG) causes recessive epidermolysis bullosa simplex type Kobner. Clin Exp Dermatol 2003;28(1):77–9.

53. Batta K, Rugg EL, Wilson NJ, et al. A keratin 14 'knockout' mutation in recessive epidermolysis bullosa simplex resulting in less severe disease. Br J Dermatol 2000;143(3):621–7.

54. Corden LD, Mellerio JE, Gratian MJ, et al. Homozygous nonsense mutation in helix 2 of K14 causes severe recessive epidermolysis bullosa simplex. Hum Mutat 1998;11(4):279–85.

55. Uttam J, Hutton E, Coulombe PA, et al. The genetic basis of epidermolysis bullosa simplex with mottled pigmentation. Proc Natl Acad Sci U S A 1996; 93(17):9079–84.

56. Harel A, Bergman R, Indelman M, et al. Epidermolysis bullosa simplex with mottled pigmentation resulting from a recurrent mutation in KRT14. J Invest Dermatol 2006;126(7):1654–7.

57. Horiguchi Y, Sawamura D, Mori R, et al. Clinical heterogeneity of 1649delG mutation in the tail domain of keratin 5: a Japanese family with epidermolysis bullosa simplex with mottled pigmentation. J Invest Dermatol 2005;125(1):83–5.

58. Hamada T, Yasumoto S, Karashima T, et al. Recurrent p.N767S mutation in the ATP2A2 gene in a Japanese family with haemorrhagic Darier disease clinically mimicking epidermolysis bullosa simplex with mottled pigmentation. Br J Dermatol 2007;157(3):605–8.

59. Gu LH, Kim SC, Ichiki Y, et al. A usual frameshift and delayed termination codon mutation in keratin 5 causes a novel type of epidermolysis bullosa simplex with migratory circinate erythema. J Invest Dermatol 2003;121(3):482–5.

60. Smith FJ, Eady RA, Leigh IM, et al. Plectin deficiency results in muscular dystrophy with epidermolysis bullosa. Nat Genet 1996;13(4):450–7.

61. Koss-Harnes D, Hoyheim B, Anton-Lamprecht I, et al. A site-specific plectin mutation causes dominant epidermolysis bullosa simplex Ogna: two identical de novo mutations. J Invest Dermatol 2002;118(1):87–93.

62. Charlesworth A, Gagnoux-Palacios L, Bonduelle M, et al. Identification of a lethal form of epidermolysis bullosa simplex associated with a homozygous genetic mutation in plectin. J Invest Dermatol 2003;121(6):1344–8.

63. Nakamura H, Sawamura D, Goto M, et al. Epidermolysis bullosa simplex associated with pyloric atresia is a novel clinical subtype caused by mutations in the plectin gene (PLEC1). J Mol Diagn 2005;7(1):28–35.

64. Fontao L, Tasanen K, Huber M, et al. Molecular consequences of deletion of the cytoplasmic domain of bullous pemphigoid 180 in a patient with predominant features of epidermolysis bullosa simplex. J Invest Dermatol 2004;122(1):65–72.

65. Jonkman MF, Pas HH, Nijenhuis M, et al. Deletion of a cytoplasmic domain of integrin beta4 causes epidermolysis bullosa simplex. J Invest Dermatol 2002;119(6):1275–81.

66. Sprecher E, Molho-Pessach V, Ingber A, et al. Homozygous splice site mutations in PKP1 result in loss of epidermal plakophilin 1 expression and underlie ectodermal dysplasia/skin fragility syndrome in two consanguineous families. J Invest Dermatol 2004;122(3):647–51.

67. Whittock NV, Haftek M, Angoulvant N, et al. Genomic amplification of the human plakophilin 1 gene and detection of a new mutation in ectodermal dysplasia/skin fragility syndrome. J Invest Dermatol 2000;115(3):368–74.

68. McGrath JA, McMillan JR, Shemanko CS, et al. Mutations in the plakophilin 1 gene result in ectodermal dysplasia/skin fragility syndrome. Nat Genet 1997;17(2):240–4.

69. Kowalczyk AP, Hatzfeld M, Bornslaeger EA, et al. The head domain of plakophilin-1 binds to desmoplakin and enhances its recruitment to desmosomes. Implications for cutaneous disease. J Biol Chem 1999;274(26):18145–8.

70. Jonkman MF, Pasmooij AM, Pasmans SG, et al. Loss of desmoplakin tail causes lethal acantholytic epidermolysis bullosa. Am J Hum Genet 2005;77(4):653–60.

71. Fine JD, Johnson L, Wright T. Epidermolysis bullosa simplex superficialis. A new variant of epidermolysis bullosa characterized by subcorneal skin cleavage mimicking peeling skin syndrome. Arch Dermatol 1989;125(5):633–8.

72. Martinez-Mir A, Liu J, Gordon D, et al. EB simplex superficialis resulting from a mutation in the type VII collagen gene. J Invest Dermatol 2002;118(3):547–9.

73. Bergman R, Harel A, Sprecher E. Dyskeratosis as a histologic feature in epidermolysis bullosa simplex-Dowling Meara. J Am Acad Dermatol 2007;57(3):463–6.

74. Fine JD. Laboratory tests for epidermolysis bullosa. Dermatol Clin 1994;12(1):123–32.

75. Yiasemides E, Walton J, Marr P, et al. A comparative study between transmission electron microscopy and immunofluorescence mapping in the diagnosis of epidermolysis bullosa. Am J Dermatopathol 2006;28(5):387–94.

76. Petronius D, Bergman R, Ben Izhak O, et al. A comparative study of immunohistochemistry and electron microscopy used in the diagnosis of epidermolysis bullosa. Am J Dermatopathol 2003;25(3):198–203.

77. Yiasemides E, Trisnowati N, Su J, et al. Clinical heterogeneity in recessive epidermolysis bullosa due to mutations in the keratin 14 gene, KRT14. Clin Exp Dermatol 2008;33(6):689–97.

78. Szeverenyi I, Cassidy AJ, Chung CW, et al. The human intermediate filament database: comprehensive information on a gene family involved in many human diseases. Hum Mutat 2008;29(3):351–60.

79. McLean WH, Smith FJ, Cassidy AJ. Insights into genotype-phenotype correlation in pachyonychia congenita from the human intermediate filament mutation database. J Investig Dermatol Symp Proc 2005;10(1):31–6.

80. Wood P, Baty DU, Lane EB, et al. Long-range polymerase chain reaction for specific full-length amplification of the human keratin 14 gene and novel keratin 14 mutations in epidermolysis bullosa simplex patients. J Invest Dermatol 2003;120(3):495–7.

81. Han S, Cooper DN, Bowden PE. Utilization of a cryptic noncanonical donor splice site in the KRT14 gene causes a mild form of epidermolysis bullosa simplex. Br J Dermatol 2006;155(1):201–3.

82. Rugg EL, Rachet-Prehu MO, Rochat A, et al. Donor splice site mutation in keratin 5 causes in-frame removal of 22 amino acids of H1 and 1A rod domains in Dowling-Meara epidermolysis bullosa simplex. Eur J Hum Genet 1999;7(3):293–300.

83. Pfendner E, Rouan F, Uitto J. Progress in epidermolysis bullosa: the phenotypic spectrum of plectin mutations. Exp Dermatol 2005;14(4):241–9.

84. Rugg EL, Horn HM, Smith FJ, et al. Epidermolysis bullosa simplex in Scotland caused by a spectrum of keratin mutations. J Invest Dermatol 2007; 127(3):574–80.

85. Pfendner EG, Sadowski SG, Uitto J. Epidermolysis bullosa simplex: recurrent and de novo mutations in the KRT5 and KRT14 genes, phenotype/genotype correlations, and implications for genetic counseling and prenatal diagnosis. J Invest Dermatol 2005;125(2):239–43.

86. Nagao-Watanabe M, Fukao T, Matsui E, et al. Identification of somatic and germline mosaicism for a keratin 5 mutation in epidermolysis bullosa simplex in a family of which the proband was previously regarded as a sporadic case. Clin Genet 2004;66(3):236–8.

87. Sybert VP, Holbrook KA, Levy M. Prenatal diagnosis of severe dermatologic diseases. Adv Dermatol 1992;7:179–209 [discussion: 210].

88. Shimizu H. Prenatal diagnosis of epidermolysis bullosa. Prenat Diagn 2006;26(13):1260–1.

89. Fassihi H, Eady RA, Mellerio JE, et al. Prenatal diagnosis for severe inherited skin disorders: 25 years' experience. Br J Dermatol 2006;154(1):106–13.

90. Mellerio JE, Weiner M, Denyer JE, et al. Medical management of epidermolysis bullosa: proceedings of the IInd International Symposium on epidermolysis bullosa, Santiago, Chile, 2005. Int J Dermatol 2007;46(8):795–800.

91. Schober-Flores C. Epidermolysis bullosa: the challenges of wound care. Dermatol Nurs 2003;15(2):135–8, 141–34.

92. Schachner L, Feiner A, Camisulli S. Epidermolysis bullosa: management principles for the neonate, infant, and young child. Dermatol Nurs 2005; 17(1):56–9.

93. Birge K. Nutrition management of patients with epidermolysis bullosa. J Am Diet Assoc 1995;95(5):575–9.

94. Mather C, Denyer J. Removing dressings in epidermolysis bullosa. Nurs Times 2008;104(14):46–8.

95. Fivenson DP, Scherschun L, Choucair M, et al. Graftskin therapy in epidermolysis bullosa. J Am Acad Dermatol 2003;48(6):886–92.

96. Falabella AF, Schachner LA, Valencia IC, et al. The use of tissue-engineered skin (Apligraf) to treat a newborn with epidermolysis bullosa. Arch Dermatol 1999;135(10):1219–22.

97. Younger IR, Priestley GC, Tidman MJ. Aluminum chloride hexahydrate and blistering in epidermolysis bullosa simplex. J Am Acad Dermatol 1990;23 (5 Pt 1):930–1.

98. Jennings JL. Aluminum chloride hexahydrate treatment of localized epidermolysis bullosa. Arch Dermatol 1984;120(10):1382.

99. Abitbol RJ, Zhou LH. Treatment of epidermolysis bullosa simplex, Weber-Cockayne type, with botulinum toxin type A. Arch Dermatol 2009;145(1): 13–5.

100. Azizkhan RG, Denyer JE, Mellerio JE, et al. Surgical management of epidermolysis bullosa: proceedings of the IInd International symposium on epidermolysis bullosa, Santiago, Chile, 2005. Int J Dermatol 2007;46(8):801–8.

101. Cagirankaya LB, Hatipoglu MG, Hatipoglu H. Localized epidermolysis bullosa simplex with generalized enamel hypoplasia in a child. Pediatr Dermatol 2006;23(2):167–8.

102. Langan SM, Williams HC. A systematic review of randomized controlled trials of treatments for inherited forms of epidermolysis bullosa. Clin Exp Dermatol 2009;34(1):20–5.

103. Weiner M, Stein A, Cash S, et al. Tetracycline and epidermolysis bullosa simplex: a double-blind, placebo-controlled, crossover randomized clinical trial. Br J Dermatol 2004;150(3):613–4.

104. Veien NK, Buus SK. Treatment of epidermolysis bullosa simplex (EBS) with tetracycline. Arch Dermatol 2000;136(3):424–5.

105. Retief CR, Malkinson FD, Pearson RW. Two familial cases of epidermolysis bullosa simplex successfully treated with tetracycline. Arch Dermatol 1999;135(8):997–8.

106. Fine JD, Eady RA. Tetracycline and epidermolysis bullosa simplex: a new indication for one of the oldest and most widely used drugs in dermatology? Arch Dermatol 1999;135(8):981–2.

107. Kerns ML, DePianto D, Dinkova-Kostova AT, et al. Reprogramming of keratin biosynthesis by sulforaphane restores skin integrity in epidermolysis bullosa simplex. Proc Natl Acad Sci U S A 2007; 104(36):14460–5.

108. Leachman SA, Hickerson RP, Hull PR, et al. Therapeutic siRNAs for dominant genetic skin disorders including pachyonychia congenita. J Dermatol Sci 2008;51(3):151–7.

109. Smith FJ, Hickerson RP, Sayers JM, et al. Development of therapeutic siRNAs for pachyonychia congenita. J Invest Dermatol 2008; 128(1):50–8.

Plectin Gene Defects Lead to Various Forms of Epidermolysis Bullosa Simplex

Günther A. Rezniczek, PhD, Gernot Walko, PhD, Gerhard Wiche, PhD*

KEYWORDS

• EBS • Plectin • Cytolinker

Within cells, multiple cytoskeletal networks (built from actin, intermediate filament (IF) subunit proteins, or tubulin) cooperate with each other to perform their diverse tasks. Accessory proteins are essential for the controlled spatiotemporal assembly and interaction of cytoskeletal filaments, their connection with various cellular components, and the generation of movement. An important family of structurally and, in part, functionally related proteins capable of interlinking different elements of the cytoskeleton are the plakins or cytolinkers.[1–5] Plakins are large proteins that were first identified on the basis of their association with IFs or IF-anchoring structures, such as desmosomes and hemidesmosomes (HDs). Thus, cytolinkers play crucial roles in maintaining cell and tissue integrity and orchestrating dynamic changes in cytoarchitecture and cell shape. With their multidomain structure and enormous size, they serve as scaffolding platforms for the assembly, positioning, and regulation of signaling complexes. Among the plakins, plectin is the best characterized and seems the most versatile.

GENE AND PROTEIN STRUCTURE

Full-length plectin has a deduced molecular mass ranging from 499 to 533 kDa, depending on the particular isoform.[6] Rotary shadowing electron microscopy of purified plectin molecules[7] revealed a dumbbell-like structure comprising a central 200-nm–long rod domain flanked by large globular domains (**Fig. 1A**). The multidomain structure of plectin was confirmed by secondary structure predictions based on complementary DNA and deduced amino acid sequences. These analyses also revealed that the rod domain is characterized by long stretches of heptad repeats, distinctive of α-helical coiled coils,[8] and exhibits a staggered strict period of 10.4 for acidic and basic residues, suggesting an energetically most favored parallel arrangement of a plectin dimer.[9] This is supported by the microscopic dimensions of plectin and gel permeation high-performance liquid chromatography data indicating a molecular mass of plectin molecules in solution of slightly more than 1.1×10^6 Da.[7,10] The structure of the 214-kDa carboxy (C)-terminal globular domain, encoded by a single very large (>6 kb) exon, is dominated by six highly homologous, approximately 300 amino acid residues–long repeat domains,[9] which also occur in different numbers in other cytolinker (plakin) protein family members, such as desmoplakin,[11] the epithelial and neuronal isoforms of BPAG1/dystonin,[12] envoplakin,[13] and epiplakin.[14,15] The amino (N)-terminal domain comprises an actin-binding domain (ABD), shared by a large superfamily of actin-binding proteins,[16] and a plakin domain containing several spectrin repeats interrupted by an SH3 domain.[5,17]

Plectin is expressed as several protein isoforms from a single gene, PLEC1, that is located on chromosome 8q24 in humans (see **Fig. 1C**).[18,19] The plectin gene locus in mouse (chromosome 15)

Department of Biochemistry and Cell Biology, Max F. Perutz Laboratories, University of Vienna, Dr.-Bohr-Gasse 9, 1030 Vienna, Austria
* Corresponding author.
E-mail address: gerhard.wiche@univie.ac.at (G. Wiche).

Dermatol Clin 28 (2010) 33–41
doi:10.1016/j.det.2009.10.004

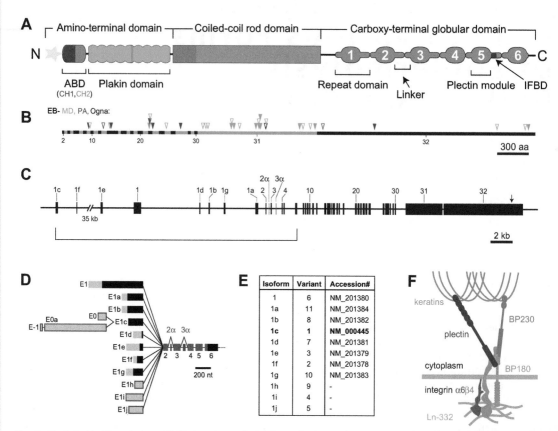

Fig. 1. Protein (*A*, *B*) and gene (*C*, *D*) structure of plectin and schematic representation of a HD (*E*). (*A*) Schematic map of the protein. The tripartite structure of plectin molecules comprises a central rod flanked by N-terminal and C-terminal (globular) domains. The N-terminal domain contains an ABD, consisting of two calponin homology (CH) domains (*dark and light orange*) and a region called plakin domain (*light green*) that consists of spectrin-like repeats and contains a SH3 domain (*dark green*). The C-terminal globular domain contains six highly homologous plectin repeat domains (*blue*), each consisting of a plectin module and a linker region, one of which harbors an IF binding domain (IFBD; *red*). Alternative splicing of plectin transcripts leads to expression of protein isoforms with different N termini (*yellow star*). (*B*) Plectin mutations. Positions of mutations described in the literature are indicated on a schematic of the protein indicating the exons (*alternating black and gray boxes*) coding for the respective part of the protein. Mutations are color-coded for the associated phenotype: EBS-MD is shown in green, EBS-PA in red, and EBS-Ogna in blue. Open triangles indicate mutations observed in a (compound) heterozygous state; full triangles represent a homozygous state. Exact positions, further details, and references for the individual mutations are given in **Table 1**. (*C*) Genomic organization of the human plectin gene. Exons are represented as black boxes, introns by lines. Plectin (exons 1c to 32) extends over approximately 60 kb. The position of the stop codon in exon 32 is indicated with an arrow. An alternative representation better suited to illustrate the alternative splice events occurring within the region marked by the bracket is shown in (*D*). (*D*) Schematic representation of alternative plectin transcripts in humans and mice. Exons are shown as boxes and splice events as lines connecting individual boxes. Alternative splicing of the 5′-end of the plectin gene gives rise to several different transcripts: eight alternative first coding exons identified in humans and mice and splicing into the common exon 2, are shown. Coding regions are shown in black; 5′ untranslated regions are gray. Two optionally spliced exons (2α and 3α, inserted between exons 2 and 3, and 3 and 4, respectively) are shown in red. Three additional noncoding exons splicing into exon 2 and three further noncoding exons upstream of exon 1c were identified in the mouse (exons with red borders). The existence of similar exons in the human plectin gene is to be expected. (*E*) Plectin isoforms and database records. The Variant numbering is based on the positioning of the first coding exon within the plectin gene (in mouse). Variants 4, 5, and 9 have not yet been identified in the human gene. Exon 1c is the most 5′ and exon 1a the most 3′ exon splicing into the common exon 2. (*F*) Schematic drawing of the structure and components of a type I HD found in (pseudo-) stratified epithelium, such as that of the skin. Plectin and BP230 mediate intracellular stabilization of the HD by binding to integrin β4 and keratin IFs. Type I HDs additionally contain the type XVII collagen BP180. The extracellular matrix ligand for integrin α6β4 is laminin 322 (Ln-322).

has been analyzed in detail,[20] revealing a genomic exon-intron organization with more than 40 exons spanning 62 kb on chromosome 15 and an unusual 5′ transcript complexity of plectin isoforms. Eleven exons (1–1j) have been identified that alternatively splice directly into a common exon 2 (which is the first exon to encode plectin's highly conserved ABD), three (−1, 0a, and 0) that are spliced upstream of exon 1c, and two additional ones (2α and 3α) that are optionally spliced within the ABD-encoding exons (2–8; see **Fig. 1D**). In a recent study, the human and rat gene loci were reanalyzed based on newly available genome sequences and compared to the mouse gene. In rat, all 11 alternative first exons identified in mouse were found, whereas in the human gene, so far, the presence of eight of these exons has been confirmed.[21] Furthermore, a rodless human plectin variant, as judged by molecular size, has been detected on the protein level.[22,23]

EXPRESSION, SUBCELLULAR LOCALIZATION, AND BINDING PARTNERS

Plectin is expressed in virtually all mammalian tissues and cell types, as has been demonstrated using antisera and a panel of monoclonal antibodies.[24,25] It is particularly prominent in various types of muscle, stratified and simple epithelia, cells forming the blood-brain barrier, and tissue layers at the interface between tissues and fluid-filled cavities, where it was found at the surfaces of kidney glomeruli, liver bile canaliculi, bladder urothelium, gut villi, ependymal layers lining the cavities of brain and spinal cord, and endothelial cells of blood vessels.[26–30] At the cellular level, plectin codistributes with different types of IFs and is located at plasma membrane attachment sites of IFs and microfilaments, such as HDs,[27,31] desmosomes,[32] Z-line structures and dense plaques of striated and smooth muscle, intercalated discs of cardiac muscle, and focal contacts.[26,33]

Ribonuclease protection experiments performed on a panel of mouse tissues and cell types, using antisense riboprobes specific for the various alternative first exons of plectin, provided clear evidence for the occurrence of tissue-specific or dominant plectin isoforms.[20,34] For example, plectin transcripts containing exon 1d were exclusively found in skeletal and heart muscle, whereas exon 1a–containing transcripts were dominant in organs rich in epithelial cell types, such as lung, small intestine, and, in particular, skin. Tissue-specific expression was characteristic also of the two optionally spliced exons, 2α and 3α, with isoforms containing exon 2α being expressed in brain,

heart, and skeletal muscle, and exon 3α being brain-specific.[20] Furthermore, the alternative first exons were found to determine the stability of gene products by controlling initiation of translation. The most intriguing finding, however, was that the short alternative N-terminal sequences encoded by the different first exons direct the various isoforms to distinct subcellular locations.[6] For instance, plectin 1a specifically associated with HD-like structures in keratinocytes,[34] plectin 1b was found associated exclusively with mitochondria,[35] and plectin 1f was concentrated in vinculin-positive structures at actin stress fiber ends.[6] Thus, it seems that each cell type (tissue) contains a unique set (proportion and composition) of plectin isoforms, as if custom-made for specific requirements of the particular cells. Concordantly, individual isoforms were found to carry out distinct and specific functions.

Consistent with its varied subcellular localization, plectin has been shown to directly interact with a variety of cytoskeletal structures and proteins. In its C-terminal domain, plectin contains a multifunctional IF-binding site that was mapped to an approximately 50 amino acid–long sequence located between the highly conserved core regions of its C-terminal repeats 5 and 6.[36] This site mediates binding to several types of IF subunit proteins, including vimentin,[36] desmin,[37] glial fibrillary acidic protein (GFAP),[38] the nuclear IF protein lamin B,[39] and type I and type II cytokeratins.[40] A highly conserved ABD close to its N terminus mediates binding not only to actin[41] but also to the integrin subunit β4,[31,42] vimentin,[43] the EF-ZZ domain of dystrophin and utrophin,[44] and binding sites for nesprin-3.[45] Additionally, the signaling molecule phosphatidylinositol-4,5-bisphosphate (PIP$_2$) binds within the ABD, regulating binding of plectin to actin.[41] Binding of integrin β4 and actin to plectin's ABD has been shown to be mutually exclusive.[6,42,46] Furthermore, the interactions of actin and integrin β4 with plectin isoform 1a are regulated in a Ca^{2+}-dependent manner by calmodulin, which binds to the CH1 domain of the ABD.[47] Additional binding sites for integrin β4[31,48] and for β-dystroglycan[44] are contained in the plakin and C-terminal domains of plectin. Direct interactions of plectin with the membrane skeleton proteins fodrin and α-spectrin,[49] the desmosomal protein desmoplakin,[32] and microtubule-associated proteins (MAP2 and MAP1 subtypes) from brain[49] have been reported. Furthermore, whole-mount electron microscopy was used to demonstrate that plectin is capable of physically linking IFs to microtubules.[50]

Recently, it has been shown that plectin not only functions as a cytolinker but also acts as a scaffold for proteins involved in signaling, anchoring them at specific sites within a cell. Such proteins include the nonreceptor tyrosine kinase Fer[51]; the receptor for activated C kinase 1 (RACK1) that is sequestered to the cytoskeleton through plectin during initial stages of cell adhesion[52]; and the γ1 subunit of the energy-controlling AMP-activated protein kinase.[53]

PLECTIN GENE MUTATIONS AND EPIDERMOLYSIS BULLOSA SIMPLEX

In 1996, several groups reported that patients suffering from epidermolysis bullosa simplex with muscular dystrophy (EBS-MD), an autosomal recessive disorder with neonatal skin blistering and delayed, progressive muscular weakness, lacked plectin expression in skin and muscle tissues due to defects in the plectin gene.[19,54–57] Based on plectin's prominence at plasma membrane junctional sites of IFs, it had been anticipated that defects in its gene would lead to such phenotypes. The direct interaction of plectin with the HD integrin subunit β4, generating a linkage between the IF cytoskeleton and the extracellular matrix (see **Fig. 1F**), provided a molecular model for the skin blistering phenotype.[31] In many cases, the responsible mutations were nonsense mutations, out-of-frame insertions, or deletions within exons 31 or 32, resulting in premature stop codons. This predicts truncated polypeptides and mRNA down-regulation through nonsense-mediated mRNA degradation. Lack of immunoreactivity of samples from such patients suggested the absence of plectin molecules. As the antibodies most commonly used were immunoreactive with the rod or C-terminal domains, however, truncated versions of plectin might still have existed. One notable mutation is 13480ins16 (homozygous), where normal levels of mRNA were found and protein was detectable, although at reduced levels.[58] EBS-MD was further found to be caused by several in-frame insertion and deletion mutations, such as homozygous 2674del9 [exon 21][55,58] or compound heterozygous 1537ins36/2674del9 [exons 14 and 21].[59] In general, the phenotypes of EBS-MD patients vary considerably in severity of skin blistering and onset of muscular dystrophy.

EBS with pyloric atresia (EBS-PA) is another HD variant that manifests as severe neonatal skin blistering and gastric abnormalities (pyloric or duodenal atresia) and frequently leads to early postnatal demise of affected individuals. Plectin mutations underlying EBS-PA comprise homozygous or compound heterozygous nonsense mutations and, in one case, a homozygous 21-bp in-frame deletion within exon 22.[60] Attempts to correlate plectin genotypes with the EBS-PA versus EBS-MD phenotypes could not provide any clues for the intriguing phenotypic differences. So far, however, no mutations causing PA have been found within the rod-encoding exon 31. Thus, the presence of rodless splice variants of plectin, which have been detected in some EBS-MD patients,[48] may be the reason for the less severe phenotype compared to EBS-PA.

Besides the recessive forms of plectin-linked EBS, one autosomal dominant form of EBS, designated EBS-Ogna, has been identified. This rare mutation was identified in a kindred near the small Norwegian town of Ogna (hence its name) and independently in a German family. It constitutes a heterozygous missense mutation, R2000W, within the rod-encoding exon 31,[61,62] apparently perturbing the function of plectin through dominant negative interference. These patients do not develop MD or show any signs of PA.

The position numbering of mutations found in the existing literature is based on different sequence database entries, and thus is confusing. The reason for this is the alternative 5′ splicing of plectin isoforms, each with its own database entry. Therefore, the authors have compiled a list of all plectin mutations published thus far (**Table 1**) and assigned numbers to the mutations based on a common reference sequence (accession no. NM_000445), plectin isoform 1c (also described as variant 1 in the databases). The positions of the mutations and resulting phenotypes are depicted in **Fig. 1B**. Thus far, no mutations in the alternative first exons have been described. Mutations that would lead to the elimination of only one specific isoform, however, are expected to be found in the future. Likely candidates are exon 1a (skin phenotype) and 1d (muscle phenotype). The authors propose that such mutations are named based on the corresponding database sequence (see **Fig. 1E**) and that the isoform or variant be indicated in that case (eg, a hypothetical mutation in exon 1a would be named R7X^{1a}).

ANIMAL MODELS OF PLECTIN-RELATED EPIDERMOLYSIS BULLOSA SIMPLEX

Several mouse models have been generated to mimic the clinical features of plectin-associated EBS. The first was a plectin-null mouse,[63] followed by a conditional knockout mouse line, where the knockout of plectin was restricted to keratin 5–expressing epithelia (K5-Cre KO),[64] and, recently,

Table 1
Plectin mutations reported in the literature

Mutation[a]	Original Designation[b]	Exon[c]	Genotype[d]	Case[e]	References
EBS-MD					
963ins3	1287ins3, 1008ins3	9	c.het. (Q1408X)	14	73
1537ins36	1541ins36	14	c.het. (2674del9)	20	59,74
2674del9	2677del9, 2719del9	21	hom.	4,20	56
2700-9del21	2745-9del21	22	c.het. (5038delG)	12	75
Q1053X	(Same)	24	c.het. (Q1936X)	9	76
Q1408X	(Same), Q1518X	31	c.het. (963ins3)	14	73
4313ins13	4359ins13	31	c.het. (4371delC)	8	77
4371delC	4416delC	31	c.het. (4313ins13)	8	77
5024del19	5069del19	31	hom.	6	78
5038delG	5083delG	31	c.het. (2700-9del21)	12	75
5103del8	5148del8	31	hom.	1	19
Q1713X	(Same)	31	c.het. (R2351X)	11	79
5264insG	5309insG, 5588insG	31	hom.	16,19	59,80
Q1910X	(Same)	31	hom.	5	54
Q1936X	(Same)	31	c.het. (Q1053X)	9	76
5821delC	5866delC	31	hom.	3	56
5854ins8	5907ins8	31	hom.	2	81
5860del2	5905del2	31	hom.	7	78
E2005X	(Same)	31	c.het. (K4460X)	13	75
R2319X	(Same)	31	hom.	18	82
R2351X	(Same)	31	c.het. (Q1665)	11	79
R2421X	(Same)	31	c.het. (12588ins4)	10,22	76
R2465X	(Same)	31	hom.	17	83
12588ins4	12633ins4	32	c.het. (R2421X)	10	76
K4460X	(Same)	32	c.het. (E2005X)	13	75
13480ins16	13803ins16	32	hom.	15	58
EBS-PA					
Q305X	(Same)	9	hom.; c.het. (1350G>A)	23,28	60,67
1350G>A	1344G>A	12	c.het. (Q305X)	23	67
1569del4	1563del4, 1567del4	14	hom.	27	60
2686del14	2727del14	21	hom.	22	66
2775del21	2769del21	22	hom.	26	60
R1189X	(Same)	27	hom.; c.het. (Q2538X)	24	67
Q2538X	(Same)	32	c.het. (R1189X)	24	67
R3029X	(Same)	32	hom.	25	60
EBS-Ogna					
R2000W	R2110W	31	het. (dominant)	29,30	62

[a] Mutations are ordered by phenotype (EBS-MD, EBS-PA, and EBS-Ogna) and position within the plectin gene. Numbers correspond to the plectin isoform 1c sequence starting with the first nucleotide of exon 1c (or the methionine encoded by the start codon of exon 1c). In the databases, this isoform is also referred to as variant 1 (GenBank accession no. NM_000445). This sequence does not include the alternatively spliced exons 2α and 3α.
[b] Designations of the mutations in the existing literature. Note the inconsistent numbering schemes.
[c] Exon harboring the mutation.
[d] Genotype of the patient, which is homozygous (hom.), heterozygous (het.), or compound heterozygous (c.het.) Mutation on the other allele is given in parentheses.
[e] The case number assigned by Pfendner and colleagues in their review on plectin mutations in EBS.[59]

a mouse line with a conditional deletion of plectin in striated muscle (MCK-Cre KO).[65] At birth, homozygous null and K5-Cre KO mice are generally not distinguishable from their heterozygote or wild-type littermates. Within 1 to 2 days after birth (occasionally even at birth), however, null mice become frail and begin to show signs of gross skin blistering, especially at fore- and hindlimbs, and in some cases around the mouth and nasal cavities.[63] In K5-Cre KO mice, skin blistering develops with a similar onset, body distribution, and severity.[64] In some cases, plectin-null and K5-Cre KO mice are born with denuded paws[64] (authors' unpublished observations), resembling aplasia cutis congenita, as was reported for the most severe cases of plectin-associated EBS-PA.[60,66,67] In plectin-null mice, blisters on the lower extremities are often hemorrhagic,[63] which, however, is not observed in K5-Cre KO mice (authors' unpublished observations). This type of bleeding might indicate a possible perturbation of vascular endothelial cells, which normally express plectin at relatively high levels.[26,29] Blistering usually occurs by cytolysis in the basal cytoplasm of basal keratinocytes, immediately above HDs[64] (authors' unpublished data), and sometimes also in perinuclear regions,[64] probably reflecting plectin's function in linking cytokeratin IFs with each other[68] and to the outer nuclear membrane.[45] Inspection of the upper gastrointestinal tract of newborn K5-Cre KO mice after at least one nursing revealed the presence of multiple blisters on their palates and in some cases also on their tongues but not in the esophagus. Thus, plectin knockout mice seem to die from malnutrition as a consequence of blistering of the oral epithelia, reducing the pups' desire for food due to pain and possibly obstruction of the oral cavity by especially large blisters or cellular debris.[64] The skin blistering phenotypes of mice lacking integrins α6 and β4 are more severe than those of plectin-null and K5-Cre KO mice. These mice show complete absence of HDs and are born with large patches of detached epidermis and generally die within a few hours after birth.[69–71] In plectin-deficient epidermis, however, HDs are still present, although their numbers are reduced and keratin IF-attachment is impaired.[63] BPAG1-null mice display only mild defects in cytokeratin IF attachment to HDs and, therefore, develop skin blisters only late during postnatal development.[72] Similar to patients suffering from EBS-MD, plectin-null mice display compromised muscle fiber integrity.[63] Mimicking the late-onset muscular dystrophy typical of EBS-MD, adult MCK-Cre KO mice develop progressive degenerative alterations in skeletal muscle, including aggregation and partial loss of desmin IF networks, detachment of the contractile apparatus from the sarcolemma, and decreased number and impaired function of mitochondria.[65]

REFERENCES

1. Wiche G. Role of plectin in cytoskeleton organization and dynamics. J Cell Sci 1998;111:2477–86.
2. Fuchs E, Karakesisoglou I. Bridging cytoskeletal intersections. Genes Dev 2001;15:1–14.
3. Leung CL, Green KJ, Liem RK. Plakins: a family of versatile cytolinker proteins. Trends Cell Biol 2002; 12:37–45.
4. Fuchs P, Wiche G. Intermediate filament linker proteins: plectin and BPAG1. In: Lennartz WJ, Lane MD, editors. Encyclopedia of biological chemistry, vol. 2. New York: Elsevier; 2004. p. 452–7.
5. Sonnenberg A, Liem RK. Plakins in development and disease. Exp Cell Res 2007;313:2189–203.
6. Rezniczek GA, Abrahamsberg C, Fuchs P, et al. Plectin 5′-transcript diversity: short alternative sequences determine stability of gene products, initiation of translation and subcellular localization of isoforms. Hum Mol Genet 2003;12(23):3181–94.
7. Foisner R, Wiche G. Structure and hydrodynamic properties of plectin molecules. J Mol Biol 1987; 198(3):515–31.
8. McLachlan AD, Stewart M. Tropomyosin coiled-coil interactions: evidence for an unstaggered structure. J Mol Biol 1975;98(2):293–304.
9. Wiche G, Becker B, Luber K, et al. Cloning and sequencing of rat plectin indicates a 466-kD polypeptide chain with a three-domain structure based on a central alpha-helical coiled coil. J Cell Biol 1991;114(1):83–99.
10. Weitzer G, Wiche G. Plectin from bovine lenses. Chemical properties, structural analysis and initial identification of interaction partners. Eur J Biochem 1987;169(1):41–52.
11. Green KJ, Parry DA, Steinert PM, et al. Structure of the human desmoplakins. Implications for function in the desmosomal plaque. J Biol Chem 1990; 265(5):2603–12.
12. Sawamura D, Li KH, Nomura K, et al. Bullous pemphigoid antigen: cDNA cloning, cellular expression, and evidence for polymorphism of the human gene. J Invest Dermatol 1991;96(6):908–15.
13. Ruhrberg C, Hajibagheri MA, Simon M, et al. Envoplakin, a novel precursor of the cornified envelope that has homology to desmoplakin. J Cell Biol 1996;134(3):715–29.
14. Fujiwara S, Takeo N, Otani Y, et al. Epiplakin, a novel member of the plakin family originally identified as a 450-kDa human epidermal autoantigen. Structure and tissue localization. J Biol Chem 2001;276(16): 13340–7.

15. Spazierer D, Fuchs P, Pröll V, et al. Epiplakin gene analysis in mouse reveals a single exon encoding a 725-kDa protein with expression restricted to epithelial tissues. J Biol Chem 2003;278(34): 31657–66.

16. Stradal T, Kranewitter W, Winder SJ, et al. CH domains revisited. FEBS Lett 1998;431(2):134–7.

17. Jefferson JJ, Ciatto C, Shapiro L, et al. Structural analysis of the plakin domain of bullous pemphigoid antigen1 (BPAG1) suggests that plakins are members of the spectrin superfamily. J Mol Biol 2007;366(1):244–57.

18. Liu CG, Maercker C, Castanon MJ, et al. Human plectin: organization of the gene, sequence analysis, and chromosome localization (8q24). Proc Natl Acad Sci U S A 1996;93(9):4278–83.

19. McLean WH, Pulkkinen L, Smith FJ, et al. Loss of plectin causes epidermolysis bullosa with muscular dystrophy: cDNA cloning and genomic organization. Genes Dev 1996;10(14):1724–35.

20. Fuchs P, Zörer M, Rezniczek GA, et al. Unusual 5' transcript complexity of plectin isoforms: novel tissue-specific exons modulate actin binding activity. Hum Mol Genet 1999;8(13):2461–72.

21. Zhang T, Haws P, Wu Q. Multiple variable first exons: a mechanism for cell- and tissue-specific gene regulation. Genome Res 2004;14(1):79–89.

22. Schröder R, Fürst DO, Klasen C, et al. Association of plectin with Z-discs is a prerequisite for the formation of the intermyofibrillar desmin cytoskeleton. Lab Invest 2000;80(4):455–64.

23. Brown MJ, Hallam JA, Liu Y, et al. Cutting edge: integration of human T lymphocyte cytoskeleton by the cytolinker plectin. J Immunol 2001;167(2):641–5.

24. Wiche G, Baker MA. Cytoplasmic network arrays demonstrated by immunolocalization using antibodies to a high molecular weight protein present in cytoskeletal preparations from cultured cells. Exp Cell Res 1982;138(1):15–29.

25. Foisner R, Feldman B, Sander L, et al. A panel of monoclonal antibodies to rat plectin: distinction by epitope mapping and immunoreactivity with different tissues and cell lines. Acta Histochem 1994;96(4):421–38.

26. Wiche G, Krepler R, Artlieb U, et al. Occurrence and immunolocalization of plectin in tissues. J Cell Biol 1983;97(3):887–901.

27. Wiche G, Krepler R, Artlieb U, et al. Identification of plectin in different human cell types and immunolocalization at epithelial basal cell surface membranes. Exp Cell Res 1984;155(1):43–9.

28. Wiche G. Plectin: general overview and appraisal of its potential role as a subunit protein of the cytomatrix. Crit Rev Biochem Mol Biol 1989;24(1): 41–67.

29. Errante LD, Wiche G, Shaw G. Distribution of plectin, an intermediate filament-associated protein, in the adult rat central nervous system. J Neurosci Res 1994;37(4):515–28.

30. Yaoita E, Wiche G, Yamamoto T, et al. Perinuclear distribution of plectin characterizes visceral epithelial cells of rat glomeruli. Am J Pathol 1996;149(1): 319–27.

31. Rezniczek GA, de Pereda JM, Reipert S, et al. Linking integrin α6β4-based cell adhesion to the intermediate filament cytoskeleton: direct interaction between the beta4 subunit and plectin at multiple molecular sites. J Cell Biol 1998;141(1):209–25.

32. Eger A, Stockinger A, Wiche G, et al. Polarisation-dependent association of plectin with desmoplakin and the lateral submembrane skeleton in MDCK cells. J Cell Sci 1997;110(Pt 11):1307–16.

33. Seifert GJ, Lawson D, Wiche G. Immunolocalization of the intermediate filament-associated protein plectin at focal contacts and actin stress fibers. Eur J Cell Biol 1992;59(1):138–47.

34. Andrä K, Kornacker I, Jörgl A, et al. Plectin-isoform-specific rescue of hemidesmosomal defects in plectin (-/-) keratinocytes. J Invest Dermatol 2003;120(2): 189–97.

35. Winter L, Abrahamsberg C, Wiche G. Plectin isoform 1b mediates mitochondrion-intermediate filament network linkage and controls organelle shape. J Cell Biol 2008;181(6):903–11.

36. Nikolic B, Mac Nulty E, Mir B, et al. Basic amino acid residue cluster within nuclear targeting sequence motif is essential for cytoplasmic plectin-vimentin network junctions. J Cell Biol 1996;134(6): 1455–67.

37. Reipert S, Steinböck F, Fischer I, et al. Association of mitochondria with plectin and desmin intermediate filaments in striated muscle. Exp Cell Res 1999; 252(2):479–91.

38. Foisner R, Leichtfried FE, Herrmann H, et al. Cytoskeleton-associated plectin: in situ localization, in vitro reconstitution, and binding to immobilized intermediate filament proteins. J Cell Biol 1988;106(3): 723–33.

39. Foisner R, Traub P, Wiche G. Protein kinase A- and protein kinase C-regulated interaction of plectin with lamin B and vimentin. Proc Natl Acad Sci U S A 1991;88(9):3812–6.

40. Steinböck FA, Nikolic B, Coulombe PA, et al. Dose-dependent linkage, assembly inhibition and disassembly of vimentin and cytokeratin 5/14 filaments through plectin's intermediate filament-binding domain. J Cell Sci 2000;113(Pt 3):483–91.

41. Andrä K, Nikolic B, Stöcher M, et al. Not just scaffolding: plectin regulates actin dynamics in cultured cells. Genes Dev 1998;12(21):3442–51.

42. Geerts D, Fontao L, Nievers MG, et al. Binding of integrin α6β4 to plectin prevents plectin association with F-actin but does not interfere with intermediate filament binding. J Cell Biol 1999;147(2):417–34.

43. Sevcik J, Urbanikova L, Kost'an J, et al. Actin-binding domain of mouse plectin. Crystal structure and binding to vimentin. Eur J Biochem 2004; 271(10):1873–84.

44. Rezniczek GA, Konieczny P, Nikolic B, et al. Plectin 1f scaffolding at the sarcolemma of dystrophic (mdx) muscle fibers through multiple interactions with beta-dystroglycan. J Cell Biol 2007;176(7): 965–77.

45. Wilhelmsen K, Litjens SH, Kuikman I, et al. Nesprin-3, a novel outer nuclear membrane protein, associates with the cytoskeletal linker protein plectin. J Cell Biol 2005;171(5):799–810.

46. Garcia-Alvarez B, Bobkov A, Sonnenberg A, et al. Structural and functional analysis of the actin binding domain of plectin suggests alternative mechanisms for binding to F-actin and integrin beta4. Structure 2003;11(6):615–25.

47. Kostan J, Gregor M, Walko G, et al. Plectin isoform-dependent regulation of keratin-integrin $\alpha6\beta4$ anchorage via Ca^{2+} calmodulin. J Biol Chem 2009; 284:18525–36.

48. Koster J, van Wilpe S, Kuikman I, et al. Role of binding of plectin to the integrin beta4 subunit in the assembly of hemidesmosomes. Mol Biol Cell 2004;15(3):1211–23.

49. Herrmann H, Wiche G. Plectin and IFAP-300K are homologous proteins binding to microtubule-associated proteins 1 and 2 and to the 240-kilodalton subunit of spectrin. J Biol Chem 1987;262(3): 1320–5.

50. Svitkina TM, Verkhovsky AB, Borisy GG. Plectin sidearms mediate interaction of intermediate filaments with microtubules and other components of the cytoskeleton. J Cell Biol 1996;135(4): 991–1007.

51. Lunter PC, Wiche G. Direct binding of plectin to Fer kinase and negative regulation of its catalytic activity. Biochem Biophys Res Commun 2002; 296(4):904–10.

52. Osmanagic-Myers S, Wiche G. Plectin-RACK1 (receptor for activated C kinase 1) scaffolding: a novel mechanism to regulate protein kinase C activity. J Biol Chem 2004;279(18):18701–10.

53. Gregor M, Zeöld A, Oehler S, et al. Plectin scaffolds recruit energy-controlling AMP-activated protein kinase (AMPK) in differentiated myofibres. J Cell Sci 2006;119(Pt 9):1864–75.

54. Chavanas S, Pulkkinen L, Gache Y, et al. A homozygous nonsense mutation in the PLEC1 gene in patients with epidermolysis bullosa simplex with muscular dystrophy. J Clin Invest 1996;98(10): 2196–200.

55. Gache Y, Chavanas S, Lacour JP, et al. Defective expression of plectin/HD1 in epidermolysis bullosa simplex with muscular dystrophy. J Clin Invest 1996;97(10):2289–98.

56. Pulkkinen L, Smith FJ, Shimizu H, et al. Homozygous deletion mutations in the plectin gene (PLEC1) in patients with epidermolysis bullosa simplex associated with late-onset muscular dystrophy. Hum Mol Genet 1996;5(10):1539–46.

57. Smith FJ, Eady RA, Leigh IM, et al. Plectin deficiency results in muscular dystrophy with epidermolysis bullosa. Nat Genet 1996;13(4):450–7.

58. Schröder R, Kunz WS, Rouan F, et al. Disorganization of the desmin cytoskeleton and mitochondrial dysfunction in plectin-related epidermolysis bullosa simplex with muscular dystrophy. J Neuropathol Exp Neurol 2002;61(6):520–30.

59. Pfendner E, Rouan F, Uitto J. Progress in epidermolysis bullosa: the phenotypic spectrum of plectin mutations. Exp Dermatol 2005;14(4):241–9.

60. Pfendner E, Uitto J. Plectin gene mutations can cause epidermolysis bullosa with pyloric atresia. J Invest Dermatol 2005;124(1):111–5.

61. Koss-Harnes D, Jahnsen FL, Wiche G, et al. Plectin abnormality in epidermolysis bullosa simplex Ogna: non-responsiveness of basal keratinocytes to some anti-rat plectin antibodies. Exp Dermatol 1997;6(1): 41–8.

62. Koss-Harnes D, Hoyheim B, Anton-Lamprecht I, et al. A site-specific plectin mutation causes dominant epidermolysis bullosa simplex Ogna: two identical de novo mutations. J Invest Dermatol 2002; 118(1):87–93.

63. Andrä K, Lassmann H, Bittner R, et al. Targeted inactivation of plectin reveals essential function in maintaining the integrity of skin, muscle, and heart cytoarchitecture. Genes Dev 1997;11(23): 3143–56.

64. Ackerl R, Walko G, Fuchs P, et al. Conditional targeting of plectin in prenatal and adult mouse stratified epithelia causes keratinocyte fragility and lesional epidermal barrier defects. J Cell Sci 2007;120(Pt 14):2435–43.

65. Konieczny P, Fuchs P, Reipert S, et al. Myofiber integrity depends on desmin network targeting to Z-disks and costameres via distinct plectin isoforms. J Cell Biol 2008;181:667–81.

66. Charlesworth A, Gagnoux-Palacios L, Bonduelle M, et al. Identification of a lethal form of epidermolysis bullosa simplex associated with a homozygous genetic mutation in plectin. J Invest Dermatol 2003;121(6):1344–8.

67. Nakamura H, Sawamura D, Goto M, et al. Epidermolysis bullosa simplex associated with pyloric atresia is a novel clinical subtype caused by mutations in the plectin gene (PLEC1). J Mol Diagn 2005;7(1):28–35.

68. Osmanagic-Myers S, Gregor M, Walko G, et al. Plectin-controlled keratin cytoarchitecture affects MAP kinases involved in cellular stress response and migration. J Cell Biol 2006;174(4):557–68.

69. Dowling J, Yu QC, Fuchs E. Beta4 integrin is required for hemidesmosome formation, cell adhesion and cell survival. J Cell Biol 1996;134(2): 559–72.

70. Georges-Labouesse E, Messaddeq N, Yehia G, et al. Absence of integrin alpha 6 leads to epidermolysis bullosa and neonatal death in mice. Nat Genet 1996;13(3):370–3.

71. van der Neut R, Krimpenfort P, Calafat J, et al. Epithelial detachment due to absence of hemidesmosomes in integrin beta 4 null mice. Nat Genet 1996;13(3):366–9.

72. Guo L, Degenstein L, Dowling J, et al. Gene targeting of BPAG1: abnormalities in mechanical strength and cell migration in stratified epithelia and neurologic degeneration. Cell 1995;81(2):233–43.

73. Bauer JW, Rouan F, Kofler B, et al. A compound heterozygous one amino-acid insertion/nonsense mutation in the plectin gene causes epidermolysis bullosa simplex with plectin deficiency. Am J Pathol 2001;158(2):617–25.

74. Uitto J, Pfendner E. Compound heterozygosity of unique in-frame insertion and deletion mutations in the plectin gene in a mild case of epidermolysis bullosa with very late onset muscular dystrophy. J Invest Dermatol 2004;122:A86.

75. Rouan F, Pulkkinen L, Meneguzzi G, et al. Epidermolysis bullosa: novel and de novo premature termination codon and deletion mutations in the plectin gene predict late-onset muscular dystrophy. J Invest Dermatol 2000;114(2):381–7.

76. Takizawa Y, Shimizu H, Rouan F, et al. Four novel plectin gene mutations in Japanese patients with epidermolysis bullosa with muscular dystrophy disclosed by heteroduplex scanning and protein truncation tests. J Invest Dermatol 1999;112(1): 109–12.

77. Dang M, Pulkkinen L, Smith FJ, et al. Novel compound heterozygous mutations in the plectin gene in epidermolysis bullosa with muscular dystrophy and the use of protein truncation test for detection of premature termination codon mutations. Lab Invest 1998;78(2):195–204.

78. Mellerio JE, Smith FJ, McMillan JR, et al. Recessive epidermolysis bullosa simplex associated with plectin mutations: infantile respiratory complications in two unrelated cases. Br J Dermatol 1997;137(6):898–906.

79. Kunz M, Rouan F, Pulkkinen L, et al. Mutation reports: epidermolysis bullosa simplex associated with severe mucous membrane involvement and novel mutations in the plectin gene. J Invest Dermatol 2000;114(2):376–80.

80. Schara U, Tücke J, Mortier W, et al. Severe mucous membrane involvement in epidermolysis bullosa simplex with muscular dystrophy due to a novel plectin gene mutation. Eur J Pediatr 2004; 163(4–5):218–22.

81. Hovnanian A, Pollack E, Hilal L, et al. A missense mutation in the rod domain of keratin 14 associated with recessive epidermolysis bullosa simplex. Nat Genet 1993;3(4):327–32.

82. Takahashi Y, Rouan F, Uitto J, et al. Plectin deficient epidermolysis bullosa simplex with 27-year-history of muscular dystrophy. J Dermatol Sci 2005;37(2): 87–93.

83. McMillan JR, Akiyama M, Rouan F, et al. Plectin defects in epidermolysis bullosa simplex with muscular dystrophy. Muscle Nerve 2007;35(1):24–35.

Epidermolysis Bullosa with Pyloric Atresia

Hye Jin Chung, MD, MS, Jouni Uitto, MD, PhD*

KEYWORDS

- Epidermolysis bullosa • Heritable skin diseases
- Blistering disorders • Molecular genetics

CLINICAL AND GENETIC HETEROGENEITY OF EB

Epidermolysis bullosa (EB) is a heterogeneous group of skin fragility syndromes with the diagnostic hallmark of blistering and erosions of the skin. Proper diagnosis and subclassification of different forms of EB can be challenging for general practitioners because of considerable phenotypic variability, as reflected by the complex classification schemes riddled with eponyms.[1] The most streamlined classification divides EB into 3 broad categories depending on the precise location of tissue separation within the cutaneous basement membrane zone, as determined by diagnostic transmission electron microscopy or by immuno-epitope mapping: (1) in the simplex forms (EBS), tissue separation takes place within the basal keratinocytes; (2) the junctional forms (JEB) show blistering within the dermal-epidermal basement membrane, frequently within the lamina lucida; and (3) in the dystrophic forms (DEB), tissue separation is below the lamina densa within the upper papillary dermis at the level of anchoring fibrils. The inheritance of different forms of EB is either autosomal dominant or autosomal recessive.[2,3] It is now known that mutations in 10 different genes expressed within the cutaneous basement membrane zone underlie the classic simplex, junctional, and dystrophic forms of EB.[4,5] The types and combinations of mutations, their consequences at the mRNA and protein levels, when placed in the context of the individuals' genetic background, including modifier genes, and the environmental trauma, all contribute to the severity of the disease, explaining the phenotypic variability in this group of disorders.

In addition to skin involvement, different forms of EB can be associated with extracutaneous manifestations; these include hair, nail, and tooth abnormalities, ocular findings, and fragility of the epithelia in upper respiratory, urogenital, and gastrointestinal tracts.[1] There are 2 rare forms of EB, one associated with late-onset muscular dystrophy (EB-MD), and another one with congenital pyloric atresia (EB-PA). EB-MD has been shown to result from mutations in the plectin gene (PLEC1), which encodes a large, approximately 500-kDa adhesion molecule.[6] In the skin, the binding partners of plectin include basal cell keratins (KRT5 and KRT14), $\alpha_6\beta_4$ integrins, and type XVII collagen/the 180-kDa bullous pemphigoid antigen, thus serving as a bridge between the intermediate filament cytoskeleton and hemidesmosomes within the basal keratinocytes (Fig. 1).[7,8] In addition to skin, plectin is expressed in various tissues, including striated muscle and gastrointestinal epithelia. Specifically, in skeletal muscle, plectin is expressed in the sarcolemma and the Z-lines, thus participating in the formation of the intermyofibrillar-desmin cytoskeleton. Consequently, expression of plectin in the skin and in the skeletal muscle explains the consequences of mutations in 2 different organ systems

The authors' original studies were supported by the US Department of Health and Human Services, National Institutes of Health/National Institute of Arthritis and Musculoskeletal and Skin Diseases grants P01 AR38923 and by the Dermatology Foundation.

Department of Dermatology and Cutaneous Biology, Jefferson Medical College, Jefferson Institute of Molecular Medicine, Thomas Jefferson University, 233 South 10th Street, Suite 450 BLSB, Philadelphia, PA 19107, USA

* Corresponding author.

E-mail address: Jouni.Uitto@jefferson.edu (J. Uitto).

doi:10.1016/j.det.2009.10.005
0733-8635/09/$ – see front matter © 2010 Elsevier Inc. All rights reserved.

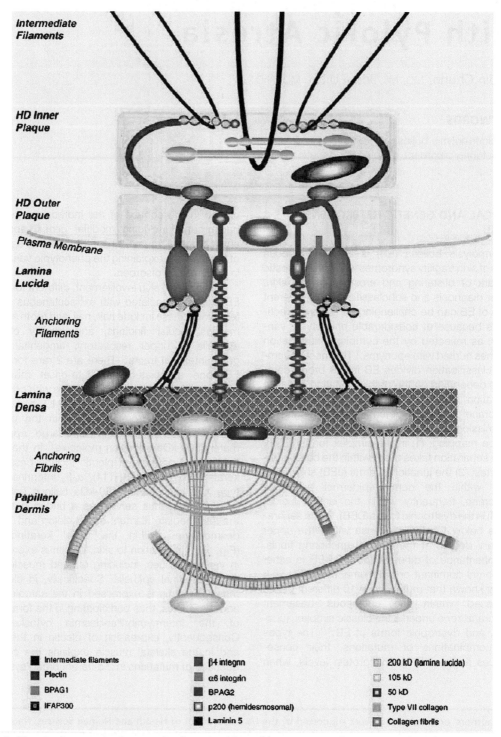

Intermediate
Filaments

HD Inner
Plaque

HD Outer
Plaque

Plasma Membrane

Lamina
Lucida

Anchoring
Filaments

Lamina
Densa

Anchoring
Fibrils

Papillary
Dermis

■ Intermediate filaments	■ β4 integrin	▨ 200 kD (lamina lucida)
■ Plectin	■ α6 integrin	☐ 105 kD
▨ BPAG1	■ BPAG2	▣ 50 kD
▣ IFAP300	☐ p200 (hemidesmosomal)	▨ Type VII collagen
	■ Laminin 5	☐ Collagen fibrils

Fig. 1. The attachment complexes at the dermal-epidermal basement membrane zone, which form a continuous network of interacting proteins necessary for stable association of epidermis and dermis at the dermal-epidermal junction. Note the presence of hemidesmosomal components, plectin, $\alpha_6\beta_4$ integrin, and the type XVII collagen/ the 180-kDa bullous pemphigoid antigen 2 (BPAG2). The critical role of the hemidesmosomal proteins in the integrity of the skin is indicated by mutations in the corresponding genes that result in dermal-epidermal separation. (*Adapted from* Pulkkinen L, Uitto J. Hemidesmosomal variants of epidermolysis bullosa. Mutations in the alpha6beta4 integrin and the 180-kD bullous pemphigoid antigen/type XVII collagen genes. Exp Dermatol 1998;7:50; with permission.)

in EB-MD, characterized by skin blistering and muscular dystrophy.[6]

Another gene/protein system harboring mutations in patients with EB-PA is the $\alpha_6\beta_4$ integrin; the corresponding subunit polypeptides of this hemidesmosomal protein are encoded by the *ITGA6* and *ITGB4* genes. This transmembrane protein is an integral part of hemidesmosomes serving a structural role in the attachment of the basal keratinocytes to the underlying basement membrane, and serving as signaling molecules. Within the intracellular milieu of basal keratinocytes, $\alpha_6\beta_4$ is linked to the cytokeratin network by plectin; the $\alpha_6\beta_4$-plectin interaction is crucial for hemidesmosome stability, and it has been proposed that this association acts as an initiation step in the assembly of hemidesmosomes.[9] The $\alpha_6\beta_4$ integrin is characteristically expressed in various epithelial tissues, including human skin and the gastrointestinal tract, in which it

functions as a receptor for laminin-332 (laminin-5), a major extracellular component of the epidermal basement membrane (see **Fig. 1**). The subunit responsible for intracellular interactions of $\alpha_6\beta_4$, including binding to plectin, is the cytoplasmic domain of the β_4 subunit, which is unusually large (approximately 1000 amino acid residues) and shares little similarity with other integrin β-subunits.[7] The β_4 cytodomain has a modular organization with 4 fibronectin type III (FnIII) domains arranged in 2 pairs of tandem repeats separated by a connecting segment region (**Fig. 2**). The N-terminal region of plectin interacts with the β_4 subunit at multiple sites. The primary contact is established between the actin binding domain of plectin and the first pair of FnIII domains and a small region of the connecting segment of β_4 polypeptide (**Figs. 2** and **3**). In the extracellular domain, β_4 integrin has a segment of cysteine-rich repeats.

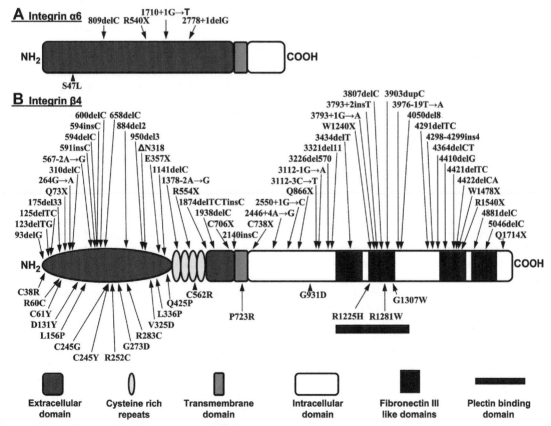

Fig. 2. The domain organizations of the α_6 integrin (*A*) and β_4 integrin (*B*) subunit polypeptides. The color-coded explanation of the domains is at the bottom of the figure. The *arrows* point to the positions of the mutations along the protein structure. Mutations above each of the schematic structures represent premature termination codon-causing mutations, whereas those below the schematic structures are missense mutations. (Note that the numbering of the mutations may differ from those in the original publications because the numbering has been adjusted to conform with the following National Center for Biotechnology Information (NCBI) database entries: ITGA6, NM-000210; ITGB4, NM-001005731.)

Mutation in EB-PA patients

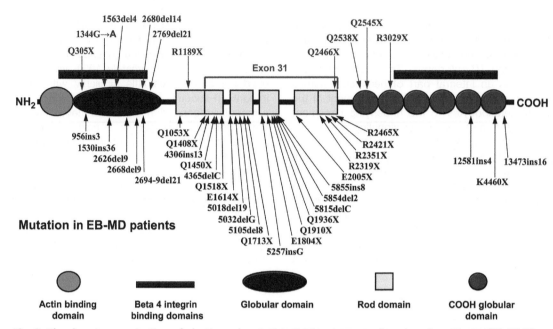

Fig. 3. The domain organization of plectin and mutations in the corresponding gene in patients with EB-PA or with EB-MD. The color code of the domain organization is at the bottom of the figure. The *arrows* point to the positions of the mutations along the plectin polypeptide. The mutations indicated above the schematic structure are those associated with EB-PA, whereas those below have been reported to result in EB-MD phenotype. Note the clustering of the mutations causing EB-MD in the rod domain that is encoded by exon 31, whereas all mutations in EB-PA patients (except one, Q2466X) are outside exon 31. (Note that the numbering of the mutations may differ from those in original publications because the numbering has been adjusted to conform with the plectin sequence in NCBI database entry NM-000445.)

The $\alpha_6\beta_4$ integrin stimulates cell migration, invasion, and survival of epithelial cells by activating signaling pathways, and these signaling functions are also coupled to disruption of the hemidesmosomal conformation. The extracellular domain of β_4 integrin interacts with the α_6 integrin, which is considerably smaller, with a small intracellular domain (see **Fig. 2**). The assembled $\alpha_6\beta_4$ integrin then interacts with laminin-332, which on the other end connects to the lamina densa of the lower portion of the cutaneous basement membrane (see **Fig. 1**). Thus, the $\alpha_6\beta_4$ integrin plays a critical role in the integral stability of the cutaneous basement membrane zone, particularly through its interactions with plectin.

EB-PA

EB-PA is a syndromic association of skin fragility and congenital gastrointestinal atresia, most frequently pyloric, although duodenal atresia with skin fragility has also been reported (**Fig. 4**).[10,11] The inheritance of EB-PA is autosomal recessive (**Fig. 5**). Although association of EB and PA is

rare, the overall incidence of PA has been reported to be less than 1% of all gastrointestinal atresias[12] and the incidence of recessively inherited junctional forms of EB has been calculated at 2.04 per 10^6.[13] Thus, the segregation of these 2 disorders must be more than coincidental.

In some cases of EB, aplasia cutis congenita (ACC) is also present (see **Fig. 4**).[10] Although congenital absence of skin is clearly a heterogenous group of disorders and can be associated with different subtypes of EB, patients with EB-PA can demonstrate widespread ulcerated lesions, frequently in the extremities, with complete absence of all layers of the skin (see **Fig. 4**). The healed ACC lesions demonstrate a smooth epidermis, proliferation of fibroblasts in loose connective tissue stroma, newly formed capillaries, and absence of adnexal structures. Although intrauterine mechanical trauma has been suggested as an explanation for the development of ACC in some patients, with or without EB, the association of PA and ACC with EB suggests a common genetic basis for pathogenesis of these complications of EB.[10]

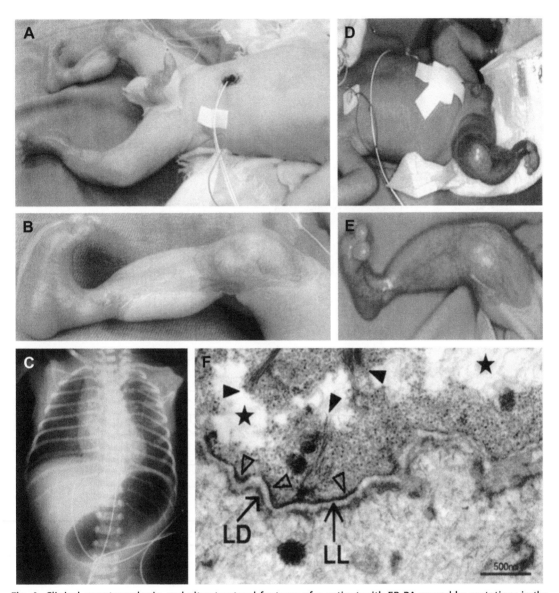

Fig. 4. Clinical, roentgenologic, and ultrastructural features of a patient with EB-PA caused by mutations in the *PLEC1* gene. (*A, B*) Note sharply demarcated ulcerations in the lower extremities of the proband. (*C*) Abdominal bubble of gas in radiograph of the proband. (*D, E*) The proband's older brother has similar, but healing cutaneous lesions. (*F*) Transmission electron microscopy reveals tissue separation within the basal cells (*stars*). Keratin filaments are sparse (*full arrowheads*) and not well associated with the hemidesmosomes, which are hypoplastic and reduced in number (*open arrowheads*). The lamina densa (LD) and lamina lucida (LL) seem intact. Original magnification: bar, 500 nm. (*Adapted from* Nakamura H, Sawamura D, Goto M, et al. Epidermolysis bullosa simplex associated with pyloric atresia is a novel clinical subtype caused by mutations in the plectin gene (PLEC1). J Mol Diagn 2005;7:30; with permission.)

The precise subclassification of the type of EB associated with PA has been confusing because ultrastructural findings of the location of skin blistering in EB-PA patients have demonstrated 2 patterns.[1] First, in most cases, tissue separation occurs within the lamina lucida, associated with small hemidesmosomal plaques and often with attenuated subbasal dense plate, observations found in classic junctional forms of EB (see **Fig. 5**). Secondly, some patients with EB-PA demonstrate intracellular tissue separation within the lower basal cell layer, just above the level of the hemidesmosomal plaque (see **Fig. 4**). The latter patients also demonstrate reduced integration of keratin filaments with hemidesmosomes. Because the tissue

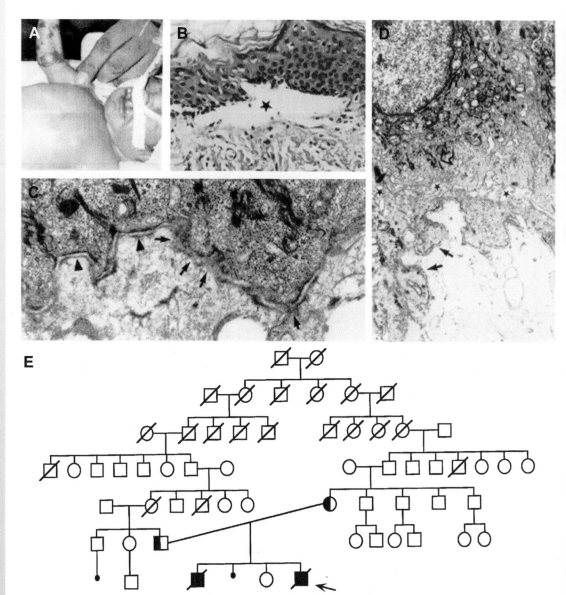

Fig. 5. Clinical, genetic, histopathological, and ultrastructural features of a patient with EB-PA. The proband (*arrow*) is the fourth child of a consanguineous mating (*E*). The proband demonstrates extensive blistering of the skin (*A*), which by histopathologic examination shows separation at the dermal-epidermal junction (*B*, the *asterisk* indicates the location of a blister). Note extensive blistering on the right arm of the proband, who also had bilateral cleft lip and cleft palate (*A*). Transmission electron microscopy of the dermal-epidermal junction reveals the presence of hemidesmosomes lacking the inner plaque (*C, arrowheads*), and segments of the basement membrane zone were morphologically perturbed (*C, arrows*). Intermediate filaments were severed from the lower portion of the basal keratinocytes and condensed perinuclearly (*D, open arrow*). (*Adapted from Pulkkinen L, Kimonis VE, Xu Y, et al. Homozygous alpha6 integrin mutation in junctional epidermolysis bullosa with congenital duodenal atresia. Hum Mol Genet 1997;6:671; with permission.*)

separation in the latter cases is within the basal cells, it has been suggested that these patients belong to the subtype of EBS. Consequently, the latest classification of inherited epidermolysis bullosa, based on the report of the Third International Consensus Meeting on Diagnosis and Classification of EB,[1] includes the existence of 2 different subtypes of EB with pyloric atresia: EBS-PA and JEB-PA. It should be noted that a previously suggested classification attempting to streamline the nomenclature of EB suggested consolidation of these 2 different forms of EB with PA in the newly proposed subgroup of "hemidesmosomal variants of EB."[14] Although this classification highlighted the molecular involvement of hemidesmosomal genes in the causes of EB-PA, together with plectin abnormalities in EB-MD and type XVII collagen/the 180-kDa bullous pemphigoid antigen in generalized atrophic benign EB (GA-BEB), the International Consensus Meeting suggested that the term "hemidesmosomal EB" not to be used.[1] Thus, EB-PA is separated into 2 distinct entities based on the ultrastructural findings of the level of tissue separation within the cutaneous basement membrane zone: EBS-PA and JEB-PA.

CLINICAL AND PATHOLOGIC FEATURES OF EB-PA

The diagnosis of EB-PA, with or without ACC, is based on clinical observations, imaging studies, histopathology, ultrastructural findings, immuno-histochemistry of the skin, and molecular diagnostics (see **Figs. 4–5; Fig. 6**).[10] As indicated earlier, the cutaneous findings include tissue separation either within the basal cells at the level of hemidesmosomes or within the lamina lucida of the dermal-epidermal basement membrane. The presence of PA is often suggested by gestational hydramnion, which can be confirmed by ultrasound and radiograph studies (see **Fig. 4**).

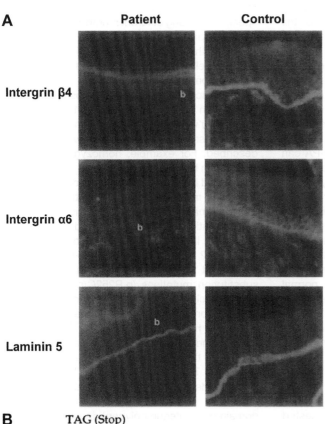

A **Patient** **Control**

Intergrin β4

Intergrin α6

Laminin 5

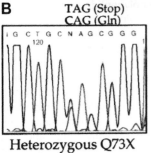

B TAG (Stop)
CAG (Gln)

Heterozygous Q73X

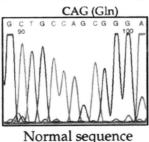

CAG (Gln)

Normal sequence

Fig. 6. Immunohistochemical analysis and mutation detection in families with EB-PA. Upper panel (*A*) illustrates immunohistochemical analysis of the skin of an affected infant with EB-PA (*left panel*), compared with an unrelated control (*right panel*). Skin sections were stained with monoclonal antibodies 3E1 recognizing integrin β_4, GoH3 recognizing integrin α_6, and GB3 recognizing intact laminin-5 (laminin-332), as indicated on the left side. Skin of the affected infant was negative for α_6 and β_4, while staining for laminin-5 was normal. The blister cavities are indicated by *b*. (*B*) A mutation in the ITGB4 gene in a patient with EB-PA (*lower panel*). Note that sequencing of the proband ITGB4 gene revealed a C→T transition mutation at nucleotide position 217 in 1 allele, resulting in change of codon for glutamine (CAG) to a stop codon (TAG) at amino acid position 73. In comparison, the control sequences are shown on the right. (*Adapted from* Pulkkinen L, Kim DU, Uitto J. Epidermolysis bullosa with pyloric atresia: novel mutations in the beta4 integrin gene (ITGB4). Am J Pathol 1998;152:162, 163; with permission.)

Histopathology of the gastrointestinal involvement can show obstruction of the esophagus by a fibrotic membrane with disappearance of the mucosal layer. Narrowing of the pylorus and proximal part of the duodenum associated with thickening of the gastric submucosal connective tissue can proceed to complete obstruction by a fibrotic membrane rich in blood vessels.[10] These findings are frequently associated with inflammation. It has been postulated that the basic pathology leading to the EB-PA-ACC phenotype involves 2 elements: (1) the integrity of the basement membrane zone and hemidesmosomes, and (2) the control of processes of fibrosis.[10] This sequence of events may be initiated by the separation of the epidermis or the intestinal mucosal layer as a result of poorly functional or absent hemidesmosomal complexes. Inflammatory responses contribute to the development of secondary fibrosis leading specifically to the obstruction of the intestinal lumina, especially in anatomically narrow spaces, such as pylorus. In support of this cascade of events are ultrastructural demonstrations of hemidesmosomal abnormalities, histologically demonstrated inflammation, and more recently, immunohistochemical demonstration of abnormalities in the expression of $\alpha_6\beta_4$ integrin or plectin.

The severity of skin involvement in EB-PA can be variable.[15–17] In some individuals, even on successful surgical correction of the pyloric or duodenal atresia, skin fragility is so severe that the affected children die from complications, such as infections or electrolyte imbalance, within a few days or weeks post partum. In other individuals, the skin fragility may be mild, and in some individuals, age-associated amelioration of the skin fragility allows them to conduct normal life activities with minor blistering tendency. In some individuals, blisters may develop only on strenuous mechanical trauma of the skin. The denuded lesions of ACC can heal in surviving individuals, with primarily cosmetic sequela.

MOLECULAR GENETICS OF EB-PA

Early immunohistochemical evidence suggested that expression of the $\alpha_6\beta_4$ integrin is reduced or completely absent in the skin of several patients affected with EB-PA (see **Fig. 6A**).[18–20] This observation was followed by cloning and sequencing of the genes encoding the 2 subunit polypeptides of the $\alpha_6\beta_4$ integrin (*ITGA6* and *ITGB4*) (see **Figs. 2** and **3**).[21,22]

The genes encoding $\alpha_6\beta_4$ integrin subunit polypeptides have been shown to harbor a large number of mutations in patients with EB-PA, most of them residing in *ITGB4* (see **Fig. 2**). Examination of the mutation database in *ITGB4* reveals a total of 70 distinct mutations in patients with skin blistering, all but 2 of whom have PA. Among these mutations, 45 were premature termination codon (PTC)-causing mutations (nonsense mutations, small insertions or deletions, or putative splice junction mutations resulting in-frame shift), which are predicted to result in the translation of shortened, and presumably nonfunctional, β_4 integrin polypeptides (see **Fig. 2B**). The generation of PTCs can also result in the absence of the corresponding protein because of accelerated mRNA decay or by the truncated polypeptides being sensitive to proteolytic degradation.[23,24] In addition, several missense mutations have been identified, and in many cases the substituted amino acid has been shown to be highly conserved through evolution of the *ITGB4* gene in different species or among different members of the human β-integrin proteins (**Fig. 7**).[25]

Among the missense mutations in *ITGB4*, there are 5 cysteine substitutions that affect the extracellular domain of the β_4 subunit (see **Fig. 2B**). Although some of the cysteine substitution mutations (such as homozygous p.C61Y) have been associated with lethal outcome,[14] nonlethal cases from consanguineous union have also been described. For example, homozygous, p.C562R mutation in the cysteine-rich region of the β_4 integrin resulted in PA noted at birth but developed only localized, mild skin blistering with subsequent tooth and nail dystrophy.[14] In addition to homozygous mutations, several compound heterozygous mutations in *ITGB4* have been described. For example, 2 nonlethal cases of EB-PA, 1 of them compound heterozygous for 2 distinct arginine substitution mutations (p.R252C/p.R1281W) and 1 for a leucine-to-proline substitution mutation, in combination with a nonsense mutation (p.L156P/p.R554X), have been reported.[14,25] The first of these 2 individuals was moderately affected at birth, but the condition considerably improved with time. The second individual had mild blistering tendency and dystrophic nails. One of the mutations (p.R1281W) affects the intracellular domain of β_4 integrin polypeptide within the putative region interacting with plectin. On the other hand, the other mutation in this individual, p.R252C, creates a new cysteine residue in the extracellular domain of β_4 integrin and may participate in the formation of new intra- or intermolecular disulfide bonds, possibly disrupting ligand binding or affecting noncovalent associations between the α_6 and β_4 integrin subunits. The missense mutations, particularly those affecting highly conserved amino acid residues within the

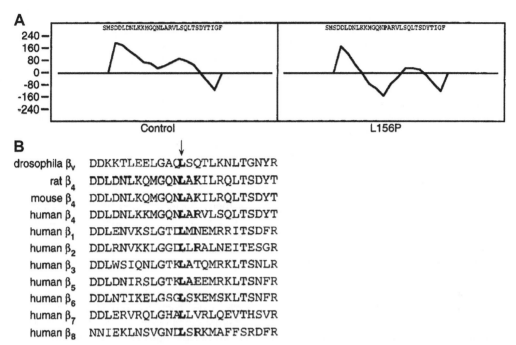

Fig. 7. Demonstration of consequences of a leucine-to-proline substitution in the amino acid position 156 of the β_4 integrin polypeptide in a patient with EB-PA. (*A*) Garnier α-helicity plot predicts that introduction of proline into position 156, in place of a leucine, disrupts the α-helix of the mutated polypeptide. (*B*) Comparison of β_4 integrin sequences in different species and between different human integrin β-chains reveals conservation of the leucine at position 156. (*Adapted from* Pulkkinen L, Bruckner-Tuderman L, August C, et al. Compound heterozygosity for missense (L156P) and nonsense (R554X) mutations in the beta4 integrin gene (ITGB4) underlies mild, nonlethal phenotype of epidermolysis bullosa with pyloric atresia. Am J Pathol 1998;152:939; with permission.)

extracellular domain of β_4 integrin, can result in conformational changes of the β_4 integrin polypeptide. For example, in a patient with p.L156P mutation, the Garnier α-helicity plot analysis has suggested that the region spanning Leu-156 has propensity for α-helix formation, and introduction of a proline residue to this position disrupts the helical conformation (see **Fig. 7**).[25] These and related observations suggest that the invariably conserved Leu-156 residue plays a critical role in the structure/function characteristics of β_4 integrin.

In addition to mutations in the *ITGB4* gene, a total of 5 mutations in the α_6 integrin subunit gene (*ITGA6*) have been reported in patients with EB-PA (see **Fig. 2A**). Examination of the *ITGA6* mutation database reveals that 4 of the total of 5 mutations are PTC-causing, and 1 is a nonsense mutation. All of them reside within the extracellular domain of the deduced protein (see **Fig. 2A**). The clinical features of the individuals with *ITGA6* mutations are largely indistinguishable from those caused by mutations in *ITGB4*, indicating that both subunit polypeptides of the $\alpha_6\beta_4$ integrin complex play a critical role in the function of this integrin.

Why the mutations in the *ITGA6* gene are less frequent than those in *ITGB4* is unknown.

As indicated earlier, ultrastructural observations on the skin lesions in EB-PA have suggested that tissue separation can occur at the level of lamina lucida or within the basal cells, thus leading to the suggestion that there are 2 subtypes: JEB-PA and EBS-PA. Although mutations in the $\alpha_6\beta_4$ integrin genes encode a transmembrane protein with intracellular and extracellular domains, most of the *ITGB4* and *ITGA6* mutations seem to be associated with lamina lucida split, suggesting that they are the primary cause of the JEB-PA subtype. In addition, deletion of a cytoplasmic domain of integrin β_4 polypeptide has been shown to cause a mild EBS without association of PA.[26] Specifically, a 2-bp deletion, c.4364delCT, in *ITGB4* resulted in in-frame skipping of 50 amino acids (p.del1450-1499) within the third fibronectin type III repeat in the cytoplasmic domain of the integrin β_4 polypeptide. This domain of integrin β_4 is believed to interact with type XVII collagen/the 180-kDa bullous pemphigoid antigen, attesting to the importance of the $\alpha_6\beta_4$ integrin in epidermal integrity.

A recent report has suggested that ITGB4 can harbor mutations that do not lead to significant skin blistering but are associated with pyloric atresia.[27] Specifically, 2 Kuwaiti siblings had PA and life-threatening intestinal desquamation, without significant skin abnormalities. Analysis of $\alpha_6\beta_4$ integrin genes identified a novel mutation in ITGB4, a homozygous deletion of a single isoleucine-1314 residue within the intracellular plectin-binding domain. Expression of α_6 and β_4 integrin within skin, duodenal, and colonic epithelium was normal or slightly reduced as detected by immunohistochemical techniques. This demonstration of a mutation within the ITGB4 gene, together with the existence of desquamated enteropathy associated with congenital PA, suggests existence of an overlap condition with JEB-PA without cutaneous signs. Although the deletion of this single amino acid (Ile1314), which resides within a fibronectin III-like domain, potentially interacting with plectin, it is unclear as to why the phenotypic expression in these patients is limited to intestinal epithelium, which does not contain hemidesmosomes. In this individual, there was evidence of mucosal inflammatory response, possibly secondary to loss of epithelial barrier function, and colocalization of IgG and C1q within the intestinal basement membrane and low-titer circulating IgG autoantibody was noted. Significant improvement in the desquamative enteropathy was noted with immune modulatory therapy, leading to the suggestion that such treatment of these patients may give significant clinical benefits in other patients also. Finally, an individual with classic features of JEB, without PA and with no history of gastrointestinal diseases, has been reported to harbor an ITGB4 mutation of critical amino acid residues leading to selected, tissue-specific manifestations in some patients.[28]

MUTATIONS IN THE PLECTIN GENE (PLEC1) CAN CAUSE EB-PA

Plectin, a 500-kDa intermediate filament-binding protein and intracellular component of hemidesmosomes, interacts with β_4 integrin (see **Fig. 1**). As indicated above, mutations in the plectin gene were originally shown to result in an autosomal recessive variant of EB with late-onset muscular dystrophy[6]; up to now, 31 mutations in the plectin gene associated with EB-MD have been reported (see **Fig. 3**). Considering the interactions of plectin and $\alpha_6\beta_4$ integrin, it was not surprising that a subset of patients with EB-PA was shown by immunohistochemical staining to have reduced or absent expression of plectin in the skin, and subsequently, 10 distinct mutations in the PLEC1 gene were demonstrated in 11 patients with EB-PA (see **Fig. 3**).[29,30] Among these patients, there are a total of 9 PTC-causing mutations, 1 mutation causes an in-frame deletion of 7 amino acids, and none of the mutations is a missense one. All these patients with EB have definite PA and none of them has been reported to develop muscular dystrophy. Most of these patients also have extensive ACC, and at least 9 of them died soon after birth.

Concerning the distribution of the mutations in the PLEC1 gene in patients with EB-PA, although the mutations in EB-MD patients are distributed along the entire length of the plectin gene, many of them cluster in exon 31, which encodes the rod domain in the middle of the protein (see **Fig. 3**). In contrast, the PLEC1 mutations in EB-PA patients, with 1 exception, are outside exon 31. This observation would provide an explanation for the phenotypic differences as a result of plectin mutations leading to EB-PA or EB-MD. Specifically, cells such as skin fibroblasts express 2 different plectin isoforms consisting of either full-length polypeptides or a rodless form generated by alternative splicing of exon 31.[31] In mutations within exon 31, the rodless isoform of plectin may be expressed, leading to milder skin manifestations, yet associated with late-onset muscular dystrophy. In PTC-causing, loss-of-function mutations outside exon 31, the full-length and the rodless isoforms of plectin are lost, thus leading to more severe cutaneous blistering phenotype associated with PA.[31] This pathomechanistic difference might provide an explanation for the genotype/phenotype correlation, resulting in 2 different phenotypes, EB-PA and EB-MD, as a result of mutations in the same gene.

CLINICAL IMPLICATIONS OF MOLECULAR GENETICS ON EB-PA

Analogous to other major forms of EB, identification of precise mutations in EB-PA has profound implications for the management of patients and counseling of families affected with these diseases. Specifically, identification of mutations in families has provided molecular confirmation of the diagnosis coupled with prognostication, and will also provide a means for prenatal testing in families at risk for recurrence of the disease.[32,33] Prenatal testing in families at risk for EB-PA has been performed from chorionic villus sampling, which can be performed as early as the 10th week of gestation.[32] As an extension of DNA-based prenatal diagnosis, it has also been suggested that immunofluorescence analysis of villus trophoblasts may provide additional prenatal information.[34] Specifically, first-trimester chorionic villi in normal pregnancies were shown to express integrin $\alpha_6\beta_4$ and plectin strongly by immunofluorescence analysis. Subsequently, in a cohort of 25 pregnancies at risk for EB-PA, 3 fetuses were predicted to be affected, a finding that was confirmed by DNA-based tests and clinical observations. As an extension of the DNA-based prenatal testing, preimplantation genetic diagnosis has been implemented for EB and related skin fragility syndromes.[35,36] Although preimplantation genetic diagnosis avoids the potential ethical issues related to termination of pregnancy, its wider adoption has been hampered by the high cost and extensive clinical involvement of the mother in preparation for the test as part of in vitro fertilization procedure. Identification of the genes and precise mutations involved in the pathomechanisms of EB-PA provides the basis for molecularly based therapies: gene therapy, protein replacement, or stem-cell based therapies.[37,38] These approaches are supported by development of animal models for different forms of EB,[39] including those generated through targeted ablation of the genes, *ITGB4*, *ITGA6*, and *PLEC1*, which harbor mutations in EB-PA.

ACKNOWLEDGMENTS

GianPaolo Guercio assisted in the preparation of this manuscript.

REFERENCES

1. Fine JD, Eady RA, Bauer EA, et al. The classification of inherited epidermolysis bullosa (EB): report of the Third International Consensus Meeting on Diagnosis and Classification of EB. J Am Acad Dermatol 2008; 58:931–50.
2. Uitto J, Richard G. Progress in epidermolysis bullosa: genetic classification and clinical implications. Am J Med Genet C Semin Med Genet 2004; 131C:61–74.
3. Uitto J, Richard G. Progress in epidermolysis bullosa: from eponyms to molecular genetic classification. Clin Dermatol 2005;23:33–40.
4. Varki R, Sadowski S, Pfendner E, et al. Epidermolysis bullosa. I. Molecular genetics of the junctional and hemidesmosomal variants. J Med Genet 2006; 43:641–52.
5. Varki R, Sadowski S, Uitto J, et al. Epidermolysis bullosa. II. Type VII collagen mutations and phenotype-genotype correlations in the dystrophic subtypes. J Med Genet 2007;44:181–92.
6. Pfendner E, Rouan F, Uitto J. Progress in epidermolysis bullosa: the phenotypic spectrum of plectin mutations. Exp Dermatol 2005;14:241–9.
7. de Pereda JM, Lillo MP, Sonnenberg A. Structural basis of the interaction between integrin alpha6-beta4 and plectin at the hemidesmosomes. EMBO J 2009;28:1180–90.
8. Andrä K, Kornacker I, Jörgl A, et al. Plectin-isoform-specific rescue of hemidesmosomal defects in plectin (-/-) keratinocytes. J Invest Dermatol 2003;120:189–97.
9. Schaapveld RQ, Borradori L, Geerts D, et al. Hemidesmosome formation is initiated by the beta4 integrin subunit, requires complex formation of beta4 and HD1/plectin, and involves a direct interaction between beta4 and the bullous pemphigoid antigen 180. J Cell Biol 1998;142:271–84.
10. Maman E, Maor E, Kachko L, et al. Epidermolysis bullosa, pyloric atresia, aplasia cutis congenita: histopathological delineation of an autosomal recessive disease. Am J Med Genet 1998;78:127–33.
11. Dang N, Klingberg S, Rubin AI, et al. Differential expression of pyloric atresia in junctional epidermolysis bullosa with ITGB4 mutations suggests that pyloric atresia is due to factors other than the mutations and not predictive of a poor outcome: three novel mutations and a review of the literature. Acta Derm Venereol 2008;88:438–48.
12. Thompson NW, Parker W, Schwartz S, et al. Congenital pyloric atresia. Arch Surg 1968;97:792–6.
13. Pfendner E, Uitto J, Fine JD. Epidermolysis bullosa carrier frequencies in the US population. J Invest Dermatol 2001;116:483–4.
14. Pulkkinen L, Uitto J. Hemidesmosomal variants of epidermolysis bullosa. Mutations in the alpha6beta4 integrin and the 180-kD bullous pemphigoid antigen/type XVII collagen genes. Exp Dermatol 1998;7:46–64.
15. Nakano A, Pulkkinen L, Murrell D, et al. Epidermolysis bullosa with congenital pyloric atresia: novel mutations in the beta 4 integrin gene (ITGB4) and genotype/phenotype correlations. Pediatr Res 2001;49:618–26.
16. Pulkkinen L, Kim DU, Uitto J. Epidermolysis bullosa with pyloric atresia: novel mutations in the beta4 integrin gene (ITGB4). Am J Pathol 1998;152:157–66.
17. Mellerio JE, Pulkkinen L, McMillan JR, et al. Pyloric atresia-junctional epidermolysis bullosa syndrome: mutations in the integrin beta4 gene (ITGB4) in two unrelated patients with mild disease. Br J Dermatol 1998;139:862–71.
18. Jonkman MF, de Jong MC, Heeres K, et al. Expression of integrin alpha 6 beta 4 in junctional epidermolysis bullosa. J Invest Dermatol 1992;99:489–96.
19. Phillips RJ, Aplin JD, Lake BD. Antigenic expression of integrin alpha 6 beta 4 in junctional epidermolysis bullosa. Histopathology 1994;24:571–6.
20. Vidal F, Aberdam D, Miquel C, et al. Integrin beta 4 mutations associated with junctional epidermolysis bullosa with pyloric atresia. Nat Genet 1995;10: 229–34.

21. Pulkkinen L, Kimonis VE, Xu Y, et al. Homozygous alpha6 integrin mutation in junctional epidermolysis bullosa with congenital duodenal atresia. Hum Mol Genet 1997;6:669–74.

22. Pulkkinen L, Kurtz K, Xu Y, et al. Genomic organization of the integrin beta 4 gene (ITGB4): a homozygous splice-site mutation in a patient with junctional epidermolysis bullosa associated with pyloric atresia. Lab Invest 1997;76:823–33.

23. Iacovacci S, Cicuzza S, Odorisio T, et al. Novel and recurrent mutations in the integrin beta 4 subunit gene causing lethal junctional epidermolysis bullosa with pyloric atresia. Exp Dermatol 2003;12:716–20.

24. Micheloni A, De Luca N, Tadini G, et al. Intracellular degradation of beta4 integrin in lethal junctional epidermolysis bullosa with pyloric atresia. Br J Dermatol 2004;151:796–802.

25. Pulkkinen L, Bruckner-Tuderman L, August C, et al. Compound heterozygosity for missense (L156P) and nonsense (R554X) mutations in the beta4 integrin gene (ITGB4) underlies mild, nonlethal phenotype of epidermolysis bullosa with pyloric atresia. Am J Pathol 1998;152:935–41.

26. Jonkman MF, Pas HH, Nijenhuis M, et al. Deletion of a cytoplasmic domain of integrin beta4 causes epidermolysis bullosa simplex. J Invest Dermatol 2002; 119:1275–81.

27. Salvestrini C, McGrath JA, Ozoemena L, et al. Desquamative enteropathy and pyloric atresia without skin disease caused by a novel intracellular beta4 integrin mutation. J Pediatr Gastroenterol Nutr 2008;47:585–91.

28. Inoue M, Tamai K, Shimizu H, et al. A homozygous missense mutation in the cytoplasmic tail of beta4 integrin, G931D, that disrupts hemidesmosome assembly and underlies Non-Herlitz junctional epidermolysis bullosa without pyloric atresia? J Invest Dermatol 2000;114:1061–4.

29. Pfendner E, Uitto J. Plectin gene mutations can cause epidermolysis bullosa with pyloric atresia. J Invest Dermatol 2005;124:111–5.

30. Nakamura H, Sawamura D, Goto M, et al. Epidermolysis bullosa simplex associated with pyloric atresia is a novel clinical subtype caused by mutations in the plectin gene (PLEC1). J Mol Diagn 2005;7:28–35.

31. Sawamura D, Goto M, Sakai K, et al. Possible involvement of exon 31 alternative splicing in phenotype and severity of epidermolysis bullosa caused by mutations in PLEC1. J Invest Dermatol 2007; 127:1537–40.

32. Pfendner EG, Nakano A, Pulkkinen L, et al. Prenatal diagnosis for epidermolysis bullosa: a study of 144 consecutive pregnancies at risk. Prenat Diagn 2003;23:447–56.

33. Fassihi H, Eady RA, Mellerio JE, et al. Prenatal diagnosis for severe inherited skin disorders: 25 years' experience. Br J Dermatol 2006;154: 106–13.

34. D'Alessio M, Zambruno G, Charlesworth A, et al. Immunofluorescence analysis of villous trophoblasts: a tool for prenatal diagnosis of inherited epidermolysis bullosa with pyloric atresia. J Invest Dermatol 2008;128:2815–9.

35. Cserhalmi-Friedman PB, Tang Y, Adler A, et al. Preimplantation genetic diagnosis in two families at risk for recurrence of Herlitz junctional epidermolysis bullosa. Exp Dermatol 2000;9:290–7.

36. Fassihi H, Grace J, Lashwood A, et al. Preimplantation genetic diagnosis of skin fragility-ectodermal dysplasia syndrome. Br J Dermatol 2006;154: 546–50.

37. Uitto J. Progress in heritable skin diseases: translational implications of mutation analysis and prospects of molecular therapies. Acta Derm Venereol 2009;89:228–35.

38. Tamai K, Kaneda Y, Uitto J. Molecular therapies for heritable blistering diseases. Trends Mol Med 2009;15:285–92.

39. Jiang QJ, Uitto J. Animal models of epidermolysis bullosa–targets for gene therapy. J Invest Dermatol 2005;124:xi–xiii.

Herlitz Junctional Epidermolysis Bullosa

Martin Laimer, MD[a],*, Christoph M. Lanschuetzer, MD[a],
Anja Diem, MD[b], Johann W. Bauer, MD[a,b]

KEYWORDS

- Herlitz epidermolysis bullosa • Laminin-332
- Mutation analysis

Junctional epidermolysis bullosa type Herlitz (JEB-H) is the autosomal recessively inherited, more severe variant of "lucidolytic" JEB. Characterized by generalized, extensive mucocutaneous blistering at birth and early lethality, this devastating condition is most often caused by homozygous null mutations in the genes *LAMA3*, *LAMB3*, or *LAMC2*, each encoding for 1 of the 3 chains of the heterotrimer laminin-332. The latter is a major adhesion protein within the basement membrane zone of the skin and mucous epithelia that provides stable anchorage of basal epithelial cells (keratinocytes) to the underlying dermis by connecting the hemidesmosomal component $\alpha6\beta4$ integrin to collagen VII containing anchoring fibrils.[1]

EPIDEMIOLOGY

Accuracy and comparability of epidemiologic data regarding the genodermatosis epidermolysis bullosa (EB), a rare "orphan" disease with complex phenotype-genotype correlations, are based on the limitation of bias by misdiagnosis, misclassification, restricted access to expert physicians with specific expertise, and differential enrolment in registries across the highly variable (clinical and genetic) spectrum of EB.[2]

In an intention to overcome these obstacles, the United States National EB Registry (US NEBR) was founded in 1986 by the National Institutes of Health. This registry became the world's largest cohort of well-characterized and monitored EB patients, and currently comprises more than 3200 patients whose demographics have been shown to closely mirror that of the entire American population, as well that of EB patient cohorts elsewhere in the world.[3] Seven percent of these EB patients have some form of JEB, of which about 20% suffer from JEB-H.[2] By extrapolation, prevalence and incidence rates of JEB-H have been estimated to be 0.07 and less than 0.41 per million, respectively.

In the following discussion on JEB-H, the authors refer to the most comprehensive and representative data provided by the US NEBR. When comparing this information with observations at the EB House Austria, an interdisciplinary clinical unit established in 2005 for state of the art medical care, academic affairs (education and training for laypersons and experts), diagnostics, and research, there is an overall corroboration/concurrence between the index populations with just one exception. In the authors' experience, which is based on 6 genetically characterized JEB-H individuals currently documented in the Austrian EB Registry (**Table 1**) and several international consultation cases, death in infancy or early childhood, despite the most aggressive therapeutic interventions, is the norm (ie, 100%). Moreover, registry data on JEB-H in general is rather believed to actually underreport mortality as infants with rapid demise may not have been referred for inclusion. This perception is in accordance with most other clinicians.[4] The authors accordingly have never observed Herlitz patients surviving beyond the first year of life (mean lifetime

[a] Division of Molecular Dermatology, Department of Dermatology, General Hospital Salzburg, Paracelsus Medical University Salzburg, Muellner Hauptstrasse 48, A-5020 Salzburg, Austria
[b] EB House Austria, Department of Dermatology, General Hospital Salzburg, Paracelsus Medical University Salzburg, Muellner Hauptstrasse 48, A-5020 Salzburg, Austria
* Corresponding author.
E-mail address: m.laimer@salk.at (M. Laimer).

Dermatol Clin 28 (2010) 55–60
doi:10.1016/j.det.2009.10.006

Table 1
Molecular characterization of JEB-H patients documented in the Austrian EB registry

Patient	Mutated Gene	Mutation	Survival Period (Months)
1	*LAMB3*	R635X/R635X	2
2	*LAMB3*	R635X/R635X	8.5
3	*LAMB3*	R635X/R635X	5.5
4	*LAMB3*	R635X/R635X	6
5	*LAMC2*	L1122X/L1122X	2.5
6	*LAMB3*	R635X/1629insG	6

5.08 months), and thus none of the long-term skin or extracutaneous complications of JEB-H disease discussed in this article when referring to Herlitz NEBR patients. Those (even within the NEBR study population very rare) cases of long-term survival may either reflect a spectrum of disease severity mediated by genetic and epigenetic factors to be further characterized, or limited/restricted diagnostic validity/validation. For optimization of the latter, molecular mutation analysis in addition to structural analyses remains the current gold standard.

CLINICAL PRESENTATION OF JEB-H
Skin

Reflecting profound mechanical fragility as the hallmark feature, at birth JEB-H patients present with extensive, generalized, recurrent and often persistent blistering, erosions, and crusting that cover not only particularly exposed skin areas (like palms and soles) but most or almost all of the body surface (**Fig. 1**). Secondary lesions following chronic, repeated (even intrauterine) tissue traumatization include atrophic scarring, webbing (intradermal scar formation between fingers and toes), contractures (typically in axillary vaults), and milia (white papules).

Consecutive pigmentary abnormalities (hyper-, hypo, de-, or mottled pigmentation) rarely also comprise EB nevi (common in non-Herlitz JEB [JEB-nH]), ie, large eruptive, asymmetric, often irregularly pigmented, highly dynamic melanocytic lesions with sharply demarcated borders that frequently arise in areas of preceding blisters and may clinically mimic malignant melanoma (see the article by Lanschuetzer and colleagues elsewhere in this issue).

Pseudosyndactyly due to repeated blistering on hands and feet, initially presenting as partial interdigital fusion, webbing, or synechiae formation, and followed by complete fusion of all of the digits to a keratinaceous cocoonlike structure, frequently causes marked functional disability,

muscle atrophy, and bone absorption.[5] Exuberant granulation tissue, typically arising symmetrically around the mouth, central face, or nose as well as on the upper back, in axillary vaults, and around nail folds, is almost pathognomonic of JEB-H. Periorificial vegetation may cause complications such as total occlusion of nares, and implies therapeutic intervention by laser and sharp dissection. Differential diagnosis from squamous cell carcinoma is sometimes challenging, and may thus necessitate continuous clinical and occasionally histopathological evaluation. In addition, onychodystrophy with thickened, yellowish, longitudinally grooved, eventually marked curved and deformed nail plates (onychogryphosis), or absence (shedding) of nails due to atrophy and scarring of the nail bed (anonychia) are common findings in JEB-H.

Despite being more prominent in JEB-nH, localized or more diffuse scarring alopecia can also be observed in the Herlitz variant. Other uncommon cutaneous manifestations of JEB-H comprise palmoplantar keratoderma and congenital absence of skin with red, angulated, flame-shaped, well demarcated, depressed patches, usually unilateral, on hands, feet, wrists, or ankles.

Therapy in general is symptomatic, with antiseptic baths and functional bandages, splints, physical therapy, and surgical corrections (with often very high peri-interventional risk), thereby emphasizing the importance of preventing blistering by cool environment, avoidance of overheating, skin lubrication, water or air mattress, and soft, nonirritating fabric clothing.

Extracutaneous Involvement

Prototypical EB lesions such as blisters and erosions, followed by strictures, contractures, and stenoses, also occur in (epithelial) tissue outside the skin, involving for example the mucous membranes of the gastrointestinal, upper respiratory, and genitourinary tracts, the kidney, and external eye. These complex affections make

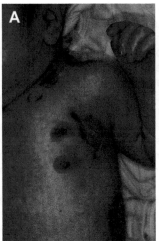
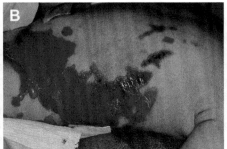
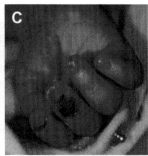

Fig. 1. (*A–C*) Junctional epidermolysis bullosa of Herlitz type (JEB-H) presenting with generalized blistering, crusted erosions, and extensive areas of denudation.

JEB-H a systemic, multidimensional disease with a considerably high morbidity and mortality.

Ophthalmic findings[6] in the Herlitz subtype include ocular surface (corneal, conjuctival) and eyelid abnormalities (blisters, erosions, and scarring), ectropion, exposure keratitis, pannus formation, limbal broadening, symblepharon, and lacrimal duct obstruction. Treatment is focused on ophthalmologic surgery and is accompanied by oral analgesics and topical antibiotics, as well as lubricants, gels, artificial tears, and bandages to reduce friction of the lids over the eye.

Upper respiratory tract involvement is a frequent phenomenon in both subtypes of JEB. The most common complications, namely chronic hoarseness, weak cry, or inspiratory stridor, are seen in up to 50% of all patients with JEB-H.[7] End-stage sequelae are laryngeal webs, stenosis, and (acute) airway obstruction due to occlusion by blisters, diffuse edema, progressive scar formation, and strictures or exuberant granulation tissue following blistering on the edges of the laryngeal cords. The cumulative risk of acute airway obstruction in JEB-H determined by analyses of the NEBR population is about 13% by as early as age 1 year. In patients surviving beyond the neonatal period, it plateaus at a risk of nearly 40% by age 6 years and thereafter decreases again, most likely due to the age-related increase in luminal diameter of airways. Consequently, early and regular surveillance is mandatory. Means of therapeutic management include dexamethasone and adrenalin nebulizers, humidified oxygen, (early elective) tracheostomy, laser and sharp dissection, or topical mitomycin C to reduce granulation tissue.

Chronic otitis media is another symptom that is more common in JEB-H patients than in the general population. Chronic otitis media is again the result of a barrier-impaired cutis and a consecutively higher risk of microbial colonization and infection. Otological therapy includes local antisepsis and topical antibacterial agents, although resistance due to long-term use is a serious concern, especially in a group of patients prone to septic complications.

Intraoral disease[8] is characterized by severe involvement of the oral soft and hard tissue, making both prophylactic and therapeutic approaches very challenging. Excessive caries results from a deficient oral hygiene due to painful peri- and intraoral blistering, erosions, and scar formation with consecutive contractures (microstomia, ankyloglossia), limited tongue mobility, and food clearance. Moreover, the specific, extremely cariogenic diet, a generally higher risk of infections such as candidiasis (reflecting the intrinsic barrier deficiency that stimulates colonization and invasiveness), as well as malnutrition (and consequent weakening of the immune system) are exacerbating factors that contribute to premature loss of teeth.

Enamel hypoplasia (pitting and furrowing of thin enamel, ultrastructurally displaying defects in prism structure and orientation) is another caries trigger and a characteristic feature of all JEB subtypes. Enamel hypoplasia is suggested to reflect a deregulated interaction of mutated adhesion proteins in the course of odontogenesis, histomorphogenesis, and cytodifferentiation. The spatially and temporally aberrant expression of mutated laminin-332 by enamel-forming ameloblasts may thus interfere with the intercellularly orchestrated regulation of enamel formation, signal transduction, cell polarity, mechanical stabilization and nutritional supply of enamel layers, enamel mineralization, orientation, and deposition at the enamel/dentin junction. The consequent disorganization and dysfunction of the basement membrane zone and the extracellular as well as enamel-forming matrix could represent the substrate of the abnormal dental architecture in JEB.

Development of highly aggressive squamous cell carcinomas was rarely reported in JEB-H patients surviving the early childhood period. Representing a dramatic long-term sequela arising most prominently in recessive dystrophic EB as early as within the second decade of life, ongoing nonhealing ulceration and consecutively permanent activation of reparative and proliferative pathways in combination with an intrinsically impaired intercellular and cell-matrix (structural as well as functional) regulation in EB are pathogenic sequences suspected to increase the risk of malignant transformation and development of tumors in the oral cavity (and skin).

Regular follow-ups by the dentist, emphasis on preventive measures (aggressive oral hygiene, fluoride substitution, reduction of cariogenic nutrition), and invasive approaches individually adopted to the patient's general condition and prognosis, including usage of stainless steel crowns to minimize enamel destruction and maintain normal spacing, restoration of enamel and dentin defects with fillings to guarantee structure and continued function of teeth, lubrication of oral tissues to reduce shear forces, and extraction of most severely affected teeth with osteolytic foci to remove continuous sources of oral infections are strategies to ameliorate the oral status of affected individuals and to allow early recognition of malignancies.

Urologic abnormalities in EB occur with the highest frequency in patients with the Herlitz variant of JEB.[9] Urethral meatus stenosis is the most common complication, observed in 11.6% of JEB-H patients within the NEBR, followed by urinary retention, hydronephrosis, and bladder hypertrophy in 9.3%, 7.0%, and 4.6%, respectively. Diverticuli within the urinary tract; scarring of the glans penis, hypospadias, epispadias; fusion of labia, narrowing of the vaginal vestibule, urinary reflux in vagina and uterine cavity; bladder-blistering, -edema, -cystitis, -infections, -extrophy, and reduced bladder capacity; ureteral stenosis, fibrosis, hydroureter; renal pelvis stenosis, pyelonephritis, recurrent urosepsis, and renal insufficiency are additional symptoms of JEB-H affecting the genitourinary tract. Dilatation, stent placement, resection, ureteral reimplantation, urethral catheterization, meatotomy,

vesicostomy, or nephrostomy tube placement are some of the surgical interventions performed aiming at symptomatic or palliative relief.

The spectrum of *gastrointestinal symptoms*[10] comprises dysphagia, esophageal stenosis or strictures, gastrointestinal reflux disease, peptic ulcer disease, and malabsorption. Constipation due to painful anal strictures and fissures, limited oral food (fiber) intake, and excessive loss of fluid through lesional skin is often exacerbated by opioid analgesia or sedatives, and may lead to life-threatening complications such as megacolon and perforation.

Together with recurrent generalized blistering and continuous transcutaneous loss of nutrients as well as a hypercatabolic state (reflecting an extraordinarily high energy consumption by wound healing, infections, and natural growth), chronic and severe gastrointestinal affection with protein-losing enteropathy can seriously compromise the nutritional status in JEB-H patients.[11] An initially good weight gain is thus usually followed by a profound failure to thrive and, together with infectious/septic and respiratory complications, is associated with a high mortality in early childhood (see later discussion). Further effects of gastrointestinal affection by EB comprise a profound multifactorial anemia (chronic blood, iron, protein loss from open wounds and erosions within intestinal tract, poor intake and absorption of iron and other nutrients) or osteoporosis/osteopenia consequent not only to chronic malnutrition and malabsorption but also immobility/immobilization and concurrent renal insufficiency. Besides mediating growth retardation and dystrophy, nutritional deficiencies further accentuate an already intrinsically impaired wound healing.

Facing this broad spectrum of serious complications, global supplementation (including specialized formula feeds, calcium and vitamin D, oral bisphosphonate therapy) is usually required in JEB-H individuals. Moreover, esophageal dilatation or gastrostomy feeding are often indicated, although these techniques harbor a significant peri-interventional risk (eg, poor healing around the entry site) and a generally high rate of recurrence. Therefore, such procedures should be regarded as part of palliative care to improve comfort and quality of life.[11]

Due to extensive disease, mortality (ie, death related to JEB-H) is very high, especially in the first year of life. Causes of premature death most commonly include recurrent infections and massive sepsis due to facilitated transcutaneous entry of *Staphylococcus aureus*, *Streptococcus*, *Candida*, or methicillin-resistant *S. aureus* via widespread skin erosions, pneumonia, respiratory failure other than pneumonia (eg, tracheolaryngeal obstruction), septic embolism, failure to thrive, and renal failure.[12] Based on calculations assessing the NEBR population, the cumulative risk of death among JEB-H children by age 1 year is 44.7%.

As any medical intervention alleviates disease symptoms and complications at best but does not ultimately limit mortality, treatment approaches in Herlitz EB should be guided by ethical principles and norms focusing on life comfort and company (see Yan and colleagues[4] for an excellent review).

DIAGNOSIS

Considering the high morbidity and mortality of JEB-H as well as the psychological and socioeconomic impact, accurate diagnosis is a prerequisite to provide best care for patients and their families. Diagnosis is largely based on clinical findings as well as immunohistochemical and ultrastructural studies, while issues like insufficiently strong genotype-phenotype correlations, limited cost effectiveness, and restricted availability are considered by several experts to currently not support DNA testing as the primary means of subclassification in EB.[13] However, clinical parameters may be highly misleading and their interpretation challenging as, for example, ("prototypic") cutaneous findings may be transient, inconsistent, or not obvious in earliest infancy when an accurate diagnosis is most often sought. For instance, JEB-H patients can have limited skin involvement, especially after cesarean delivery, and appropriate growth in early life, thereby being sometimes indistinguishable in clinical terms from children suffering from JEB-nH.[4] Only immunohistochemistry and mutation analysis provide a means to clarify the differentiation between the Herlitz and non-Herlitz variant, thereby affecting strategies of management and diagnostic approaches. The extension of the mutation database of a given gene further allows one to better correlate the genotype-phenotype relationship and provides prognostic markers for the progress of the disease. Apart from investigative studies as a precondition for the currently promising gene-therapeutic perspective (see articles elsewhere in this issue), mutation analysis profiling is of great value in prenatal (fetal skin biopsy, chorionic villus sampling, and amniocentesis) and preimplantation genetic diagnosis, carrier testing, and genetic counseling.

In *routine light microscopy*, JEB (just like dystrophic EB) variants appear as "subepidermal" cell-poor blisters with the periodic acid Schiff–positive basement membrane detectable along the floor of the blister. Skin biopsies should be performed on freshly induced blisters, as reepithelialization of intact blisters may lead to false results.[4]

Antigen mapping of clinically uninvolved skin (inner aspect of the upper arm) reveals absent or markedly reduced laminin-332.

If immunomapping is inconclusive, *electron microscopy* (EM) reveals cleavage occurring through the lamina lucida.[14] Hemidesmosomes in JEB-H are small, rudimentary, or absent, and the close association with keratin intermediate filaments is reduced. Despite the limited availability of equipment and skilled microscopists with experience in EB, EM thus still retains a preeminent position in determining the precise level of tissue separation and visualized ultrastructural analysis.

DNA extracted from peripheral blood mononuclear or buccal cells or fetal tissue (chorionic microvilli sample, cultured amnion cells) is used for *mutation analysis*. Genetically heterogeneous, JEB-H is caused by homozygous null mutations or frame-shift mutations with premature termination codons in *LAM* genes, leading to non-sense associated mRNA decay or truncated nonfunctional proteins with biallelic loss of laminin-332.[15] As 2 recurrent mutations in *LAMB3*, R635X and R42X, account for almost 60% of the mutant *LAMB3* alleles, restriction enzyme digests are the first approach to molecular profiling in JEB-H.

The Herlitz variant is usually inherited as an autosomal recessive trait from heterozygous healthy parents to 25% of their offspring. Of note, the reported higher incidence of uniparental isodisomy in JEB-H, describing 2 identical copies of a single homolog, allows 2 copies of a recessive mutation (or both homologs of a pair of chromosomes, which refers to "uniparental heterodisomy") to be transmitted from just one heterozygous carrier parent. Molecular mechanisms for this phenomenon include trisomic rescue, duplication of monosomy, gamete complementation, or somatic recombination.[16] Thus, molecular analysis of each parent of a child with autosomal disease must be routinely performed to identify a hidden isodisomy and to properly counsel the couple. In contrast to the classic autosomal recessive pattern of inheritance with a 25% recurrence risk for future pregnancies, an autosomal recessive condition caused by uniparental disomy, resulting from sporadic event(s) that occur in the gamete(s) or zygote, has a negligible risk of recurrence.[16]

SUMMARY

The JEB-H subtype usually presents as a very severe and clinically diverse variant of the EB group of mechanobullous genodermatoses. Morbidity and mortality due to cutaneous as well as numerous extracutaneous manifestations are very high, necessitating optimized protocols for early (including prenatal) diagnosis and palliative care. Especially for this dramatic disease, gene therapy remains the most promising perspective.

ACKNOWLEDGMENTS

The authors thank Dr Rudolf Hametner for providing the clinical photographs.

REFERENCES

1. Castori M, Floriddia G, De Luca N, et al. Herlitz junctional epidermolysis bullosa: laminin-5 mutational profile and carrier frequency in the Italian population. Br J Dermatol 2008;158:38–44.

2. Fine JD. Epidemiology of inherited epidermolysis bullosa. In: Fine JD, Hintner H, editors. Life with epidermolysis bullosa (EB): etiology, diagnosis, multidisciplinary care and therapy. Wien-New York: Springer; 2008. p. 24–9.

3. Fine JD, Johnson LB, Suchindran C, et al. The national epidermolysis bullosa registry. In: Fine JD, Bauer EA, McGuire J, et al, editors. Epidermolysis bullosa. Clinical, epidemiologic, and laboratory findings of the national epidermolysis bullosa registry. Baltimore (MD): The Johns Hopkins University Press; 1999. p. 79–100.

4. Yan EG, Paris JJ, Ahluwalia J, et al. Treatment decision-making for patients with the Herlitz subtype of junctional epidermolysis bullosa. J Perinatol 2007;26:307–11.

5. Fine JD. Musculoskeletal deformities. In: Fine JD, Hintner H, editors. Life with epidermolysis bullosa (EB): etiology, diagnosis, multidisciplinary care and therapy. Wien-New York: Springer; 2008. p. 177–84.

6. Stoiber J. Ophthalmologic aspects of EB. In: Fine JD, Hintner H, editors. Life with epidermolysis bullosa (EB): etiology, diagnosis, multidisciplinary care and therapy. Wien-New York: Springer; 2008. p. 132–42.

7. Laimer M. Ear, nose and throat complications. In: Fine JD, Hintner H, editors. Life with epidermolysis bullosa (EB): etiology, diagnosis, multidisciplinary care and therapy. Wien-New York: Springer; 2008. p. 143–9.

8. Laimer M, Nischler E. Intraoral disease. In: Fine JD, Hintner H, editors. Life with epidermolysis bullosa (EB): etiology, diagnosis, multidisciplinary care and therapy. Wien-New York: Springer; 2008. p. 150–66.

9. Fine JD. Other internal complications. In: Fine JD, Hintner H, editors. Life with epidermolysis bullosa (EB): etiology, diagnosis, multidisciplinary care and therapy. Wien-New York: Springer; 2008. p. 185–96.

10. Nischler E. Gastrointestinal complications. In: Fine JD, Hintner H, editors. Life with epidermolysis bullosa (EB): etiology, diagnosis, multidisciplinary care and therapy. Wien-New York: Springer; 2008. p. 167–76.

11. Haynes L. Nutritional support for children with epidermolysis bullosa. In: Fine JD, Hintner H, editors. Life with epidermolysis bullosa (EB): etiology, diagnosis, multidisciplinary care and therapy. Wien-New York: Springer; 2008. p. 258–77.

12. Fine JD. Premature death in EB. In: Fine JD, Hintner H, editors. Life with epidermolysis bullosa (EB): etiology, diagnosis, multidisciplinary care and therapy. Wien-New York: Springer; 2008. p. 197–203.

13. Lanschuetzer CM, Fine JD. Classification and molecular basis of hereditary epidermolysis bullosa. In: Fine JD, Hintner H, editors. Life with epidermolysis bullosa (EB): etiology, diagnosis, multidisciplinary care and therapy. Wien-New York: Springer; 2008. p. 6–23.

14. Eady RAJ. Electron microscopy for the diagnosis of EB. In: Fine JD, Hintner H, editors. Life with epidermolysis bullosa (EB): etiology, diagnosis, multidisciplinary care and therapy. Wien-New York: Springer; 2008. p. 43–53.

15. Klausegger A, Bauer JW. Mutation analysis. In: Fine JD, Hintner H, editors. Life with epidermolysis bullosa (EB): etiology, diagnosis, multidisciplinary care and therapy. Wien-New York: Springer; 2008. p. 54–64.

16. Castori M, Floriddia G, Pisaneschi E, et al. Complete maternal isodisomy causing reduction to homozygosity for a novel LAMB3 mutation in Herlitz junctional epidermolysis bullosa. J Dermatol Sci 2008; 51:58–61.

Collagen XVII

Cristina Has, MD*, Johannes S. Kern, MD

KEYWORDS

- Collagen XVII • Epidermolysis bullosa • Bullous pemphigoid
- Dermal-epidermal junction • Epidermal adhesion

COLLAGEN XVII

Collagen XVII was initially identified as the 180-kDa bullous pemphigoid antigen (BP180),[1] and several years later its role in inherited junctional epidermolysis bullosa non-Herlitz (JEB-other, MIM #226650) was identified.[2,3] The role of collagen XVII in both autoimmune and genetic blistering disorders demonstrates its relevance to dermal-epidermal adhesion. Collagen XVII is a major structural component of the hemidesmosome (HD), a highly specialized multiprotein complex that mediates the anchorage of basal epithelial cells to the underlying basement membrane in stratified, pseudostratified, and transitional epithelia (Fig. 1A).[4,5] Collagen XVII is expressed in skin, oral mucosa, ocular conjunctiva, epithelial basement membrane of the cornea, upper esophagus, transitional epithelium of the bladder, and widely in the brain, located primarily in the soma and proximal axons of neurons.[4,6] Furthermore, during embryonic development collagen XVII is expressed during the first trimester in syncytial and cytotrophoblastic cells of normal placenta and in epithelial cells of amniotic membranes[7]; it contributes to embryonic cardiogenesis,[8] regulates ameloblast differentiation, and is essential for normal formation of Tomes' processes.[9] Sequence analysis for collagen XVII orthologs from other species revealed a particularly high level of evolutionary conservation. For example, at protein level human collagen XVII shows an overall homology of 86% with murine collagen XVII.

Collagen XVII is a homotrimeric type II transmembrane protein consisting of 3 180-kDa collagen alpha-1(XVII) chains. Each chain is 1497 amino acids long and has a globular N-terminal intracellular domain of 466 amino acids, a short hydrophobic transmembrane stretch of 23 amino acids, and an extracellular C-terminus 1008 amino acids long (Fig. 1B). The intracellular domain, part of the HD plaque, has no similarities to other proteins, and interacts with integrin β4, plectin, and BP230. The extracellular domain contains 15 collagen domains. These domains are made up of Gly-X-Y tripeptide repeats with very high proline content at the X and Y positions, and are separated by noncollagenous regions. Collagen XVII extracellular domain contributes to the structure of anchoring filaments in the lamina lucida of the basement membrane, and contains at least one loop structure in the lamina densa. Collagen XVII serves as a cell surface receptor for extracellular matrix proteins; its ligands are laminin 332 and integrin α6 (see Fig. 1A, B).[4,5] Further binding partners are still to be identified. The juxtamembranous noncollagenous NC16A region is likely to be important for trimerization and subsequent triple-helix folding in the N → C terminal direction.[10] A particular interest was dedicated to this domain because 80% to 90% of bullous pemphigoid and pemphigoid gestationis patients' sera targets epitopes within the NC16A domain.[11]

The extracellular domain of collagen XVII can undergo proteolytic processing, resulting in the formation of a 120-kDa fragment (designated as LAD-1), and subsequent cleavage to a second soluble form of 97 kDa (designated as 97-LAD or LABD97) (see Fig. 1B). The constitutive shedding, which results in the 120-kDa ectodomain, is mediated by ADAM-9, ADAM-10, and ADAM-17 (TACE).[12] This shedding seems to be dependent on the conformation of the NC16A domain and the steric availability of the cleavage site.[13] The

This work was supported in part by a grant from the German Research Foundation DFG (HA 5663/1-1) to C.H.
Department of Dermatology, University Medical Center Freiburg, Hauptstr. 7, 79104 Freiburg, Germany
* Corresponding author.
E-mail address: cristina.has@uniklinik-freiburg.de (C. Has).

Dermatol Clin 28 (2010) 61–66
doi:10.1016/j.det.2009.10.007

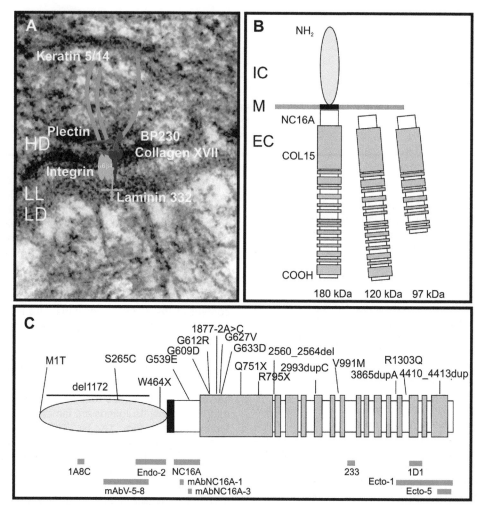

Fig. 1. (A) Transmission electron microscopy representing the dermal-epidermal junction zone with a part of a basal keratinocyte, a hemidesmosome (HD), the lamina lucida (LL), the lamina densa (LD), as well as anchoring fibrils and collagenous fibrils in the upper dermis. Schematically the most important structural hemidesmosomal proteins are represented, including collagen XVII. (B) Collagen XVII with the intracellular (IC, in *grey*), transmembranous (M, in *black*), and extracellular domains (EC). The collagenous domains are depicted in *violet*. Shedding leads to the formation of the 120-kDa soluble collagen XVII ectodomain and to a 97-kDa fragment. (C) The collagen XVII polypeptide: published mutations discussed in this review are represented. Underneath, the regions recognized by domain-specific antibodies (in *green*) available to date are depicted. The antibodies 1A8C (amino acids [aa] 155–163[38]), Endo-2 (aa 367–466[39]), and mAbV-5–8 (aa 234–398[40]) target epitopes within the intracellular domain; NC16A (aa 490–566[41]), mAbNC16A-1 (aa 515–523[16]), and mAbNC16A-3 (aa 545–557[16]) recognize specifically the NC16A domain, while 233 (aa 1118–1143[38]), 1D1 (aa 1357–1387[38]), Ecto-5 (aa 1447–1497[39]) and Ecto-1 (aa 1292–1497[42]) are directed against the C-terminus of collagen XVII.

regulation is complex: the membrane microenvironment, namely the organization of lipid rafts—cholesterol- and sphingolipids-enriched microdomains within the plasma membrane—may be involved.[14] The extracellular phosphorylation of collagen XVII by ecto-casein kinase 2 is also likely to play a role.[15] The cleavage of collagen XVII occurs in the NC16A domain between the amino acid residues 528 and 547. However, the precise site and the biologic functions of the soluble constitutively shed 120-kDa ectodomain remain elusive. There is evidence that the ectodomain is incorporated in the basement membrane and may have cell adhesion properties. It is also predicted that the cleavage process itself may be important for regulation of keratinocyte detachment from the basement membrane in the process of differentiation and migration.[12] The cleavage of the extracellular domain of collagen XVII, which results in formation of a 97-kDa fragment, seems to be dependent, at least in vitro, on plasmin.[16] The biologic relevance of this is not well understood. Nevertheless, shedding is clinically relevant because the 120-kDa ectodomain (LAD-1) and the 97-kDa form (LABD97) are targets for autoantibodies in the autoimmune disease linear IgA bullous dermatosis.[11]

In vitro experiments demonstrated that absence of collagen XVII has important consequences on cell behavior. Tasanen and colleagues[17] reported that collagen XVII null keratinocytes had a migratory phenotype. The collagen XVII-deficient cells develop lamellipodia on different substrates and show improved spreading on laminin 111, but normal adhesion. This finding implicates collagen XVII in the stabilization of keratinocytes and inhibition of their migration. However, by using another model with different experimental conditions and substrates, Qiao and colleagues[18] showed recently that siRNA COL17A1 knockdown of HaCaT keratinocytes led to reduced adhesion and migration, and implicated the p38MAPK-signaling pathway in this abnormal migratory behavior. Collagen XVII may have a role in the formation of HD through its intracellular domain interacting with HD proteins, and also in the establishment of anchoring filaments through binding its ectodomain to laminin 332, an event that may control cell motility.[17]

THE COLLAGEN XVII GENE AND THE MOLECULAR PATHOLOGY OF JUNCTIONAL EPIDERMOLYSIS BULLOSA-OTHER
The Spectrum of COL17A1 Mutations

The collagen alpha-1(XVII) chain is encoded by the COL17A1 gene, which spans 52 kb of the genome and is located on the long arm of chromosome 10 (10q24.3). This gene's mutations are associated with a nonlethal subtype of JEB, designated as JEB-other in the revised classification of epidermolysis bullosa (EB).[3] COL17A1 has a split structure consisting of 56 exons and short introns.

Mutations in the COL17A1 gene have been uncovered in several patients with JEB-other; 77 different mutations have been identified, the vast majority of which are nonsense and splicing mutations, deletions and insertions, leading to formation of premature termination codons, mRNA decay, and absence of collagen XVII expression (reviewed in Fig. 1C).[19,20] Only few missense mutations have been described: p.M1T affects the Start codon; p.G609D, p.G612R, p.G627V, and p.G633D are glycine substitutions; p.S265C, p.G539E, p.V991M, and p.R1303Q are amino acid substitutions (see Fig. 1C). In skin samples of JEB-other patients with homozygous or compound heterozygous COL17A1 mutations, indirect immunofluorescence mapping demonstrates cleavage in the lamina lucida of the basement membrane and reduced or absent collagen XVII staining (for antibodies see Fig. 1C). Transmission electron microscopy shows splitting in the lamina lucida of the basement membrane of the epidermis and reduced or hypoplastic HDs.[3]

Studies of the molecular consequences of COL17A1 mutations in patients with JEB were helpful in understanding the biochemical properties of collagen XVII. For example, the glycine substitutions have been carefully investigated. As in the case of other collagens, glycine substitutions located in the largest collagenous domain of collagen XVII, Col15, interrupt triple helix formation. This process leads to partial unfolding of the ectodomain, which decreases thermal stability, causes intracellular accumulation, and affects posttranslational modifications.[21–24]

The C-terminal truncation mutation 4410_4413dupCATT (see Fig. 1C) impairs N-glycosylation of the ectodomain, 77 amino acids proximal to the C-terminus. This process leads to intracellular accumulation, indicating that N-glycosylation of the ectodomain is required for the targeting of collagen XVII to the plasma membrane.[25]

Genotype-Phenotype Correlations

Genotype-phenotype correlations are not well established in JEB-other caused by COL17A1 mutations. The spectrum of phenotypes ranges from mild localized blistering, with mild accompanying symptoms, to severe generalized blistering with universal alopecia, nail dystrophy, and enamel hypoplasia. Despite the fact that most mutations lead to premature termination codons, their consequences and the resulting phenotypes are difficult to predict, and require analyses on mRNA and protein level. Also, the presence of mosaicisms can interfere with the severity of the phenotype.[26–28]

In some cases nonsense mutations can cause mild phenotypes because of alternative splicing mechanisms. For example, the mutation p.R795X (see Fig. 1C) in exon 33—a frequent mutation in Italian patients—led to alternatively spliced COL17A1 mRNA that entirely lacked exon 33. This situation allowed for residual synthesis and expression of collagen XVII at the cutaneous basement membrane zone.[29] In the case of a mildly affected patient with the mutation p.Q751X (see Fig. 1C), the deleterious effect similarly was skirted by deleting exon 30 containing the premature termination codon. The reading frame was restored, resulting in a 36-nucleotides shorter transcript, deleting 12 amino acids from the Col15 domain.[30] Also, in the case of glycine substitutions there are no clear-cut genotype-phenotype correlations, but patients seem to be less affected than patients with null mutations.[21] Of note, the mutation p.G627V was shown to act in a dominant fashion, giving rise to severe dental enamel hypoplasia or JEB-other in the heterozygous patients.[31–33] However, the investigators did not exclude the presence of a heterozygous large deletion on the second allele, which cannot be detected by routine mutation detection strategies.[33]

A particular constellation was described in the case of the 1172-bp in-frame deletion from the intracellular domain of the collagen XVII polypeptide (see **Fig. 1**C). This constellation led to intraepidermal skin cleavage and phenotypic features of EB simplex.[34] Surprisingly, a similar situation with intraepidermal cleavage at the level above the cytoplasmic attachment plaque of the HD was reportedly due to the mutation c.1877-2A>C at the acceptor splice site of intron 21 (see **Fig. 1**C) in the ectodomain of collagen XVII.[35]

Heterozygous carriers of *COL17A1* mutations may have enamel defects, demonstrating that reduced amounts or mutated collagen XVII might be sufficient for dermal-epidermal stability, but not for proper teeth development.[20]

Revertant Mosaicism

In a recent Dutch cohort of 14 JEB-other patients, the surprisingly high number of 5 patients showed revertant mosaicism.[28] The clinical hallmarks of this genetic event are homogeneously pigmented apparently unaffected skin areas that are surrounded by skin that is susceptible to blistering. Patients may present with an atypically mild phenotype. Different genetic mechanisms—intragenic crossover, second-site mutation, mitotic gene conversion, or back mutation—may occur in one single patient.[26,27] In the future these patients might profit from cell therapy with autologous revertant cells.[36]

MOUSE MODEL

Col17-knockout (*Col17*[m−/−]) mice were generated and demonstrated phenotypic features closely resembling human JEB-other. At birth, blisters and erosions were easily mechanically inducible or emerged spontaneously. Adult mice had genital erosions, hemorrhagic blisters around the digits, and diffuse, nonpigmented hair growth associated with hair loss. *Col17*[m−/−] showed growth retardation and most of them died within 2 weeks of birth. Skin of the mice demonstrated subepidermal blistering, absence of collagen XVII

immunofluorescence staining, and small and abnormally shaped HDs.[37]

Major Role of Collagen XVII in Tooth Enamel Formation

Col17-knockout mice also showed aberrant enamel prisms, increased molar wear, abnormal teeth color, and decreased mineral deposition. The differentiation of ameloblasts was delayed, with irregularly shaped Tomes' processes and changed secretion of enamel matrix as a result.[9] The Col17-knockout mouse model therefore helped to establish that collagen XVII plays a role in the regulation of ameloblast differentiation, and that its absence leads to enamel malformations. These results explain the phenotype of enamel hypoplasia in JEB-other patients, and demonstrate that it is a consequence of the gene defect.

REFERENCES

1. Stanley JR, Hawley-Nelson P, Yuspa SH, et al. Characterization of bullous pemphigoid antigen: a unique basement membrane protein of stratified squamous epithelia. Cell 1981;24(3):897–903.
2. McGrath JA, Gatalica B, Christiano AM, et al. Mutations in the 180-kD bullous pemphigoid antigen (BPAG2), a hemidesmosomal transmembrane collagen (COL17A1), in generalized atrophic benign epidermolysis bullosa. Nat Genet 1995;11(1):83–6.
3. Fine JD, Eady RA, Bauer EA, et al. The classification of inherited epidermolysis bullosa (EB): report of the Third International Consensus Meeting on Diagnosis and Classification of EB. J Am Acad Dermatol 2008; 58(6):931–50.
4. Van den Bergh F, Giudice GJ. BP180 (type XVII collagen) and its role in cutaneous biology and disease. Adv Dermatol 2003;19:37–71.
5. Koster J, Borradori L, Sonnenberg A. Hemidesmosomes: molecular organization and their importance for cell adhesion and disease. In: Beissert T, Nelson CF, editors. Handbook of experimental pharmacology, vol. 165. Berlin: Springer; 2004. p. 245–67.
6. Seppanen A, Suuronen T, Hofmann SC, et al. Distribution of collagen XVII in the human brain. Brain Res 2007;1158:50–6.
7. Huilaja L, Hurskainen T, Autio-Harmainen H, et al. Pemphigoid gestationis autoantigen, transmembrane collagen XVII, promotes the migration of cytotrophoblastic cells of placenta and is a structural component of fetal membranes. Matrix Biol 2008; 27(3):190–200.
8. Kondo J, Kusachi S, Ninomiya Y, et al. Expression of type XVII collagen alpha 1 chain mRNA in the mouse heart. Jpn Heart J 1998;39(2):211–20.

9. Asaka T, Akiyama M, Domon T, et al. Type XVII collagen is a key player in tooth enamel formation. Am J Pathol 2009;174(1):91–100.

10. Areida SK, Reinhardt DP, Muller PK, et al. Properties of the collagen type XVII ectodomain. Evidence for N- to C-terminal triple helix folding. J Biol Chem 2001;276(2):1594–601.

11. Mihai S, Sitaru C. Immunopathology and molecular diagnosis of autoimmune bullous diseases. J Cell Mol Med 2007;11(3):462–81.

12. Franzke CW, Tasanen K, Schumann H, et al. Collagenous transmembrane proteins: collagen XVII as a prototype. Matrix Biol 2003;22(4):299–309.

13. Franzke CW, Tasanen K, Borradori L, et al. Shedding of collagen XVII/BP180: structural motifs influence cleavage from cell surface. J Biol Chem 2004; 279(23):24521–9.

14. Zimina EP, Bruckner-Tuderman L, Franzke CW. Shedding of collagen XVII ectodomain depends on plasma membrane microenvironment. J Biol Chem 2005;280(40):34019–24.

15. Zimina EP, Fritsch A, Schermer B, et al. Extracellular phosphorylation of collagen XVII by ecto-casein kinase 2 inhibits ectodomain shedding. J Biol Chem 2007;282(31):22737–46.

16. Hofmann SC, Voith U, Schonau V, et al. Plasmin plays a role in the in vitro generation of the linear IgA dermatosis antigen LADB97. J Invest Dermatol 2009;129(7): 1730–9.

17. Tasanen K, Tunggal L, Chometon G, et al. Keratinocytes from patients lacking collagen XVII display a migratory phenotype. Am J Pathol 2004;164(6):2027–38.

18. Qiao H, Shibaki A, Long HA, et al. Collagen XVII participates in keratinocyte adhesion to collagen IV, and in p38MAPK-dependent migration and cell signaling. J Invest Dermatol 2009;129(9):2288–95.

19. Pasmooij AM, Pas HH, Jansen GH, et al. Localized and generalized forms of blistering in junctional epidermolysis bullosa due to COL17A1 mutations in the Netherlands. Br J Dermatol 2007;156(5):861–70.

20. Murrell DF, Pasmooij AM, Pas HH, et al. Retrospective diagnosis of fatal BP180-deficient non-Herlitz junctional epidermolysis bullosa suggested by immunofluorescence (IF) antigen-mapping of parental carriers bearing enamel defects. J Invest Dermatol 2007;127(7):1772–5.

21. Vaisanen L, Has C, Franzke C, et al. Molecular mechanisms of junctional epidermolysis bullosa: col 15 domain mutations decrease the thermal stability of collagen XVII. J Invest Dermatol 2005; 125(6):1112–8.

22. Tasanen K, Floeth M, Schumann H, et al. Hemizygosity for a glycine substitution in collagen XVII: unfolding and degradation of the ectodomain. J Invest Dermatol 2000;115(2):207–12.

23. Tasanen K, Eble JA, Aumailley M, et al. Collagen XVII is destabilized by a glycine substitution

24. Huilaja L, Hurskainen T, Autio-Harmainen H, et al. Glycine substitution mutations cause intracellular accumulation of collagen XVII and affect its post-translational modifications. J Invest Dermatol 2009;129(9):2302–6.

25. Franzke CW, Has C, Schulte C, et al. C-terminal truncation impairs glycosylation of transmembrane collagen XVII and leads to intracellular accumulation. J Biol Chem 2006;281(40):30260–8.

26. Jonkman MF, Scheffer H, Stulp R, et al. Revertant mosaicism in epidermolysis bullosa caused by mitotic gene conversion. Cell 1997;88(4):543–51.

27. Pasmooij AM, Pas HH, Deviaene FC, et al. Multiple correcting COL17A1 mutations in patients with revertant mosaicism of epidermolysis bullosa. Am J Hum Genet 2005;77(5):727–40.

28. Jonkman MF, Pasmooij AM. Revertant mosaicism—patchwork in the skin. N Engl J Med 2009;360(16): 1680–2.

29. Ruzzi L, Pas H, Posteraro P, et al. A homozygous nonsense mutation in type XVII collagen gene (COL17A1) uncovers an alternatively spliced mRNA accounting for an unusually mild form of non-Herlitz junctional epidermolysis bullosa. J Invest Dermatol 2001;116(1):182–7.

30. Pasmooij AM, van Zalen S, Nijenhuis AM, et al. A very mild form of non-Herlitz junctional epidermolysis bullosa: BP180 rescue by outsplicing of mutated exon 30 coding for the COL15 domain. Exp Dermatol 2004;13(2):125–8.

31. McGrath JA, Gatalica B, Li K, et al. Compound heterozygosity for a dominant glycine substitution and a recessive internal duplication mutation in the type XVII collagen gene results in junctional epidermolysis bullosa and abnormal dentition. Am J Pathol 1996;148(6):1787–96.

32. Olague-Marchan M, Twining SS, Hacker MK, et al. A disease-associated glycine substitution in BP180 (type XVII collagen) leads to a local destabilization of the major collagen triple helix. Matrix Biol 2000; 19(3):223–33.

33. Almaani N, Liu L, Dopping-Hepenstal PJ, et al. Autosomal dominant junctional epidermolysis bullosa. Br J Dermatol 2009;160(5):1094–7.

34. Fontao L, Tasanen K, Huber M, et al. Molecular consequences of deletion of the cytoplasmic domain of bullous pemphigoid 180 in a patient with predominant features of epidermolysis bullosa simplex. J Invest Dermatol 2004;122(1):65–72.

35. Pasmooij AM, van der Steege G, Pas HH, et al. Features of epidermolysis bullosa simplex due to mutations in the ectodomain of type XVII collagen. Br J Dermatol 2004;151(3):669–74.

36. Gostynski A, Deviaene FC, Pasmooij AM, et al. Adhesive stripping to remove epidermis in junctional

epidermolysis bullosa for revertant cell therapy. Br J Dermatol 2009;161(2):444–7.

37. Nishie W, Sawamura D, Goto M, et al. Humanization of autoantigen. Nat Med 2007;13(3):378–83.

38. Di Zenzo G, Grosso F, Terracina M, et al. Characterization of the anti-BP180 autoantibody reactivity profile and epitope mapping in bullous pemphigoid patients. J Invest Dermatol 2004;122(1): 103–10.

39. Franzke CW, Tasanen K, Schacke H, et al. Transmembrane collagen XVII, an epithelial adhesion protein, is shed from the cell surface by ADAMs. EMBO J 2002;21(19):5026–35.

40. Olaru F, Mihai S, Petrescu I, et al. Generation and characterization of monoclonal antibodies against the intracellular domain of hemidesmosomal type XVII collagen. Hybridoma (Larchmt) 2006;25(3): 158–62.

41. Schumann H, Baetge J, Tasanen K, et al. The shed ectodomain of collagen XVII/BP180 is targeted by autoantibodies in different blistering skin diseases. Am J Pathol 2000;156(2):685–95.

42. Schacke H, Schumann H, Hammami-Hauasli N, et al. Two forms of collagen XVII in keratinocytes. A full-length transmembrane protein and a soluble ectodomain. J Biol Chem 1998;273(40):25937–43.

Non-Herlitz Junctional Epidermolysis Bullosa

Kim B. Yancey, MD[a],*, Helmut Hintner, MD[b]

KEYWORDS

- Genetic disease • Epidermal adhesion • Blistering disease
- Generalized atrophic benign epidermolysis bullosa
- Herlitz disease

Epidermolysis bullosa (EB) is the term applied to a heterogeneous group of inherited blistering diseases in which minor trauma leads to blistering of skin and mucous membranes.[1] Three major groups of EB have been defined according to the level of blister formation that occurs in epidermal basement membrane (BM): (1) EB simplex, in which blisters form within basal keratinocytes; (2) junctional EB (JEB), in which blisters form within the lamina lucida of the epidermal BM; and (3) dystrophic EB, in which blisters form below the lamina densa. These 3 major groups are further divided into several subtypes based on their pattern of inheritance, morphology of lesions, or the distribution of involvement. The severity of these diseases ranges from mild, with almost no functional impairment, to devastating, with life-threatening complications and fatal outcomes. Junctional EB (JEB) represents a group of disorders characterized by autosomal recessive inheritance (though a rare exception has recently been reported[2]) and manifestation of disease activity at birth (in almost all subtypes). The various types of JEB are summarized in **Table 1**. Most EB classification schemes place emphasis on distinguishing Herlitz from non-Herlitz forms of JEB, because the former typically has a far less favorable prognosis (hence its prior designation as EB lethalis or the gravis variant of generalized JEB). Several variant forms of non-Herlitz JEB (nH JEB) are currently recognized (see **Table 1**). This review focuses on nH JEB generalized, nH JEB localized, nH JEB inversa, and nH JEB late onset (EB progressive),

as entities currently classified as other JEB variants are detailed elsewhere in this monograph.

HISTORY

In 1935, Herlitz[3] described a form of EB that was lethal in infancy. When the skin of patients with this form of EB was evaluated by electron microscopy, a subepidermal blister was evident within the plane of the lamina lucida.[4] Early on, therefore, JEB was considered synonymous with Herlitz disease. The grim prognosis for this disease made it remarkable when, in 1976, Hashimoto and colleagues[5] described a patient with JEB who survived to adulthood. The proband was a 38 year-old man who displayed generalized blistering of skin and mucous membranes since birth, atrophy in areas of repeated blistering, alopecia, dystrophic nails, loss of teeth, and blister formation within the lamina lucida. Of note, this patient had 2 siblings who died in their first days of life due to blistering and associated complications. Hashimoto named this form of JEB the Disentis type, based on the place of birth of these Swiss patients. Four more patients with similar clinical and electron microscopic features were subsequently described in 1979 by Anton-Lamprecht and Schnyder.[6] The dramatically different prognosis in these patients prompted a new appellation for this subtype of JEB, namely EB atrophicans generalisata mitis. In 1982, Hintner and Wolff[7] described 8 additional patients with

This work was supported in part by NIH Grant R01 AR048982 (KBY).

[a] Department of Dermatology, University of Texas Southwestern Medical Center in Dallas, 5323 Harry Hines Boulevard, Dallas, TX 75390-9069, USA

[b] Department of Dermatology, Paracelsus Medical University Salzburg, Muellner-Hauptstr. 48, A-5020 Salzburg, Austria

* Corresponding author.

E-mail address: kim.yancey@utsouthwestern.edu (K.B. Yancey).

Dermatol Clin 28 (2010) 67–77
doi:10.1016/j.det.2009.10.008

Table 1
Types of junctional EB

Subtype	Disease Gene	Protein Target
H JEB	LAMA3, LAMB3, LAMC2	Laminin 332
nH JEB	COL17A1	Collagen XVII
	LAMA3, LAMB3, LAMC2	Laminin 332
nH JEB, localized	COL17A1	Collagen XVII
JEB, inversa	LAMA3, LAMB3, LAMC2	Laminin 332
JEB, progressiva	?	?
JEB with pyloric atresia	ITGA6, ITGB4	Integrin subunits α_6 and β_4 respectively

nonlethal JEB and anglicized the previous term to generalized atrophic benign epidermolysis bullosa (GABEB). More patients were subsequently described, including additional European cases as well as patients from the United States, Asia, and Northern Africa.[8,9] Accordingly, nH JEB is now recognized as a sporadic disease that occurs worldwide.

LABORATORY FINDINGS
Light Microscopy

Light microscopy studies of early lesional skin from patients with nH JEB typically show subepidermal blisters with no signs of inflammation.[1] Induced blisters have the same histologic appearance as early trauma-induced blisters. In periodic acid Schiff (PAS)-stained sections, the BM is found on the blister floor, while intact keratinocytes form the roof. Although light microscopy studies are helpful in the evaluation of these patients, more specialized techniques are currently used to establish the plane of blister formation in these patients' skin.

Transmission Electron Microscopy

Transmission electron microscopy of skin from patients with nH JEB identifies a blister cleavage plane within the electron lucent lamina lucida subregion of epidermal BM. Whereas immunofluorescence mapping studies can establish this finding, transmission electron microscopy studies offer the potential to identify other relevant findings in the skin of nH JEB patients, namely, a potential reduction in the number or size of hemidesmosomes in epidermal BM (**Table 2**).[10,11] However, it should be kept in mind that patients with nH JEB may show a spectrum of ultrastructural findings in their skin; findings perhaps dependent on corresponding mutations in disease genes, patient age, regional variations of skin samples, degree of

disease activity in the skin sample under study, or other variables yet to be defined. Transmission electron microscopy of skin from patients with EB is a highly specialized investigation best performed in an experienced reference laboratory (several are enumerated by Fine and colleagues).[1]

Immunofluorescence Mapping Studies

The level of blister formation in skin from EB patients can also be defined by immunofluorescence (IF) mapping studies.[12] These studies typically use cryopreserved skin harvested (best by shave/saucerization techniques) from fresh spontaneous or friction-induced blisters. Using monoclonal antibodies directed against reference landmark adhesion proteins that reside in epidermal BM (eg, bullous pemphigoid antigen 1 [BPAG1], type IV collagen, type VII collagen, and so forth), it is usually possible to determine with accuracy whether the plane of cleavage in lesional skin resides within basal keratinocytes (all markers on floor of blister), the lamina lucida (BPAG1 on roof of blister, collagen IV and VII on floor of blister), or the sublamina densa region (all markers on roof of blister). IF mapping studies offer the additional advantage in that inclusion of additional monoclonal antibodies directed against candidate "disease-proteins" (eg, monoclonal antibodies vs type XVII collagen [often altered in patients with nH JEB], monoclonal antibodies vs type VII collagen [altered in patients with dystrophic EB]) has the potential to identify defects in the relative expression or distribution of adhesion proteins within the epidermal BM of patient skin.[13,14] Indeed, identifying a candidate disease protein (and hence, its corresponding disease gene) greatly facilitates DNA mutational analyses. Prior studies have demonstrated that IF mapping studies are as reliable diagnostically as transmission electron microscopy for the classification of patients with EB.[1] Moreover, there are numerous

Table 2
Ultrastructural alterations in patients with JEB

JEB Type	TEM Cleavage Plane	TEM, Other Observations	IF Mapping Studies	Alterations in Structural Proteins
H JEB	Lamina lucida	Decreased or absent HDs and/ or SBDPs	BPAG1 roof; collagens IV and VII, base	Laminin 332 absent (or markedly decreased)
nH JEB	Lamina lucida	HDs within normal limits, or decreased in size and number	BPAG1, roof; collagens IV and VII, base	Type XVII collagen absent (or notably decreased) Laminin 332 attenuated or markedly decreased
JEB with pyloric atresia	Lamina lucida	Small plaques in HDs; attenuated SBDPs common	BPAG1 roof; collagens IV and VII, base	Integrin $\alpha_6\beta_4$ absent or markedly decreased

Abbreviations: BPAG1, bullous pemphigoid antigen 1; HDs, hemidesmosomes; IF, immunofluorescence; SBDPs, sub-basal dense plaques; TEM, transmission electron microscopy.

university-based and commercial laboratories that can perform this testing.[1] A summary overview of what IF mapping studies typically show in nH JEB patients is shown in **Table 2**.

Mutational Analysis

The ultimate means of determining precise defects in patients with EB resides in mutational analysis of genes encoding epidermal BM-associated structural proteins.[9,15] In addition, identification of mutations responsible for disease in a given patient also has relevance to defining: (a) the exact mode of disease inheritance; (b) what defects require correction (or modulation) by gene therapy; and (c) data sets required for prenatal or preimplantation diagnostics. As noted earlier, the clinical and genetic heterogeneity of EB (especially junctional forms of EB) coupled with the labor-intensive character of mutational analyses places great emphasis on IF mapping and screening studies to narrow candidates for genetic testing. At present, several research laboratories and commercial vendors offer mutational analysis for EB patients.[1]

In JEB, the majority of mutations identified to date in both Herlitz and non-Herlitz forms of disease have resided in the 3 genes, *LAMA3*, *LAMB3*, and *LAMC2*, that encode the α, β, and γ subunits, respectively, of laminin 332.[15,16] Most mutations in patients with H JEB are nonsense mutations in *LAMA3*, *LAMB3*, or *LAMC2* that result in the formation of premature termination codons (PTC). In turn,

such PTCs elicit nonsense-mediated mRNA decay or synthesis of truncated (or nonfunctional) laminin subunit polypeptides. The correlate observation in IF mapping studies of skin from patients with H JEB is complete (or near complete) absence of laminin 332 expression in epidermal BM.

In nH JEB, patients may demonstrate mutations in *COL17A1*, the gene encoding type XVII collagen (also termed bullous pemphigoid antigen 2 [BPAG2] or BP180), or the genes encoding laminin 332.[8,15–19] In the subset of nH JEB patients with *COL17A1* defects, mutations have traditionally been shown to consist of insertions, deletions, or nonsense mutations that result in PTCs, nonsense-mediated mRNA decay, and complete absence of collagen XVII expression in epidermal BM.[15–17] However, exceptions to this paradigm exist, as evidenced by one patient who carried one *COL17A1* allele harboring a dominantly inherited mutation encoding a glycine substitution and one *COL17A1* allele bearing a mutation encoding a PTC.[15] In nH JEB patients with laminin 332 gene mutations, it is not uncommon for patients to carry a PTC on one allele and a missense or in-frame splice site mutation on the alternate allele. Such alterations have been thought to result in production of small amounts of truncated or altered subunit polypeptides that retain the ability to be incorporated with laminin 332 heterotrimers within hemidesmosome-anchoring filament complexes. This interpretation is consistent with IF mapping studies that show diminished expression of laminin 332 within the

Table 3
Genetic abnormalities in patients with nH JEB

Gene	Types of Mutations	Corresponding Protein
COL17A1	Nonsense, missense, insertion, deletion, or splice site mutations that often result in PTCs on both COL17A1 alleles	Type XVII collagen (bullous pemphigoid antigen 2 [BPAG2], BP180)
LAMA3 LAMB3 LAMC2	Nonsense, missense, insertion, deletion, or splice site mutations that often result in a PTC on one allele and missense mutations or in frame insertions/deletions on the other allele	Laminin 332 (also termed laminin 5, epiligrin, nicein, kalinin, or the BM600 antigen)

Abbreviation: PTCs, premature termination codons.

epidermal BM of patients with nH JEB. In nH JEB (and H JEB as well), the majority of the mutations identified to date reside within LAMB3.

A recent study examining mutations in 265 patients carrying a preliminary diagnosis of JEB generally confirmed the summary observations outlined herein along with several unexpected findings.[15] For example, several patients harboring mutations causing PTCs in genes encoding laminin 332 displayed a relatively mild phenotype that contrasted notably with that traditionally seen in patients with H JEB. In addition, this study identified several patients with an H JEB phenotype that carried no mutations in LAMA3, LAMB3, or LAMC2 but instead harbored PTC causing mutations in COL17A1. These patients not only had disease characterized by greater relative severity but also an increased risk of lethality. Additional summary information about genetic alterations in patients with nH JEB is presented in **Table 3**.

CLINICAL MANIFESTATIONS

nH JEB in adults is characterized by generalized blisters in a distribution that predominates in sites exposed to friction, trauma, or heat. These patients typically demonstrate atrophic scars, hypopigmentation, or hyperpigmentation at sites of healed blisters as well as incomplete alopecia, dystrophic nails, mild mucous membrane involvement, dental abnormalities, and (in selected patients) melanocytic nevi at sites of prior blisters (**Figs. 1–5** and **Table 4**). However, infants and children with nH JEB often fail to demonstrate many of these clinical manifestations and may appear to resemble patients with other forms of EB.[1,8] Accordingly, it is important to carefully establish the type (and subtype, if possible) of EB present

in neonates and infants by transmission electron microscopy, IF mapping studies, or (if feasible) mutational analysis (**Fig. 6**).[20] It is also important to acknowledge that mild (or severe) disease early in life may be characterized by the opposite phenotype in adults. Finally, it should be noted

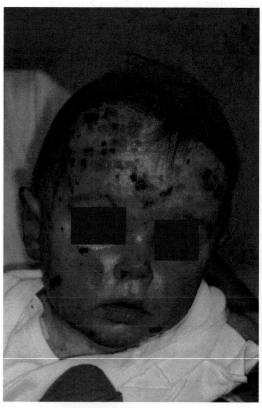

Fig. 1. A 1-year-old child with nH JEB (mutation, COL17A1: 2188C>T, homozygous; protein: R730X).

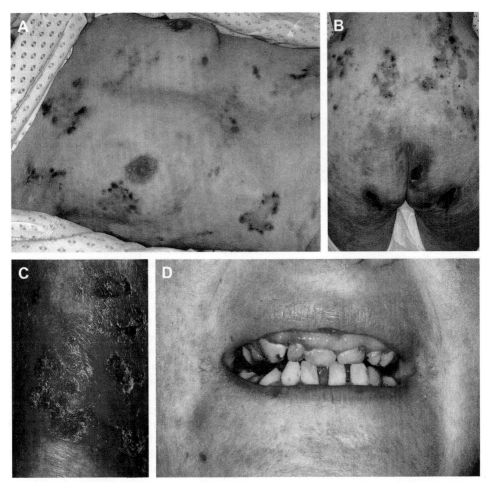

Fig. 2. A 43-year-old patient with nH JEB. (*A* and *B*) Generalized blistering; (*C*), a nonhealing, superinfected wound; (*D*) misshaped teeth with caries (mutation, *LAMB3*: 3009C>T/1903C>T; protein R635X).

that although nH JEB is generally less severe than H JEB, fatalities (especially in neonates) are not uncommon among patients with the former diagnosis. Indeed, a recent study examining cause-specific risks of childhood death in patients with EB in the United States found that patients with all forms of JEB have a relatively high risk of death by age 1 year.[21] This risk increases continuously to age 15, being higher among patients with H JEB than those with nH JEB. In this large study, sepsis, failure to thrive, and respiratory failure were the major causes of death in children with JEB.[21]

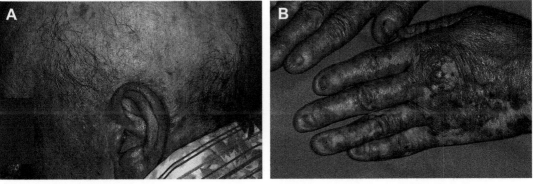

Fig. 3. A 65-year-old patient with nH JEB. (*A*) Baldness; (*B*) lack of fingernails and onychodystrophy (mutation, *COL17A1*: 4003delTC, homozygous).

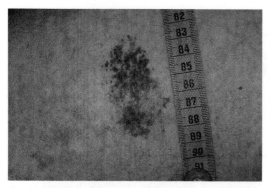

Fig. 4. A14-year-old patient with nH JEB displaying an EB-associated melanocytic nevus (mutation, *COL17A1*: 4003delTC, homozygous).

nH JEB, Generalized

Blisters in patients with nH JEB, generalized are typically 0.5 to 3 cm² and filled with serous or hemorrhagic fluid. Blister formation is augmented by elevated environmental temperature or hyperhidrosis. Blisters may progress to form superficial ulcers, crusted lesions, fissures, or deep ulcers. Recurrent blistering leads to atrophy sometimes accompanied by pigmentary disturbances and erythema that result in a poikilodermatous appearance. Recurrent blistering may also give rise to faint stellate scars. Severe scarring and milia are rare.[1,8,20]

Hair loss is an important characteristic of nH JEB, generalized.[7,20] Scalp hair growth in these

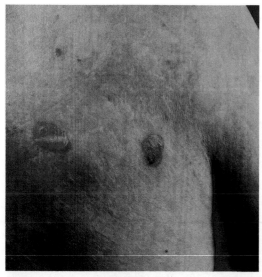

Fig. 5. A 65-year-old patient with nH JEB showing blisters, erosions, crusts, and stellate scars on the upper back (mutation, *COL17A1*: 4003 del TC, homozygous).

patients appears to be normal in childhood, but by the end of the first or second decade, alopecia becomes apparent. Scalp hair loss is typically diffuse, though generally incomplete. Such hair loss is typically progressive and permanent. This type of alopecia has been referred to as atrophic because of the gross loss of hair follicles as well as atrophic changes that are apparent in these patients' surrounding epidermis. Female patients may develop a "male" pattern of diffuse alopecia. Baldness can be pronounced by the third or fourth decade, prompting patients to wear a wig. In addition to scalp alopecia, patients may show partial loss of eyebrows and eyelashes. Body hair is also decreased, and pubic as well as axillary hair is scant or does not fully develop. Failure to develop secondary sexual hair has not been linked to endocrinologic abnormalities in the few patients who have been studied to date.[7]

Nail dystrophy is regarded as a typical manifestation of nH JEB.[1] Some affected infants have been reported to have nail alterations at birth. Nails, like hair, show progressive changes, becoming increasingly dystrophic (or absent) with age. Nails may be shed after subungual blistering. Although initially the nails may regrow normally, they typically become thickened, dome-shaped, or onychogryphotic after repeated trauma.[22] The relative severity of nail dystrophy in nH JEB is variable.

Mucous membrane involvement in patients with nH JEB, generalized tends to be more notable in infancy and early childhood. All mucous membranes appear to be susceptible. Patients with nH JEB, generalized commonly have oral erosions and may demonstrate similar lesions of the nasal mucosa.[5,7,20] The extent of oral erosions is usually moderate compared with that seen in dystrophic EB, and usually does not result in scarring or ankyloglosia. Hoarseness (or a weak cry in children) is an alarming finding in patients with JEB because it often signifies airway obstruction that has the potential to prove fatal. Tracheolaryngeal stenosis or obstruction occurs almost exclusively in the junctional forms of EB, with most cases developing in the first 2 years of life. A recent analysis of patients enrolled in the United States EB Registry between 1986 and 2002 found that tracheolaryngeal stenosis or stricture arose in approximately 40% and 12% of patients with H JEB and nH JEB, respectively.[23] This study concluded that elective tracheostomy should be considered for JEB patients showing evidence of airway compromise. Patients with nH JEB, generalized are also at risk for esophageal webs, esophageal structures, and urogenital alterations.[8,24] Involvement of the urinary tract has been

Table 4
Common clinical manifestations of nH JEB

nH JEB, generalized

Generalized blisters at birth or soon thereafter

Lesional sites tend to heal with atrophic scars, milia, hypo- and/or hyperpigmentation

Mucosal lesions that are most pronounced in infancy and childhood

Progressive yet incomplete alopecia (scalp, body, and anogenital regions)

Dystrophic (or absent) nails

Dental enamel hypoplasia and an increased incidence of caries

Risk of ocular, nasal, laryngeal, tracheal, and genitourinary involvement

Risk of gastrointestinal involvement (including stricture formation)

Anemia

Growth retardation

Features that contrast from those seen in patients with H JEB: low incidence of granulation tissue, squamous cell carcinoma, and death secondary to EB

nH JEB, localized

Localized blisters at birth or soon thereafter

Dystrophic (or absent) nails

Dental enamel hypoplasia and an increased incidence of caries

nH JEB, inverse

Blisters at birth or soon thereafter

Lesions predominate in intertringinous sites

Lesional sites tend to heal with atrophic scars, milia, hypo- and/or hyperpigmentation

Some risk for oral mucosal lesions

Dystrophic (or absent) nails

Dental enamel hypoplasia and an increased incidence of caries

Some risk for gastrointestinal involvement (including stricture formation)

nH JEB, progressive

Blisters develop in young adulthood or later

Dystrophic (or absent) nails

Dental enamel hypoplasia and an increased incidence of caries

An absence of dermatoglyphs

Hyperhidrosis

postulated to result in renal dysfunction in several patients.[14,25] Fortunately, patients with nH JEB seem to have a relatively low incidence of cardiomyopathy, a complication more commonly seen in patients with Hallopeau Siemens recessive dystrophic EB.[26] Corneal blisters, erosions, and scars have been observed in patients with nH JEB.[27,28] Symblepharon and ectropion formation seems to occur more commonly in patients with H JEB than in individuals with nH JEB.

Dental abnormalities are typically observed in patients with nH JEB.[1,7,8,29,30] Patients exhibit generalized enamel hypoplasia that manifests as pitting of the teeth or as a thin enamel with furrows. As a consequence and possibly because of difficulty in oral hygiene, patients with nH JEB are susceptible to severe caries. Many of these patients lose all of their teeth early in life.

An inconstant feature of nH JEB, generalized is the development of large melanocytic nevi at sites of prior blisters.[7,31] These lesions have been observed as early as 2 years of age. Such nevi are round or oval, and grow rapidly within the confines of prior blisters. Nevi may attain the size of an adult palm. Some lesions demonstrate a darker rim as if nevus cells have become trapped in the sharp angle of the blister. After months, the nevi become uniformly black or develop different shades of brown to black. After several years, the surfaces of these nevi change from flat to papillomatous; these lesions also often become lighter in color later in life. Such nevi are not

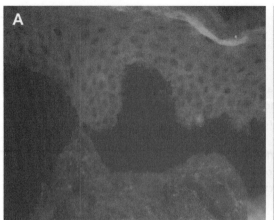
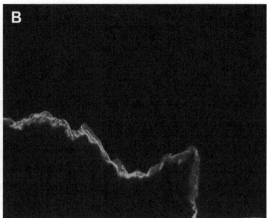

Fig. 6. Antigen mapping in a patient with nH JEB. (*A*) Complete lack of expression of type XVII collagen in epidermal BM; (*B*) Normal expression of laminin 332 in epidermal BM (mutation, *COL17A1*: 3666delG, homozygous).

specific to patients with nH JEB in that similar lesions have also been observed in patients with the 2 other major types of EB (ie, EB simplex and dystrophic EB).

It is uncommon for patients with nH JEB, generalized to develop squamous cell carcinoma, though it has been reported.[32] The overall risk for mortality due to EB in nH JEB patients is lower than that noted for patients with H JEB, JEB with pyloric atresia, and recessive dystrophic EB. However, a recent study of 140 randomly selected children who were representative of all major EB subtypes found that approximately 15% of children with nH JEB had a parental daily pain assessment score exceeding 5 on a 10-point scale. A comparable percentage (ie, approximately 15%) was scored as being free of daily pain.[33]

nH JEB, Localized

As this designation implies, nH JEB, localized is characterized by localized disease of lesser extent (and in additional respects, lesser severity) than nH JEB, generalized.[1] Like the latter, nH JEB, localized is characterized by autosomal recessive inheritance, onset at birth, dystrophic (or absent) nails, dental enamel hypoplasia, and a tendency for the development of severe caries. Unlike nH JEB, generalized, patients with nH JEB, localized typically do not demonstrate extensive atrophic scars, hair loss, anemia, impairments in growth and development, ocular abnormalities, or alterations affecting the gastrointestinal, genitourinary, or respiratory tracts.

nH JEB, Inversa

This clinical variant of nH JEB displays disease that is predominantly located in intertriginous areas, and typically displays an overall extent that exceeds that observed in patients with nH JEB, localized.[1] Like patients with nH JEB, generalized, patients with nH JEB, inversa typically demonstrate blisters, milia, atrophic scars, dystrophic (or absent) nails, dental enamel hypoplasia, and (to a lesser extent) dental caries and gastrointestinal abnormalities.

nH JEB, Progressiva

This rare variant of form of nH JEB typically presents as a mild form of JEB in young adulthood (in marked contrast to presentation at birth as noted in other forms of JEB).[1] Though of lesser severity than nH JEB, generalized, patients with nH JEB, progressiva typically display dystrophic (or absent) nails, dental enamel hypoplasia, hyperhidrosis, and an absence of dermatoglyphs (ridged skin patterns found on fingers, palms, toes, and soles).

MANAGEMENT

The management of patients with nH JEB is a long-term endeavor aimed at alleviating cutaneous and extracutaneous manifestations of disease. Management includes intensive care of affected infants, treatment and prevention of wounds, care of potentially serious complications, education of patient and parents, and provision of psychosocial support.[1,34,35]

Infancy is the most serious period for management, because a number of infant fatalities have been reported.[1,34,35] It is important that nH JEB be correctly diagnosed based on clinical, histologic, ultrastructural, or immunohistologic features of the disease. Extreme care must be used to avoid trauma to the skin of the infant, with gentle handling and avoidance of adhesives. nH JEB patients require close monitoring for evidence of secondary infections, imbalances of fluids and electrolytes, and potential complications resulting from systemic absorption of topical medications. Nutritional support and airway management are of the highest priority. Salient issues relating to the care of patients (infants, children, and adults) is presented in **Table 5** and described elsewhere in this monograph series.

In addition to the traditional approaches outlined earlier and in **Table 5**, several new molecular approaches are being applied to the management of patients with EB and other intractable inherited skin diseases. For example, Mavilio and colleagues[36] recently transduced epidermal stem cells from an adult affected by *LAMB3*-deficient nH JEB with a retroviral vector expressing a corresponding normal cDNA to prepare genetically engineered and corrected keratinocytes. These cells were expanded ex vivo, characterized, grown as epidermal sheets, and grafted back onto the skin of the affected individual. Synthesis and proper assembly of normal levels of functional laminin 332 were observed and yielded neoepidermis in this patient, who has now remained stable for more than 3 years. Additional gene therapy approaches as well as the use of agents to modulate or correct abnormal mRNAs, replace defective proteins, or introduce

Table 5
Principles and themes regarding the management of patients with nH JEB

Guiding principles

Prevent the development of blisters

Prevent the development of secondary bacterial infections

Aggressively treat infections to prevent cellulitis, sepsis, and other complications

Promote wound healing

Aggressively treat complications (eg, esophageal strictures, etc)

Maintain nutritional support

Maintain physical functionalities

Provide emotional support to patients and their family members

Specific (and nonexperimental) supportive measures

Do not place tape on skin

Regular use of mild soaps, cleansers, antimicrobial washes

Carefully deflate and drain large blisters; leave roof in place

Application of antibiotic ointments or disinfecting agents to wounds (avoid neomycin)

Use of wet compresses (+/− bacteriostatic agents) on colonized wounds

Cushioned clean (or sterile) non adherent dressings

Synthetic and/or hydrocolloid dressings over wounds on pressure points

Use of elastic mesh (and/or tubular gauze) to secure dressings

Use of tub soaks (or water vapor sources) to assist with removal of dressings

Liberal use of systemic antibiotics in the face of fever and/or infection

Appropriate use of analgesics and antipruritics

Consider topical analgesics for painful fissures

Stool softeners (avoid mineral oil and harsh laxatives)

Oral hygiene measures to preserve dentition, including use of fluoride

Supplemental minerals and vitamins as indicated

Correction of anemia (especially before any surgical intervention)

Careful use of padded hand splits in selected patients

Regular examinations to identify and treat complicated wounds and skin cancers

Rehabilitative physical, speech, and vocational therapy as indicated

Regular evaluation of EB-associated melanocytic nevi

bone marrow–derived stem cells that have the ability to home to damaged skin, produce protein(s) of interest, and ameliorate skin fragility are currently under study, development, and application.[37,38]

Finally, an important aspect of the care of patients with nH JEB lies in educating patients and parents about the disease. Parents of an affected child need to know that this disease has a genetic basis and that the risk for disease in further offspring is 1 in 4. Options for prenatal and preimplantation diagnosis should be discussed. At each encounter, information about the management of the disease should be presented in a progressive manner and reinforced in subsequent visits. In addition, the family should be educated about the initial signs and symptoms indicating potential complications. The parents as well as the child will need some form of psychosocial support to help deal with issues related to this chronic, disfiguring disease. Organizations such as the Dystrophic Epidermolysis Bullosa Research Association provide important information and support for families dealing with inherited blistering diseases. It should be kept in mind that with adequate care, most children with nH JEB grow normally, attend school, reach adulthood, and lead productive lives.

REFERENCES

1. Fine JD, Eady RAJ, Bauer EA, et al. The classification of inherited epidermolysis bullosa (EB): report of the Third International Consensus Meeting on diagnosis and Classification of EB. J Am Acad Dermatol 2008;58:931–50.
2. Almaani N, Liu L, Dopping-Hepenstal PJ, et al. Autosomal dominant junctional epidermolysis bullosa. Br J Dermatol 2009;160:1094–7.
3. Herlitz G. Kongenitaler, nicht syphilitischer Pemphigus: Eine Uebersicht nebst Beschreibung einer neuen Krankheitsform. Acta Paediatr 1935;7:315–71 [in German].
4. Pearson RW. Studies on the pathogenesis of epidermolysis bullosa. J Invest Dermatol 1962;39:551–75.
5. Hashimoto I, Schnyder UW, Anton-Lamprecht I. Epidermolysis bullosa hereditaria with junctional blistering in an adult. Dermatologica 1976;152:72–86.
6. Anton-Lamprecht I, Schnyder U. Zur ultrastruktur der epidermolysen mit junktionaler blasenbildung. Dermatologica 1979;159:377–82 [in German].
7. Hintner H, Wolff K. Generalized atrophic benign epidermolysis bullosa. Arch Dermatol 1982;118:375–84.
8. Darling TN, Bauer JW, Hintner H, et al. Generalized atrophic benign epidermolysis bullosa. Adv Dermatol 1997;13:87–119.
9. Pulkkinen L, Uitto J. Mutation analysis and molecular genetics of epidermolysis bullosa. Matrix Biol 1999;18:29–42.
10. Tidman MJ, Eady RAJ. Hemidesmosome heterogeneity in junctional epidermolysis bullosa revealed by morphometric analysis. J Invest Dermatol 1986;86:51–6.
11. McMillan JR, McGrath JA, Tidman MJ, et al. Hemidesmosomes show abnormal association with the keratin filament network in junctional forms of epidermolysis bullosa. J Invest Dermatol 1998;110:132–7.
12. Hintner H, Stingl G, Schuler G, et al. Immunofluorescence mapping of antigenic determinants within the dermal epidermal junction in mechanobullous disorders. J Invest Dermatol 1981;76:113–8.
13. Pohla-Gubo G, Lazarova Z, Giudice GJ, et al. Diminished expression of the extracellular domain of bullous pemphigoid antigen 2 (BPAG2) in the epidermal basement membrane of patients with generalized atrophic benign epidermolysis bullosa. Exp Dermatol 1995;4:199–206.
14. Jonkman MF, de Jong MC, Heeres K, et al. 180-kD bullous pemphigoid antigen (BP180) is deficient in generalized atrophic benign epidermolysis bullosa. J Clin Invest 1995;95:1345–52.
15. Varki R, Sadowski S, Pfendner E, et al. Epidermolysis bullosa 1: molecular genetics of the junctional and hemidesmosomal variants. J Med Genet 2006;43:641–52.
16. Nakano A, Chao S-C, Pulkkinen L, et al. Laminin 5 mutations in junctional epidermolysis bullosa: molecular basis of Herlitz vs non-Herlitz phenotypes. Hum Genet 2002;110:41–51.
17. Bauer JW, Lanschuetzer C. Type XVII collagen gene mutations in junctional epidermolysis bullosa and prospects for gene therapy. Clin Exp Dermatol 2003;28:53–60.
18. McGrath JA, Gatalica B, Christiano AM, et al. Mutations in the 180-kD bullous pemphigoid antigen (BPAG2), a transmembrane hemidesmosomal collagen (COL17A1), in generalized atrophic benign epidermolysis bullosa. Nat Genet 1995;11:83–6.
19. McGrath JA, Darling T, Gatalica B, et al. A homozygous deletion mutation in the gene for the 180-kDA bullous pemphigoid antigen (BPAG2) in a family with generalized atrophic benign epidermolysis bullosa. J Invest Dermatol 1996;106:771–4.
20. Jonkman MF, de Jong MC, Heeres K, et al. Generalized atrophic benign epidermolysis bullosa: either the 180-kD bullous pemphigoid antigen or laminin 5 is deficient. Arch Dermatol 1996;132:145–50.
21. Fine JD, Johnson LB, Weiner M, et al. Cause-specific risks of childhood death in inherited epidermolysis bullosa. J Pediatr 2008;152:276–80.
22. Bruckner-Tuderman L, Schnyder UW, Baran R. Nail changes in epidermolysis bullosa: clinical and

pathogenetic considerations. Br J Dermatol 1995; 132:339–44.

23. Fine JD, Johnson LB, Weiner M, et al. Tracheolaryngeal complications of inherited epidermolysis bullosa: cumulative experience of the national epidermolysis bullosa registry. Laryngoscope 2007;117:1652–60.

24. Rubin AI, Moran K, Fine JD, et al. Urethral meatal stenosis in junctional epidermolysis bullosa: a rare complication effectively treated with a novel and simple modality. Int J Dermatol 2007;46:1076–7.

25. Yamada Y, Dekio S, Jidoi J, et al. Epidermolysis bullosa atrophicans generalisata mitis: report of a case with renal dysfunction. J Dermatol 1990; 17:690–5.

26. Fine JD, Hall M, Weiner M, et al. The risk of cardiomyopathy in inherited epidermolysis bullosa. Br J Dermatol 2008;159:677–82.

27. Lin AN, Murphy F, Brodie SE, et al. Review of ophthalmic findings in 2004 patients with epidermolysis bullosa. Am J Ophthalmol 1994;118: 384–90.

28. Fine JD, Johnson LB, Weiner M, et al. Eye involvement in inherited epidermolysis bullosa: experience of the National Epidermolysis Bullosa Registry. Am J Ophthalmol 2004;138:254–62.

29. McGrath JA, Gatalica B, Li K, et al. Compound heterozygosity for a dominant glycine substitution and a recessive internal duplication mutation in the type XVII collagen gene results in junctional epidermolysis bullosa and abnormal dentition. Am J Pathol 1996;148:1787–96.

30. Wright JT, Fine JD. Hereditary epidermolysis bullosa. Semin Dermatol 1994;13:102–7.

31. Bauer JW, Schaeppi H, Kaserer C, et al. Large melanocytic nevi in hereditary epidermolysis bullosa. J Am Acad Dermatol 2001;44:577–84.

32. Mallipeddi R, Keane FM, McGrath JA, et al. Increased risk of squamous cell carcinoma in junctional epidermolysis bullosa. J Eur Acad Dermatol Venereol 2004;18:521–6.

33. Fine JD, Johnson LB, Weiner M, et al. Assessment of mobility, activities and pain in different subtypes of epidermolysis bullosa. Clin Exp Dermatol 2004;29: 122–7.

34. Fine JD, Bauer EA, McGuire J, et al, editors. Epidermolysis bullosa: clinical, epidemiologic, and laboratory advances and the findings of the National Epidermolysis Bullosa Registry. Baltimore (MD): Johns Hopkins University Press; 1999.

35. Fine JD, Hintner H, editors. Life with epidermolysis bullosa: etiology, diagnosis, multidisciplinary care and therapy. Vienna: Springer-Verlag; 2009.

36. Mavilio F, Pellegrini G, Ferrari S, et al. Correction of junctional epidermolysis bullosa by transplantation of genetically modified epidermal stem cells. Nat Med 2006;12:1397–402.

37. Tolar J, Ishida-Yamamoto A, Riddle M, et al. Amelioration of epidermolysis bullosa by transfer of wild-type bone marrow cells. Blood 2009;113: 1167–74.

38. Tamai K, Kaneda Y, Uitto J. Molecular therapies for heritable blistering diseases. Trends Mol Med 2009;15:285–92.

Adhesion and Migration, the Diverse Functions of the Laminin α3 Subunit

Kevin J. Hamill, PhD[a],*, Amy S. Paller, MD[b],
Jonathan C.R. Jones, PhD[c]

KEYWORDS

- Basement membrane • Cell adhesion
- Cell migration • Laminins

The laminins are a secreted family of heterotrimeric molecules essential for basement membrane (BM) formation, structure, and function.[1,2] Through the study of blistering skin diseases, it is now well established that the α3 subunit of laminins-332, -321, and -311 plays an important role in mediating epidermal-dermal integrity and is essential for the skin to withstand mechanical stresses.[3] These laminins, however, also regulate cell migration and mechanosignal transduction.[4–8] The precise mechanisms involved in cell migration and signaling are not yet fully clarified. This article provides an overview of the gene, transcripts, and protein structures of laminin α3, and briefly discusses the proposed functions for the α3 subunit–containing laminins.

LAMA3 GENE STRUCTURE AND EXPRESSION REGULATION

The human *LAMA3* gene encodes 76 exons from 318 kb of genomic DNA at chromosomal location 18q11.2 (**Fig. 1**A).[9,10] Isolation of cDNA clones has revealed the presence of two major transcripts: *LAMA3A* and *LAMA3B* (**Fig. 1**B). Both of these transcripts share a common 3′ end that includes exons 40 through 76. Through alternate promoter usage, however, their 5′ ends are markedly different. *LAMA3A*, encoding laminin α3A, is expressed from a promoter within intron 38 and its protein product is encoded by exons 39 to 76 (5175 bp open reading frame, encoding 1724 amino acids, calculated molecular weight 190 kDa (see **Fig. 1**B)). *LAMA3B* is much longer, consisting of exons 1 to 38 and the common 3′ exons 40 to 76; exon 39 is skipped (10002 bp open reading frame, encoding 3333 amino acids, calculated molecular weight 366 kDa (see **Fig. 1**B)).[9–12] In addition, at the message level about 20% of keratinocyte *LAMA3B* has exon 10 skipped. This shorter isoform has been termed "laminin α3B2," whereas the full length transcript encodes laminin α3B1 (see **Fig. 1**B).[10]

Testing of the promoter regions for both *LAMA3* transcripts reveals them to be responsive to typical epithelial-mesenchymal transcription factors: epidermal growth factor, keratinocyte growth factor, insulin-like growth factor-1, thymosin beta 4, interferon-γ, transforming growth factor-α and -β1, and tumor necrosis factor-α.[13–17]

Work in the Jones laboratory is supported by grant RO1 AR054184 (JCRJ) from the National Institutes of Health.

[a] Department of Cell and Molecular Biology, Feinberg School of Medicine, Northwestern University, 303 East Chicago Avenue, Tarry 8-746, Chicago, IL 60611, USA
[b] Departments of Dermatology and Cell and Molecular Biology, Feinberg School of Medicine, Northwestern University, 303 East Chicago Avenue, Tarry 8-746, Chicago, IL 60611, USA
[c] Departments of Dermatology and Pediatrics, Feinberg School of Medicine, Northwestern University, 676 North Street Clair, Suite 1600, Chicago, IL 60611, USA
* Corresponding author.
E-mail address: k-hamill@northwestern.edu (K.J. Hamill).

Dermatol Clin 28 (2010) 79–87
doi:10.1016/j.det.2009.10.009

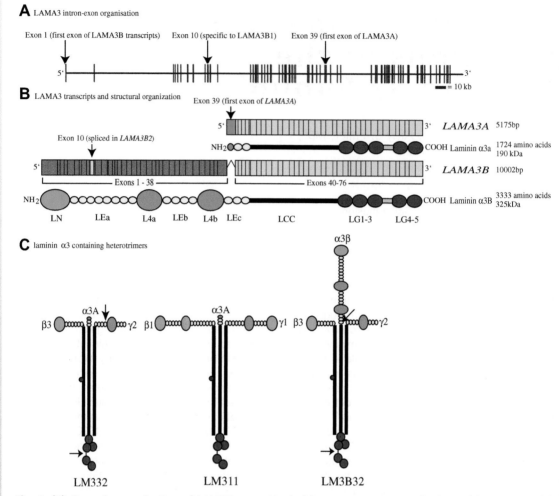

Fig. 1. (A) Genomic organization of LAMA3 gene. Vertical bars represent exons, horizontal line introns. (B) LAMA3A and LAMA3B transcript organization. Blue exons, common to both transcripts. Orange, specific to LA-MA3A. Gray, specific to LAMA3B. Pink, specific to LAMA3B2. Below each transcript is a diagrammatic representation of the domain architecture. LN, laminin N terminal domain; LE, laminin-type epidermal growth factor–like repeats; L4, globular domain; LCC, laminin coiled coil domain; LG, laminin globular domains. (C) Laminin α3 containing heterotrimer structure. Color scheme of conserved domains as in B, with purple, Lβ- laminin β chain globular domain. Arrows in LM332 and LM3B32 indicate processing points discussed in the text.

Both promoters also contain acute-phase reactant sequences and interleukin-6 binding sequences, both of which are found in many proteins upregulated at sites of trauma.[18]

Through RNase protection assays on total RNA from adult human tissues, Doliana and colleagues[12] have investigated the expression pattern of *LAMA3A* and *LAMA3B*. Spleen, stomach, kidney, skeletal muscle, pancreas, and adrenal gland express similar levels of both transcripts, whereas the salivary gland expresses only *LAMA3A*. Placenta expresses the highest *LA-MA3A* message, whereas the uterus expresses the highest *LAMA3B* message.[12] In situ reverse transcriptase polymerase chain reaction of human embryonic tissues reveals positive staining for *LAMA3* (not *LAMA3/B* specific) message in developing tubules and developing comma-shaped bodies of the kidney, in epithelial cells of the developing lung, in the basal layer of developing skin at gestational week 6.5, and in all layers of the epidermis from gestational week 8 onward.[19]

LAMININ α3A/B SUBUNIT DOMAIN ARCHITECTURE AND ASSEMBLY ISOFORMS

The laminin family of proteins shares a common architecture with regions of conserved protein folding.[20] Laminins are secreted as heterotrimeric cross-shaped molecules consisting of one α, one β, and one γ subunit that assemble intracellularly through a coiled-coil domain termed the "LCC" (formerly known as "domains I and II"). In laminin α subunits, this LCC is followed by five globular domains (termed "LG1–5"). The link between LG3 and 4 is slightly extended in the laminin α3 subunit relative to other laminin α subunits, and is the site of an extracellular processing event (see later).[21–23] In the laminin α3A subunit, the LCC is preceded by a short stretch of rodlike, laminin-type epithelial growth factor-like domains (LE, formerly domain V). In contrast, the amino terminus of laminin α3B subunit is much longer, consisting of an approximately 250 amino acid laminin N-terminal domain (LN domain, previously domain VI), which has been shown to be important for higher-order network formation through copolymerization and self-polymerization.[24,25] The LN domain is followed by three stretches of rodlike LE domains (of eight, four, and three repeats, respectively), which are interspersed by two approximately 250 amino acid globular domains (termed "L4a" and "L4b," previously domain IV (see **Fig. 1B**)).[20]

The functionality of individual laminin subunits depends not only on their own domain composition but also on that of the laminin subunits with which they associate. In terms of laminin α3A subunit, the most abundant and most studied isoform is laminin 332, comprising laminin α3A, β3, and γ2 (LM332, formerly known as "laminin 5/kalinin/epiligrin/ladsin" (**Fig. 1C**)).[21,26] In addition, laminin α3A associates with laminin β1 and γ1 forming LM311 (laminin 6, k-laminin (see **Fig. 1C**)) and, from co-immunoprecipitation data, with β2 and γ1 to form LM321 (laminin 7 (see **Fig. 1C**)).[2,21,27] The expression profile LM332, as expected, roughly matches that of its constituent mRNAs. Immunofluorescence staining for LM332 in adult tissues gives positive results in the BM of glomeruli and tubuli in kidney, the BM of alveoli, bronchioli and bronchi in lung, in the dermal-epidermal junction of skin, corneal BM, and in the enteric BM zone of the small intestine under the intestinal epithelium.[19,28]

Laminin heterotrimer formation proceeds by a βγ dimer stage and seems to be dependent on sequences toward the C-terminus of the LCC.[29–31] In theory, the laminin α3B subunit should be capable of associating with the same repertoire of β and γ laminin subunits as α3A. Although immunohistologic analyses have suggested the presence of LM3B11 in the BM of blood vessels,[32] only LM3B32 has been studied in any detail to date (see **Fig. 1C**). Interestingly, although βγ dimers require α laminin subunit incorporation to drive secretion, there is evidence that laminin α subunits can be secreted

independently of trimerization; the functional significance of this observation is yet to be established.[29]

Human LM332 is secreted as a 460-kDa species that is subsequently processed to a predominant 440-kDa form in keratinocytes maintained in low calcium medium (0.035 mM) and to a predominant 400-kDa form in keratinocytes maintained at higher concentrations of calcium (1 mM).[33] These size shifts are caused by processing of the C-terminus of the α3A subunit, which removes LG domains 4 and 5 and converts it from approximately 190 kDa to 165 kDa, and processing of the γ2 subunit toward its N-terminus, converting it from a 155-kDa form to 105 kDa.[33] LM332 containing the 165-kDa α3A and 105-kDa γ2 processed subunits is sometimes termed "mature" (matLM332). Processing of the laminin α3B subunit converts it from approximately 325 kDa to an approximately 280-kDa mature form.[25] An additional minor product of 145 kDa, which is recognized by laminin α3 antibodies, has also been identified in extracts from human amnion, with the secondary processing occurring at the N-terminus, just before the LCC.[33] Interestingly, in vitro studies have demonstrated that laminin α3A in LM311 is processed at a much lower rate than when it is incorporated into LM332, which may be relevant with regards to some of the functional differences between these heterotrimers (discussed later).[34]

THE FUNCTION OF THE LAMININ α3 SUBUNIT IN CELLULAR ADHESION

In epithelial cells LM332 is able to interact with two integrins, α6β4 and α3β1, and thereby is of central importance in the function of the two major forms of dermal-epidermal junctions: hemidesmosomes and focal adhesions.[35–38]

Hemidesmosome Formation

Hemidesmosomes are specialized adhesion structures that provide linkage from LM332 to the intermediate filament cytoskeleton. This linkage is established through the association of the extracellular domains of α6β4 integrin with the laminin α3 subunit and through binding of the intracellular tail of β4 integrin to the plakin molecule plectin (HD1). Plectin, in turn, interacts with the keratin cytoskeleton.[39–41] Adhesion is further strengthened through the association with the transmembrane protein, bullous pemphigoid antigen 2 (collagen XVIII), which also interacts with LM332 and by binding to β4 integrin of a second plakin molecule termed BPAG1e

(BP230), which acts to strengthen the link to the keratins.[42–44]

Carboxy terminal processing of laminin α3A may regulate the assembly of hemidesomsomes. Specifically, in tissue culture, only the matrix of cell lines that contain a C-terminally processed form of laminin α3A supports formation of hemidesmosomes.[22] Furthermore, treatment with plasmin of an extracellular matrix rich in LM332, but containing an unprocessed α3A laminin subunit that fails to support hemidesmosome formation, results in laminin α3A processing and conversion of that matrix to one that is competent to induce HD assembly.[22] In addition to plasmin, all of the bone morphogenetic protein-1 isoenzymes (mammalian tolloid, mammalian tolloid–like-1 and -2) have been shown to be capable of processing the laminin α3A subunit to 165 kDa and the laminin γ2 subunit to 105 kDa in vitro.[45,46] The skin of mice deficient for mammalian tolloid–bone morphogenetic protein-1 exhibits defects in hemidesomsomes,[46] suggesting the importance of such processing for hemidesmosome formation.

The importance in vivo of laminin α3 in dermal-epidermal adhesion is dramatically exemplified by skin blistering at the dermal-epidermal junction from mutation of the LAMA3 gene in patients with junctional epidermolysis bullosa, in which hemidesmosomes are either entirely undetectable ultrastructurally or are reduced in number and aberrant (see discussion of junctional epidermolysis bullosa elsewhere in this issue).

Focal Contact Formation

In contrast to hemidesmosomes, which provide a link from LM332 to the keratin cytoskeleton, focal adhesions provide a link from LM332 to the actin cytoskeleton through interaction of the laminin α3 subunit with α3β1 integrin.[37,47] α3β1 Integrin, in turn, interacts with a number of linker molecules, which mediate the association of the actin cytoskeleton with the cell surface.[48] Moreover, α3β1 integrin also interacts with molecules involved in signal transduction.[37,49,50] In cultured epidermal cells, α3β1 integrin is found clustered at the site of focal adhesions.[37] In intact skin, focal adhesions are not obvious and are likely transient matrix adhesion points that are assembled by actively moving cells.[37] The identification of mutations in FERMT1, a gene encoding a focal contact protein termed "Kindlin-1," have recently been demonstrated as pathogenic in another form of epidermolysis bullosa associated with photosensitivity, the Kindler syndrome subtype. These data suggest that the LM332-α3β1-actin linkage may

also be required for maintenance of epithelia-dermal attachment integrity; however, whether the skin fragility of Kindler syndrome is a direct result of loss of LM332-α3β1 integrin linkage or indirect, caused by disruption of HDs in Kindlin-1–deficient skin, requires further investigation.[51–53]

THE LAMININ α3 SUBUNIT IN CELL MIGRATION AND WOUND HEALING

There is considerable evidence that LM332 is an important regulator of cell migration.[4,6,7,13,54,55] Histologically, LM332 is deposited into the provisional BM of healing wound beds within 8 hours of wounding.[56] Moreover, in squamous cell carcinoma (SCC) an upregulation of LM332 correlates with poor prognosis as a result of increased metastatic potential.[57] The precise mechanisms through which laminins with an α3 subunit regulate cell migration is controversial, particularly with respect to the roles of α3β1 and α6β4 integrin, and the functional significance of LM332 proteolytic processing.[4,58]

Historically, α3β1 integrin has been thought to promote cellular migration, whereas α6β4 integrin, because of its ability to nucleate hemidesmosome formation, has long been believed to retard migration by promoting stable adhesion.[37,59] A recent paper has suggested, however, that the α3β1 integrin–LM332 interaction may actually slow wound healing rates, specifically that α3 integrin–deficient keratinocytes migrate with increased velocity and persistence relative to controls.[58] Furthermore, there are accumulating data suggesting that α6β4 integrin positively regulates skin cell migration.[4,60,61]

Processing and Regulation of Motility and Proliferation

The role of proteolytic processing of LM332 in regulating its function requires further clarification. The processed form of LM332 is known to be present in mature, unwounded skin, whereas the unprocessed form is deposited at the leading edge of acute wounds or in culture equivalents.[22,33,62] As previously described, laminin α3 subunit processing is required for hemidesmosome formation.[63] Similarly, using an antibody to LG4/5 domain of laminin α3, Frank and Carter[6] showed that migrating keratinocytes deposit unprocessed laminin α3 in a linear trail that marks the path of migration.

Interestingly, the presence of the released LG4/5 region also seems to aid deposition of LM332 or its incorporation into the BM. Processing could drive a localized increase in LM332 concentration, which in turn may enhance integrin clustering and signaling activities.[64,65] Consistent with this, the level of LM332 deposition in SCCs correlates well with their invasive potential.[55,65,66] Given that the unprocessed form of the laminin α3A subunit is predominantly found in SCC, whereas only the mature, processed subunit is present in unwounded skin, the Marinkovich group has generated an antibody specific for the LG4/5 region of the laminin α3A subunit that might specifically target SCC cells therapeutically.[66] Indeed, in a mouse model of humanized SCC, treatment with LG4/5 antibodies induced a significant decrease in tumor volume without causing skin fragility.[66]

The C-terminus of the laminin α3 subunit may also activate cell proliferative responses. Function-inhibiting antibodies to the laminin α3 LG domain inhibit proliferation of epithelial cells and decrease the level of p42/p44 MAPK activity.[47] Ligation of either of its integrin-binding partners may be responsible for initiation of this response. Ligation of α6β4 integrin by LM332 induces phosphorylation of the β4 cytoplasmic domain. The Shc adaptor protein binds to these phosphorylated tyrosines and is subsequently tyrosine phosphorylated. On phosphorylation, Shc recruits Grb2 (which is stably associated with the Ras-GTP exhange factor mSOS) and this leads to activation of the Ras-Erk and Rac-Jnk MAPK pathways.[60,67,68] Similarly, function-blocking antibodies to integrin α3 and β1 also block proliferation and MAPK phosphorylation. Further, laminin α3 subunit antibody-induced inhibition of proliferation can be rescued through treatment with β1 activating antibodies, indicating that α3β1 integrin likely mediates signals initiated by LM332 that control growth and drive proliferation.[47]

Laminin γ2 subunit processing is also an important regulator of LM332 function. The second stretch of LE repeats in the laminin γ2 subunit has been shown to be capable of interacting with epidermal growth factor and it has been proposed that the amino terminal processing of the laminin γ2 subunit exposes this region and allows this interaction to occur, thereby triggering cell motility.[69]

LM332 Deposition

A critical aspect of appropriate cell migration is the ability to move in a polarized manner and this ability is dependent on the exogenous ligand presented to cells; in one study approximately 50% of cultured epithelial cells displayed a polarized phenotype when plated on LM332, compared with only approximately 11% when plated onto collagen.[6] The precise way LM332 is deposited,

rather than deposition alone, however, is most important in supporting directed keratinocyte migration.[4]

The involvement of both α3β1 integrin and α6β4 integrin in LM332 deposition has been made apparent through analyses of LM332 matrix patterns in keratinocytes deficient in either α3 integrin or β4 integrin.[4,70] Specifically, keratinocytes derived from α3 integrin null mice deposit LM332 into spikes and arrowhead patterns, compared with more diffuse arcs in wild-type keratinocytes.[70] Furthermore, α3 integrin deficient keratinocytes are unable to reorganize precoated LM332 into ring structures in the same way as do wild-type cells.[70] In comparison, migrating human cells deficient in integrin β4 deposit LM332 in circular arrays, as compared with the linear trails deposited by migrating wild-type keratinocytes.[4] Moreover, the precise way LM332 is deposited into the matrix is dominant with regards to motile behavior, because plating β4-deficient cells onto the LM332 trails deposited by wild-type cells restores their migration patterns, whereas plating wild-type cells onto the circular tracks laid down by β4-deficient cells leads to a circular motility phenotype.[4]

Multiple further studies have implicated a role for the actin cytoskeleton in determining the specific arrangement of LM332 in the matrix of cultured keratinocytes. Inhibition of actomyosin contraction in wild-type cells, either through drug treatment or through introduction of dominant negative forms of the Rac, Rho, and Cdc42 small GTPases, leads to an aberrant organization of LM332.[4,71] It has also been observed that reorganization of precoated LM332 occurs in regions that have been extended over by filopodia and lamellipodia.[70] The different ability of α3β1 and α6β4 integrins to activate RhoGTPase family members plays a role in their mediating deposition of LM332. Specifically, α3 integrin has been implicated in the activation of RhoA, whereas β4 integrin regulates Rac activity.[4,60,72,73] In the case of α6β4 this regulation likely is caused by formation of a complex with Rac, because Rac can be co-immunoprecipiated with β4 integrin and the activity level of Rac is decreased in β4-deficient cells.[4,74] Downstream of Rac, activity of the actin severing and remodeling protein cofilin is also reduced in β4-deficient cells.[4] Rac and cofilin activity are intrinsically linked to directed migration through their ability to nucleate and drive extension of lamellipodia; the α6β4 integrin-Rac association may provide a means of spatially restricting this signaling.[75,76] Intriguingly, recent data indicate that the interaction of β4 integrin with Rac, and Rac activation, is dependent on BPAG1e and further, that BPAG1e knockdown cells show a loss of front-rear polarity.[77] These results are somewhat surprising because both $\alpha6\beta4$ integrin and BPAG1e are hemidesmosomal components and have been thought to be primarily involved in stable adhesion rather than migration.[43]

OTHER LAMININS WITH AN $\alpha3$ SUBUNIT
LM311

To this point the data discussed refer almost exclusively to laminin $\alpha3A$ as part of LM332. In various tissues including bronchial epithelial cells laminin $\alpha3a$ associates with $\beta1$ and $\gamma1$ to form LM311 (laminin 6).[2] Recently, a distinct mechanosignaling function for laminin $\alpha3A$ within this context has been demonstrated using rat primary alveolar endothelial cells grown on elastomer membranes and stretched to mimic deformation during breathing. Alveolar endothelial cells secrete a fibrous matrix enriched for LM311, perlecan, and nidogen secreted in cable-like structures.[8] Stretching of alveolar endothelial cells on this matrix leads to activation of p42/p44 MAPK, whereas treatment with function-blocking antibodies to laminin $\alpha3$ decreases MAPK phosphorylation by 40%. Similarly, α-dystroglycan antibody inhibition or shRNA knockdown leads to an approximately 30% or approximately 50% decrease, respectively, whereas antibodies to integrin $\alpha3$ and $\beta1$ have no affect.[8] These data implicate LM311 as having a role in stretch-induced signaling, and further, that this signaling involves the cell surface receptor dystroglycan.

In addition to mechanosignalling in the lung, LM311 and LM321 can be isolated from skin and human amnion BM. Isolated LM311 has cell adhesive and cell migration supporting activities but both of these are significantly less than that observed for LM332.[34] Most strikingly in junctional epidermolysis bullosa patients with mutations in LAMB3, LM311 is still produced but is unable to provide sufficient adhesive capability to prevent blister formation.[65] From rotary shadowed images of complexes it seems that LM332 and LM311 interact by their short (amino terminal) arms and there could be cooperativity of actions.[27,34] Compared with the other laminin heterotrimers, LM332 is significantly different in that its short arms are much shorter and that both the $\alpha3A$ and $\gamma2$ chains lack the amino terminal LN domain through which other laminins form order network structures (see **Fig. 1**B).[25,78] Association in the BM of LM332 with LM311 and LM321 may enable the construction of a more cohesive, integrated network of laminins, which may lead to an increased ability to withstand stresses.

LM3B32

An additional, longer form of the laminin $\alpha3$ subunit is also derived from the LAMA3 gene, laminin $\alpha3B$, which differs from the laminin $\alpha3A$ subunit in the length of its amino terminus (see **Fig. 1**B). The greatest functional significance of this is likely to be the presence of the LN domain, which may allow self-polymerization and copolymerization with other LN domain–containing laminins (similarly LM311-LM321 may also be able to form higher-order networks because of the presence of the LN domain containing $\beta1$-2 and $\gamma1$ chains).[25,78] Interestingly, one of the few studies that has been performed of laminin $\alpha3B$ function has demonstrated significantly higher cell adhesion activities and cell migration–promoting activities for LM3B32 compared with LM332.[79] In addition to the activities of the intact molecule, proteolytic processing of the amino terminus releases a 190-kDa fragment that, through interaction with $\alpha3\beta1$ integrin, promotes adhesion, migration, and proliferation.[79] These data present the interesting possibility that two regions of the same protein, separated by 100 + nm long rod domain, are capable of stimulating the same processes through ligation of the same integrin. Further research is required to shed light onto the regulation and transition between the N and C terminal-mediated signaling responses of LM3B32.

SUMMARY

Analyses of blistering skin diseases and epithelial cells in culture have shed considerable light on the functions of the laminin $\alpha3$ subunit. It is now apparent that the $\alpha3$ subunit is a multifunctional molecule with roles in adhesion, motility, and signaling. Much is now known about its processing and its receptor binding, and researchers are beginning to dissect how such processing and interactions regulate behavior of cells in a variety of tissues. Further work is needed on defining how the laminin $\alpha3$ subunit functions in a tissue context. In addition, very little is known about some of the functions of those laminin trimers that contain splice variants or proteolytically cleaved versions of the laminin $\alpha3$ subunit. These represent interesting avenues of future investigation.

REFERENCES

1. Sugawara K, Tsuruta D, Ishii M, et al. Laminin-332 and -511 in skin. Exp Dermatol 2008;17(6):473–80.
2. Marinkovich MP, Lunstrum GP, Keene DR, et al. The dermal-epidermal junction of human skin contains

a novel laminin variant. J Cell Biol 1992;119(3): 695–703.

3. Nievers MG, Schaapveld RQ, Sonnenberg A. Biology and function of hemidesmosomes. Matrix Biol 1999;18(1):5–17.

4. Sehgal BU, DeBiase PJ, Matzno S, et al. Integrin beta4 regulates migratory behavior of keratinocytes by determining laminin-332 organization. J Biol Chem 2006;281(46):35487–98.

5. Budinger GR, Urich D, DeBiase PJ, et al. Stretch-induced activation of AMP kinase in the lung requires dystroglycan. Am J Respir Cell Mol Biol 2008;39(6):666–72.

6. Frank DE, Carter WG. Laminin 5 deposition regulates keratinocyte polarization and persistent migration. J Cell Sci 2004;117(Pt 8):1351–63.

7. Kariya Y, Miyazaki K. The basement membrane protein laminin-5 acts as a soluble cell motility factor. Exp Cell Res 2004;297(2):508–20.

8. Jones JC, Lane K, Hopkinson SB, et al. Laminin-6 assembles into multimolecular fibrillar complexes with perlecan and participates in mechanical-signal transduction via a dystroglycan-dependent, integrin-independent mechanism. J Cell Sci 2005;118(Pt 12): 2557–66.

9. Ryan MC, Tizard R, VanDevanter DR, et al. Cloning of the LamA3 gene encoding the alpha 3 chain of the adhesive ligand epiligrin. Expression in wound repair. J Biol Chem 1994;269(36):22779–87.

10. McLean WH, Irvine AD, Hamill KJ, et al. An unusual N-terminal deletion of the laminin alpha3a isoform leads to the chronic granulation tissue disorder laryngo-onycho-cutaneous syndrome. Hum Mol Genet 2003;12(18):2395–409.

11. Vidal F, Baudoin C, Miquel C, et al. Cloning of the laminin alpha 3 chain gene (LAMA3) and identification of a homozygous deletion in a patient with Herlitz junctional epidermolysis bullosa. Genomics 1995;30(2):273–80.

12. Doliana R, Bellina I, Bucciotti F, et al. The human alpha3b is a 'full-sized' laminin chain variant with a more widespread tissue expression than the truncated alpha3a. FEBS Lett 1997;417(1):65–70.

13. Amano S, Akutsu N, Ogura Y, et al. Increase of laminin 5 synthesis in human keratinocytes by acute wound fluid, inflammatory cytokines and growth factors, and lysophospholipids. Br J Dermatol 2004;151(5):961–70.

14. Kainulainen T, Hakkinen L, Hamidi S, et al. Laminin-5 expression is independent of the injury and the microenvironment during reepithelialization of wounds. J Histochem Cytochem 1998;46(3):353–60.

15. Korang K, Christiano AM, Uitto J, et al. Differential cytokine modulation of the genes LAMA3, LAMB3, and LAMC2, encoding the constitutive polypeptides, alpha 3, beta 3, and gamma 2, of human laminin 5 in epidermal keratinocytes. FEBS Lett 1995;368(3):556–8.

16. Virolle T, Monthouel MN, Djabari Z, et al. Three activator protein-1-binding sites bound by the Fra-2.JunD complex cooperate for the regulation of murine laminin alpha3A (lama3A) promoter activity by transforming growth factor-beta. J Biol Chem 1998;273(28):17318–25.

17. Sosne G, Xu L, Prach L, et al. Thymosin beta 4 stimulates laminin-5 production independent of TGF-beta. Exp Cell Res 2004;293(1):175–83.

18. Ferrigno O, Virolle T, Galliano MF, et al. Murine laminin alpha3A and alpha3B isoform chains are generated by usage of two promoters and alternative splicing. J Biol Chem 1997;272(33):20502–7.

19. Miosge N, Kluge JG, Studzinski A, et al. In situ-RT-PCR and immunohistochemistry for the localisation of the mRNA of the alpha 3 chain of laminin and laminin-5 during human organogenesis. Anat Embryol (Berl) 2002;205(5–6):355–63.

20. Aumailley M, Bruckner-Tuderman L, Carter WG, et al. A simplified laminin nomenclature. Matrix Biol 2005;24(5):326–32.

21. Marinkovich MP, Verrando P, Keene DR, et al. Basement membrane proteins kalinin and nicein are structurally and immunologically identical. Lab Invest 1993;69(3):295–9.

22. Goldfinger LE, Stack MS, Jones JC. Processing of laminin-5 and its functional consequences: role of plasmin and tissue-type plasminogen activator. J Cell Biol 1998;141(1):255–65.

23. Tsubota Y, Mizushima H, Hirosaki T, et al. Isolation and activity of proteolytic fragment of laminin-5 alpha3 chain. Biochem Biophys Res Commun 2000;278(3):614–20.

24. Cheng YS, Champliaud MF, Burgeson RE, et al. Self-assembly of laminin isoforms. J Biol Chem 1997; 272(50):31525–32.

25. Garbe JH, Gohring W, Mann K, et al. Complete sequence, recombinant analysis and binding to laminins and sulphated ligands of the N-terminal domains of laminin alpha3B and alpha5 chains. Biochem J 2002;362(Pt 1):213–21.

26. Miyazaki K, Kikkawa Y, Nakamura A, et al. A large cell-adhesive scatter factor secreted by human gastric carcinoma cells. Proc Natl Acad Sci U S A 1993;90(24):11767–71.

27. Champliaud MF, Lunstrum GP, Rousselle P, et al. Human amnion contains a novel laminin variant, laminin 7, which like laminin 6, covalently associates with laminin 5 to promote stable epithelial-stromal attachment. J Cell Biol 1996;132(6): 1189–98.

28. Tuori A, Uusitalo H, Burgeson RE, et al. The immunohistochemical composition of the human corneal basement membrane. Cornea 1996;15(3):286–94.

29. Yurchenco PD, Quan Y, Colognato H, et al. The alpha chain of laminin-1 is independently secreted and drives secretion of its beta- and gamma-chain

partners. Proc Natl Acad Sci U S A 1997;94(19): 10189–94.

30. Nomizu M, Utani A, Beck K, et al. Mechanism of laminin chain assembly into a triple-stranded coiled-coil structure. Biochemistry 1996;35(9):2885–93.

31. Utani A, Nomizu M, Timpl R, et al. Laminin chain assembly: specific sequences at the C terminus of the long arm are required for the formation of specific double- and triple-stranded coiled-coil structures. J Biol Chem 1994;269(29):19167–75.

32. Kariya Y, Mori T, Yasuda C, et al. Localization of laminin alpha3B chain in vascular and epithelial basement membranes of normal human tissues and its down-regulation in skin cancers. J Mol Histol 2008; 39(4):435–46.

33. Marinkovich MP, Lunstrum GP, Burgeson RE. The anchoring filament protein kalinin is synthesized and secreted as a high molecular weight precursor. J Biol Chem 1992;267(25):17900–6.

34. Hirosaki T, Tsubota Y, Kariya Y, et al. Laminin-6 is activated by proteolytic processing and regulates cellular adhesion and migration differently from laminin-5. J Biol Chem 2002;277(51):49287–95.

35. Rousselle P, Lunstrum GP, Keene DR, et al. Kalinin: an epithelium-specific basement membrane adhesion molecule that is a component of anchoring filaments. J Cell Biol 1991;114(3):567–76.

36. Carter WG, Ryan MC, Gahr PJ. Epiligrin, a new cell adhesion ligand for integrin alpha 3 beta 1 in epithelial basement membranes. Cell 1991;65(4):599–610.

37. Carter WG, Kaur P, Gil SG, et al. Distinct functions for integrins alpha 3 beta 1 in focal adhesions and alpha 6 beta 4/bullous pemphigoid antigen in a new stable anchoring contact (SAC) of keratinocytes: relation to hemidesmosomes. J Cell Biol 1990;111(6 Pt 2):3141–54.

38. Zamir E, Geiger B. Components of cell-matrix adhesions. J Cell Sci 2001;114(Pt 20):3577–9.

39. Koster J, van Wilpe S, Kuikman I, et al. Role of binding of plectin to the integrin beta4 subunit in the assembly of hemidesmosomes. Mol Biol Cell 2004;15(3):1211–23.

40. Rousselle P, Aumailley M. Kalinin is more efficient than laminin in promoting adhesion of primary keratinocytes and some other epithelial cells and has a different requirement for integrin receptors. J Cell Biol 1994;125(1):205–14.

41. Jones JC, Hopkinson SB, Goldfinger LE. Structure and assembly of hemidesmosomes. Bioessays 1998;20(6):488–94.

42. Gagnoux-Palacios L, Gache Y, Ortonne JP, et al. Hemidesmosome assembly assessed by expression of a wild-type integrin beta 4 cDNA in junctional epidermolysis bullosa keratinocytes. Lab Invest. 1997;77(5):459–68.

43. Koster J, Geerts D, Favre B, et al. Analysis of the interactions between BP180, BP230, plectin and the integrin alpha6beta4 important for hemidesmosome assembly. J Cell Sci 2003;116(Pt 2):387–99.

44. Schaapveld RQ, Borradori L, Geerts D, et al. Hemidesmosome formation is initiated by the beta4 integrin subunit, requires complex formation of beta4 and HD1/plectin, and involves a direct interaction between beta4 and the bullous pemphigoid antigen 180. J Cell Biol 1998;142(1):271–84.

45. Amano S, Scott IC, Takahara K, et al. Bone morphogenetic protein 1 is an extracellular processing enzyme of the laminin 5 gamma 2 chain. J Biol Chem 2000;275(30):22728–35.

46. Veitch DP, Nokelainen P, McGowan KA, et al. Mammalian tolloid metalloproteinase, and not matrix metalloprotease 2 or membrane type 1 metalloprotease, processes laminin-5 in keratinocytes and skin. J Biol Chem 2003;278(18):15661–8.

47. Gonzales M, Haan K, Baker SE, et al. A cell signal pathway involving laminin-5, alpha3beta1 integrin, and mitogen-activated protein kinase can regulate epithelial cell proliferation. Mol Biol Cell 1999;10(2): 259–70.

48. Zamir E, Geiger B. Molecular complexity and dynamics of cell-matrix adhesions. J Cell Sci 2001; 114(Pt 20):3583–90.

49. Critchley DR. Focal adhesions: the cytoskeletal connection. Curr Opin Cell Biol 2000;12(1):133–9.

50. Wozniak MA, Modzelewska K, Kwong L, et al. Focal adhesion regulation of cell behavior. Biochim Biophys Acta 2004;1692(2–3):103–19.

51. Ashton GH, McLean WH, South AP, et al. Recurrent mutations in kindlin-1, a novel keratinocyte focal contact protein, in the autosomal recessive skin fragility and photosensitivity disorder, Kindler syndrome. J Invest Dermatol 2004;122(1):78–83.

52. Siegel DH, Ashton GH, Penagos HG, et al. Loss of kindlin-1, a human homolog of the *Caenorhabditis elegans* actin-extracellular-matrix linker protein UNC-112, causes Kindler syndrome. Am J Hum Genet 2003;73(1):174–87.

53. Jobard F, Bouadjar B, Caux F, et al. Identification of mutations in a new gene encoding a FERM family protein with a pleckstrin homology domain in Kindler syndrome. Hum Mol Genet 2003;12(8): 925–35.

54. Kinumatsu T, Hashimoto S, Muramatsu T, et al. Involvement of laminin and integrins in adhesion and migration of junctional epithelium cells. J Periodontal Res 2009;44(1):12–28.

55. Baba Y, Iyama KI, Hirashima K, et al. Laminin-332 promotes the invasion of oesophageal squamous cell carcinoma via PI3K activation. Br J Cancer 2008;98(5):974–80.

56. Lampe PD, Nguyen BP, Gil S, et al. Cellular interaction of integrin alpha3beta1 with laminin 5 promotes gap junctional communication. J Cell Biol 1998; 143(6):1735–47.

57. Marinkovich MP. Tumour microenvironment: laminin 332 in squamous-cell carcinoma. Nat Rev Cancer 2007;7(5):370–80.

58. Margadant C, Raymond K, Kreft M, et al. Integrin alpha3beta1 inhibits directional migration and wound re-epithelialization in the skin. J Cell Sci 2009; 122(Pt 2):278–88.

59. Sonnenberg A, Calafat J, Janssen H, et al. Integrin alpha 6/beta 4 complex is located in hemidesmosomes, suggesting a major role in epidermal cell-basement membrane adhesion. J Cell Biol 1991; 113(4):907–17.

60. Mercurio AM, Rabinovitz I, Shaw LM. The alpha 6 beta 4 integrin and epithelial cell migration. Curr Opin Cell Biol 2001;13(5):541–5.

61. Pullar CE, Baier BS, Kariya Y, et al. beta4 integrin and epidermal growth factor coordinately regulate electric field-mediated directional migration via Rac1. Mol Biol Cell 2006;17(11):4925–35.

62. Aumailley M, El Khal A, Knoss N, et al. Laminin 5 processing and its integration into the ECM. Matrix Biol 2003;22(1):49–54.

63. Goldfinger LE, Hopkinson SB, deHart GW, et al. The alpha3 laminin subunit, alpha6beta4 and alpha3-beta1 integrin coordinately regulate wound healing in cultured epithelial cells and in the skin. J Cell Sci 1999;112(Pt 16):2615–29.

64. Schatzmann F, Marlow R, Streuli CH. Integrin signaling and mammary cell function. J Mammary Gland Biol Neoplasia 2003;8(4):395–408.

65. Sigle RO, Gil SG, Bhattacharya M, et al. Globular domains 4/5 of the laminin alpha3 chain mediate deposition of precursor laminin 5. J Cell Sci 2004; 117(Pt 19):4481–94.

66. Tran M, Rousselle P, Nokelainen P, et al. Targeting a tumor-specific laminin domain critical for human carcinogenesis. Cancer Res 2008;68(8):2885–94.

67. Mainiero F, Murgia C, Wary KK, et al. The coupling of alpha6beta4 integrin to Ras-MAP kinase pathways mediated by Shc controls keratinocyte proliferation. Embo J 1997;16(9):2365–75.

68. Jonkman MF. Hereditary skin diseases of hemidesmosomes. J Dermatol Sci 1999;20(2):103–21.

69. Schenk S, Hintermann E, Bilban M, et al. Binding to EGF receptor of a laminin-5 EGF-like fragment liberated during MMP-dependent mammary gland involution. J Cell Biol 2003;161(1):197–209.

70. deHart GW, Healy KE, Jones JC. The role of alpha3-beta1 integrin in determining the supramolecular organization of laminin-5 in the extracellular matrix of keratinocytes. Exp Cell Res 2003;283(1):67–79.

71. DeHart GW, Jones JC. Myosin-mediated cytoskeleton contraction and Rho GTPases regulate laminin-5 matrix assembly. Cell Motil Cytoskeleton 2004;57(2):107–17.

72. Rabinovitz I, Mercurio AM. The integrin alpha6beta4 functions in carcinoma cell migration on laminin-1 by mediating the formation and stabilization of actin-containing motility structures. J Cell Biol 1997; 139(7):1873–84.

73. Nguyen BP, Ren XD, Schwartz MA, et al. Ligation of integrin alpha 3beta 1 by laminin 5 at the wound edge activates Rho-dependent adhesion of leading keratinocytes on collagen. J Biol Chem 2001; 276(47):43860–70.

74. Russell AJ, Fincher EF, Millman L, et al. Alpha 6 beta 4 integrin regulates keratinocyte chemotaxis through differential GTPase activation and antagonism of alpha 3 beta 1 integrin. J Cell Sci 2003;116(Pt 17): 3543–56.

75. Nobes CD, Hall A. Rho, rac, and cdc42 GTPases regulate the assembly of multimolecular focal complexes associated with actin stress fibers, lamellipodia, and filopodia. Cell 1995;81(1):53–62.

76. Yang N, Higuchi O, Ohashi K, et al. Cofilin phosphorylation by LIM-kinase 1 and its role in Rac-mediated actin reorganization. Nature 1998;393(6687):809–12.

77. Hamill KJ, Hopkinson SB, DeBiase P, et al. BPAG1e maintains keratinocyte polarity through beta4 integrin-mediated modulation of Rac1 and cofilin activities. Mol Biol Cell 2009;20(12):2954–62.

78. Odenthal U, Haehn S, Tunggal P, et al. Molecular analysis of laminin N-terminal domains mediating self-interactions. J Biol Chem 2004;279(43): 44504–12.

79. Kariya Y, Yasuda C, Nakashima Y, et al. Characterization of laminin 5B and NH2-terminal proteolytic fragment of its alpha3B chain: promotion of cellular adhesion, migration, and proliferation. J Biol Chem 2004;279(23):24774–84.

Laryngo-onycho-cutaneous Syndrome

Heather Irina Cohn, BS, MD[a,b],
Dédée F. Murrell, MA, BMBCh, FAAD, MD[b,c],*

KEYWORDS

- Laryngo-onycho-cutaneous syndrome • LOC • JEB-LOC
- LOGIC • Shabbir disease • JEB-O

Our understanding of the pathogenesis of laryngo-onycho-cutaneous (LOC) syndrome, now classified as a subtype of junctional epidermolysis bullosa, other (JEB-O), has come a long way since the earliest documented case by Shabbir in 1986. In a concerted effort to elucidate the disease origin and chain of events leading to LOC syndrome (previously termed, laryngeal and ocular granulation tissue in children from the Indian subcontinent [LOGIC] syndrome and Shabbir disease), more than a dozen articles have been published. LOC syndrome was appropriately reclassified as a subtype of JEB based on its clinical features being similar to JEB and its association, in the majority of patients from the Punjab, with a unique mutation affecting the N terminus of the α3 chain of LM332. Although LOC syndrome is now a subtype of JEB-O, aptly termed JEB-LOC, it is important to acknowledge JEB-LOC has a distinct clinicopathologic appearance and molecular fingerprint. Therefore, the intricacies of the JEB-LOC subtype are discussed in this article with regard to disease presentation, pathogenesis, management, and prognosis.

DISEASE PRESENTATION

Described mainly in the offspring of consanguineous Muslim families originating in the Punjabi region of Pakistan and India, JEB-LOC is rare and has an autosomal recessive inheritance.[2,5,6] Few JEB-LOC cases have been reported in the absence of consanguineous coupling.[5-7] It is characterized by an altered cry at birth, erosions, nail abnormalities, and aberrant production of granulation tissue, resulting in conjunctival and laryngeal granulomatous papules.[2,5-7] Patients are diagnosed in the first few months of infancy and the disease progresses with multiple cutaneous manifestations. JEB-LOC patients acquire facial erosions originating from short-lived blistering, conjunctival papules, and teeth deformities (ie, notched teeth) (**Fig. 1**). In contrast to the excessive erosions and bulla formation described in other JEB subtypes, patients with JEB-LOC have minimal blistering and extensive granulation formation.[1] The conjunctival lesions start in the lateral portion of the eye and result in symblepharon. The conjunctival granulation tissue often leads to total palpebral occlusion and blindness. Conjunctival granulation tissue is rare outside this variant.[1,4]

DISEASE PATHOGENESIS

The biology of the two laminin A3 isoforms is reviewed in detail in the article by Hamill and colleagues elsewhere in this issue. In most JEB-LOC cases, in patients of Punjabi origin, there is

Work was funded by the Dystrophic Epidermolysis Bullosa Research Association of Australia (to D.F. Murrell), by the Research Infrastructure Support Services Ltd funded under the Commonwealth Government's National Collaborative Research Infrastructure Strategy (to D.F. Murrell), by a Foerderer Fellowship (to H.I. Cohn), and by a Dubbs Scholar Fellowship (to H.I. Cohn).

[a] Department of Dermatology and Cutaneous Biology, Jefferson Medical College, Thomas Jefferson University, Bluemle Life Sciences Building, 233 South 10th Street, Suite 450, Philadelphia, PA 19107, USA
[b] Department of Dermatology, St George Hospital, St George Clinical School, Kogarah, NSW 2217, Australia
[c] University of New South Wales, St George Clinical School, St George Hospital, Kogarah (Sydney), NSW 2050, Australia
* Corresponding author. Department of Dermatology, St George Hospital, University of New South Wales, Gray Street, Kogarah, Sydney, NSW 2217, Australia.
E-mail address: d.murrell@unsw.edu.au (D.F. Murrell).

Dermatol Clin 28 (2010) 89–92
doi:10.1016/j.det.2009.10.010

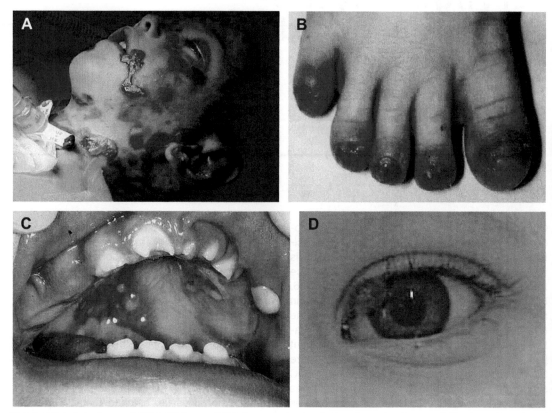

Fig. 1. Clinical features of JEB-LOC form of JEB: laryngeal granulation tissue leading to asphyxia and trachyostomy and granulation tissue on erosions (*A*); nail dystrophy with blistering under the nails (*B*); amelogenesis imperfecta with notching of incisors and oral erosions (*C*) and conjunctival granulation tissue (*D*).

a homozygous recessive mutation in *LAMA3A*, leading to the foreshortening of a critical portion of the N terminus of the α3 chain laminin-5 trimer (**Fig. 2**).[3,8] Studies suggest that extracellular matrix homeostasis is altered when the basal keratinocytes secrete the abbreviated α3 chain.[9] This aberrant microenvironment provides a venue for erosion along the mucosal membranes, including the nail bed, and throughout the larynx. The tissue localization of the laminin α3A corresponds to the clinical manifestations of JEB-LOC: with LM332 this applies to the skin, nail, and mucous membrane fragility, but with LM311 (another laminin containing the α3A variant, which is present in the lungs) the JEB-LOC patients also are susceptible to pneumonia.[10] The conjunctival involvement is another striking feature of the JEB-LOC variant. Expression studies of the relative amounts of LAMA3A versus LAMA3B might assist in explaining this, as one study of the conjunctiva in LOC syndrome found the granulating cells to be mainly fibroblastic in origin and to have reduced p63 expression.[11] Missense mutations in the tumor suppressor gene encoding p63 lead to ankyloblepharon in Hay-Wells (ankyloblepharon–ectodermal

dysplasia–clefting) syndrome,[12] so reduced p63 in LOC syndrome might be related to the limbal margin granulation overgrowth in JEB-LOC.

Similar to other junctional subtypes of EB, immunofluorescence mapping exhibits avidity to type IV collagen below the blister and BP180 above the blister in patients with the JEB-LOC variant. JEB-LOC diverges molecularly from other JEB subtypes, however, in that laminin α3, β3, and γ2 antibody studies may have normal luminous intensity compared with control tissues.[4]

The first non-Punjabi case was a white boy with nonconsanguineous parents of Irish descent, who had overlapping clinical features of JEB and JEB-LOC (**Table 1**), with the conjunctival papules.[4] He had a paternal *LAMA3* splice mutation, which would have affected the C terminus, which is common to the LAMA3A and LAMA3B variants, and a maternal exon 39 I17N missense mutation,[9] affecting only the *LAMA3A* variant, with consequent JEB-LOC features. The isoleucine is highly conserved in evolution, suggesting it has an important function in the protein. It changes from hydrophobic to hydrophilic (asparagine), which is likely to affect the protein's conformation and interactions. This overlap case

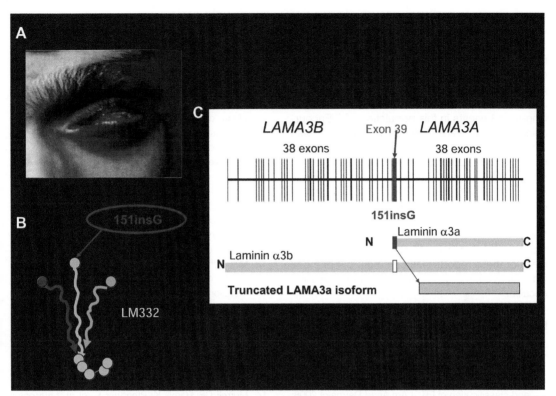

Fig. 2. Pathogenesis of JEB-LOC: (*A*) the conjunctival granulation tissue; (*B*) diagram of the triple helix of LM332 with the laminin α3A variant in anchoring filaments and the site of the founder frameshift mutation 151insG in most cases of Punjabi descent; (*C*) representation of the isoforms of the LAMA3 gene, showing the shorter LAMA3a version which contains exon 39, the site of the 151insG mutation, and the longer LAMA3b version, in which exons 40–76 are identical to LAMA3a. The frameshift leads to a downstream initiation codon, such that only the first approximately 50 amino acids from the N terminus of laminin α3A are missing. (Part A from McLean WH, Irvine AD, Hamill KJ, et al. An unusual N-terminal deletion of the laminin α3a isoform leads to the chronic granulation tissue disorder laryngo-onycho-cutaneous syndrome. Hum Mol Genet 2003;2(18):2395–409; with permission.)

provided the first proof that JEB-LOC was a variant of JEB[4,13–15] after much earlier speculation.[7]

MANAGEMENT AND PROGNOSIS

Further details about management of clinical complications of JEB-LOC common to other subtypes of JEB are mentioned in this issue by Hamill et al. High childhood mortality is seen with this variant of JEB.[2,4–6] Erosions, granulation tissue, nail dystrophy, conjunctival eye lesions, laryngeal involvement, enamel hypoplasia, and ulcers tend to be unresponsive to chemical therapeutics.[2,4–6] Tracheostomy, gastrostomy, and

Table 1
Comparison of clinical features of junctional epidermolysis bullosa and laryngo-onycho-cutaneous syndrome

	Junctional Epidermolysis Bullosa	Laryngo-onycho-cutaneous Syndrome
Erosions	+++	+
Granulation tissue	++	++
Nail dystrophy	+++	+++
Conjunctival eye lesions	±	+++
Laryngeal involvement	+++	+++
Enamel defects	+++	++

Scale of severity: ±, absent/minimal; +, mild; ++, moderate; +++, extensive.

suprapubic catheterization are all surgical interventions performed throughout the first decade of life to halt the resulting laryngeal, gastrointestinal, and urethral strictures, respectively. Death can ensue via fatal respiratory obstruction and pneumonia. Antibiotics, corticosteroids, dapsone, and antituberculosis therapeutics have minimal long-term benefits in this population.[2,4–6] Encouraging results were achieved, however, with vascular laser therapy for laryngeal involvement in our non-Punjabi patient with JEB-LOC in the face of respiratory obstruction.[4,16] What is unique about management of JEB-LOC is the severe eye involvement; thalidomide has been trialed to reduce granulation tissue[17] and amniotic membrane transplantation has been used to reduce ocular scarring.[18] Death in childhood in many of these reports was common, but of those who survived, many had remission in the second decade.[2,4–6]

REFERENCES

1. Fine JD, Eady RA, Bauer EA, et al. The classification of inherited epidermolysis bullosa (EB): report of the Third International Consensus Meeting on diagnosis and classification of EB. J Am Acad Dermatol 2008; 58(6):931–50.

2. Shabbir G, Hassan M, Kazmi A. Laryngo-onycho-cutaneous syndrome: a study of 22 cases. Biomedica 1986;2:15–25.

3. McLean WH, Irvine AD, Hamill KJ, et al. An unusual N-terminal deletion of the laminin alpha3a isoform leads to the chronic granulation tissue disorder laryngo-onycho-cutaneous syndrome. Hum Mol Genet 2003;12(18):2395–409.

4. Figueira EC, Crotty A, Challinor CJ, et al. Granulation tissue in the eyelid margin and conjunctiva in junctional epidermolysis bullosa with features of laryngo-onycho-cutaneous syndrome. Clin Experiment Ophthalmol 2007;35(2):163–6.

5. Ainsworth JR, Spencer AF, Dudgeon J, et al. Laryngeal and ocular granulation tissue formation in two Punjabi children: LOGIC syndrome. Eye 1991;5(Pt 6):717–22.

6. Ainsworth JR, Shabbir G, Spencer AF, et al. Multi-system disorder of Punjabi children exhibiting spontaneous dermal and submucosal granulation tissue formation: LOGIC syndrome. Clin Dysmorphol 1992;1(1):3–15.

7. Phillips RJ, Atherton DJ, Gibbs ML, et al. Laryngo-onycho-cutaneous syndrome: an inherited epithelial defect. Arch Dis Child 1994;70(4):319–26.

8. Hamill K. [PhD Thesis]. Dundee University; 2006.

9. Hamill KJ, McLean WH. The alpha-3 polypeptide chain of laminin 5: insight into wound healing responses from the study of genodermatoses. Clin Exp Dermatol 2005;30(4):398–404.

10. Aumailley M, Bruckner-Tuderman L, Carter WG, et al. A simplified laminin nomenclature. Matrix Biol 2005;24(5):326–32.

11. Atkinson SD, Moore JE, Shah S, et al. P63 expression in conjunctival proliferative diseases: pterygium and laryngo-onycho-cutaneous (LOC) syndrome. Curr Eye Res 2008;33(7):551–8.

12. McGrath JA, Duijf PH, Doetsch V, et al. Hay-Wells syndrome is caused by heterozygous missense mutations in the SAM domain of p63. Hum Mol Genet 2001;10(3):221–9.

13. Murrell D. Eyelid granulomas in late onset Herlitz Junctional epidermolysis bullosa. Paper presented at Proceedings of the International Symposium on Epidermolysis Bullosa, Institute for Child Health, London, 2003.

14. Murrell DF, Hamill K, Pfendner E, et al. Late onset herlitz junctional epidermolysis bullosa mimicking laryngo-onycho-cutaneous syndrome Aust Soc Derm Research [abstract]. J Invest Dermatol 2005; 125(A10).

15. Murrell D. Studies in blistering diseases [MD Thesis]. University of New South Wales, Sydney; 2006.

16. Murrell DF, Pasmooij AM, Pas HH, et al. Retrospective diagnosis of fatal BP180-deficient non-Herlitz junctional epidermolysis bullosa suggested by immunofluorescence (IF) antigen-mapping of parental carriers bearing enamel defects. J Invest Dermatol 2007;127:1772–5.

17. Strauss RM, Bate J, Nischal KK, et al. A child with laryngo-onychocutaneous syndrome partially responsive to treatment with thalidomide. Br J Dermatol 2006;155(6):1283–6.

18. Moore JE, Shah S, Kumar V, et al. Follow up of patients with ocular scarring secondary to LOC syndrome treated by amniotic membrane transplantation. Br J Ophthalmol 2005;89(8):939–41.

Type VII Collagen: The Anchoring Fibril Protein at Fault in Dystrophic Epidermolysis Bullosa

Hye Jin Chung, MD, MS, Jouni Uitto, MD, PhD*

KEYWORDS

- Epidermolysis bullosa • Type VII collagen
- Anchoring fibrils • Heritable blistering diseases

THE COLLAGEN FAMILY OF PROTEINS

Collagens, the major extracellular matrix components in most vertebrate tissues, comprise a superfamily of proteins.[1] A total of 29 genetically distinct collagens have been described so far in vertebrate tissues and designated by Roman numerals I to XXIX in order of their discovery.[2,3] The collagen molecules consist of 3 subunit polypeptides, so-called α-chains, and whereas some collagens are homotrimers, others can be heterotrimers containing 2, or even 3, genetically distinct subunit polypeptides. Consequently, there are well over 40 genes in vertebrate tissues that encode the subunits polypeptides of different, genetically distinct collagen molecules.[1,2]

A characteristic structural feature of all collagens is the presence of a protein domain in triple-helical conformation that provides stability to these molecules to serve as structural building blocks providing integrity to connective tissues. The triple-helical conformation resists nonspecific proteolysis, such as digestion with pepsin. The folding of the individual α-chains into the triple-helical conformation is predicated on the characteristic primary sequence, consisting of repeating Gly-X-Y triplet sequences. In some collagens, such as in type I collagen, the most abundant collagen in the skin and bones, the central collagenous domain of individual α-chains, contains an uninterrupted Gly-X-Y repeat segment spanning approximately 1000 amino acids. In some collagens, such as in type IV (the basement membrane collagen) and type VII (the anchoring fibril collagen), the Gly-X-Y repeat sequence contains imperfections that interrupt the triple-helical conformation.[1] These interruptions then provide flexibility to the rodlike collagen molecules and also provide sites susceptible to nonspecific proteolytic cleavage of the primary sequence.

On the basis of their fiber architecture in tissues, the genetically distinct collagens have been divided into different subgroups.[1] Collagens types I, II, III, V, and X align into large extracellular fibrils and are designated as fibril-forming collagens. Type IV collagen is arranged in an interlacing network within the basement membranes, whereas type VI collagen forms distinct microfibrils and type VII forms anchoring fibrils. Fibril-associated collagens with interrupted triple helices (FACIT) collagens[4] include types IX, XII, XIV, XIX, XX, and XXI. Several of the latter types of collagens associate with larger collagen fibers and serve as molecular bridges, stabilizing the organization of the extracellular matrix.

The major collagens in human skin are types I and III, which account for approximately 80% and 10% of the total bulk of collagen, respectively

Department of Dermatology and Cutaneous Biology, Jefferson Medical College, and Jefferson Institute of Molecular Medicine, Thomas Jefferson University, 233 South 10th Street, Suite 450 BLSB, Philadelphia, PA 19107, USA

* Corresponding author.

E-mail address: jouni.uitto@jefferson.edu (J. Uitto).

Dermatol Clin 28 (2010) 93–105
doi:10.1016/j.det.2009.10.011

(Table 1). These 2 collagens associate to form broad extracellular fibers characteristic of human dermis. Type V collagen is present in most connective tissues, including the dermis where it represents less than 5% of the total collagen. In the dermis, type V collagen is located on the surface of the large collagen fibers formed by type I and III collagens, and type V collagen regulates the lateral growth of these fibers. Another major collagen in the skin is type IV collagen, present within the dermal-epidermal junction and in the vascular basement membranes.

In addition to these major collagens, human skin contains several minor collagens that demonstrate spatially restricted location, yet they play a critical role in providing integral stability to the skin (see Table 1). One of them is type VII collagen, the major, if not exclusive, component of anchoring fibrils.[5] Another one is type XVII collagen, a transmembrane collagen in type II topography.[6] Type XVII collagen resides in hemidesmosomes complexed with α6β4 integrin, plectin, and laminin-332 (laminin-5).[7] Finally, type XXIX collagen has been recently reported to be a putative epidermal collagen with the highest level of expression in suprabasal layers.[3] This collagen has been suggested to play a role in atopic dermatitis but its characterization is currently incomplete.

THE BIOLOGY OF TYPE VII COLLAGEN

Type VII collagen was initially described as an extended, unusually long molecule, hence the original designation as long-chain (LC) collagen.[8] Rotary shadowing electron microscopy of type VII collagen molecules synthesized and secreted by human keratinocytes in culture revealed a long, 424-nm, triple-helical domain and flanking noncollagenous sequences (Fig. 1A). The amino-terminal domain was particularly noticeable, with individual α-chains contributing an extended arm. Simultaneously, visualization of type VII collagen isolated by limited pepsin proteolysis of amniotic membranes revealed a 780-nm dimer of 2 identical molecules in antiparallel orientation, with a 60-nm overlap stabilized by disulfide bonds (Fig. 1B, C).[5] Further proteolytic digestion with pepsin revealed that type VII collagen molecules consist of a central collagenous, triple-helical segment flanked by the noncollagenous NC-1 and NC-2 domains. Subsequent cloning of the human type VII collagen gene and the corresponding complementary DNA (cDNA) indicated that the initially synthesized type VII collagen subunit polypeptide, the pro-α1(VII) chain is a complex modular protein consisting of a central, 1530-amino acid triple-helical domain (Fig. 2A).[9,10] However, unlike interstitial collagens, the repeating Gly-X-Y sequence is

Table 1
Genetic heterogeneity of collagen in human skin

Collagen Type	Chain Composition	Supramolecular Assembly	Tissue Distribution[b]
I	$[\alpha1(I)]_2\alpha2(I)$	Fibrillar	Dermis, bone, tendons
III	$[\alpha1(III)]_3$	Fibrillar	Fetal dermis, blood vessels, GI tract
IV	$[\alpha1(IV)]_2\alpha2(IV)^a$	Basement membrane	Ubiquitous
V	$[\alpha1(V)]_2\alpha2(V)^a$	Fibrillar	Ubiquitous
VI	$\alpha1(VI)\alpha2(VI)\alpha3(VI)^a$	Microfibrils	Ubiquitous
VII	$[\alpha1(VII)]_3$	Anchoring fibrils	Anchoring fibrils (see table 2)
VIII	$[\alpha1(VIII)]_3$	Network forming	Endothelia
XIII	$[\alpha1(XIII)]_3$	Transmembrane	Ubiquitous, including epidermis
XIV	$[\alpha1(XIV)]_3$	FACIT	Skin, cornea
XV	$[\alpha1(XV)]_3$	Basement membrane	Ubiquitous
XVII	$[\alpha1(XVII)]_3$	Transmembrane	Hemidesmosomes in skin, cornea, mucous membrane
XXIX	Unknown	Unknown	Epidermis

[a] Additional α-chains have been identified.
[b] Distribution in the skin and other major tissues is indicated; lesser amounts may be present in other tissues.

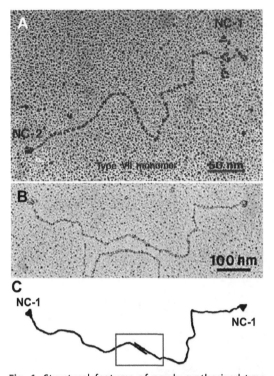

Fig. 1. Structural features of newly synthesized type VII collagen. (*A*) Rotary shadowing image of a type VII collagen molecule synthesized and secreted by human keratinocytes in culture. Note the central collagenous domain, flanked by noncollagenous NC-1 and NC-2 sequences. (*B*) Identification of NC-1 domains at both ends of a type VII collagen dimer molecule, as visualized by a monoclonal anti-type VII collagen antibody in rotary shadowing image. Note that the dimer has an overlapping region of the carboxy-terminal ends of the 2 molecules, as schematically illustrated in (*C*). (*Adapted from* Sakai LY, Keene DR, Morris NP, et al. Type VII collagen is a major structural component of anchoring fibrils. J Cell Biol 1986;103:1577–86, and Burgeson RE. Type VII collagen, anchoring fibrils, and epidermolysis bullosa. J Invest Dermatol 1993;101:252–5; with permission.)

interrupted by 19 imperfections because of insertions or deletions of amino acids in the Gly-X-Y repeat sequence. In the middle of the triple-helical domain, there is a 39-amino acid noncollagenous "hinge" region that is susceptible to proteolytic digestion with pepsin. The amino-terminal NC-1 domain of type VII collagen (NC-1[VII]), approximately 145 kDa in size, consists of submodules with homology to known adhesive proteins, including segments with homology to cartilage matrix protein, 9 consecutive fibronectin type III-like (FN-III) domains, a segment with homology to the A domain of von Willebrand factor, and a short cysteine and proline-rich region.[11] The

carboxy-terminal noncollagenous domain, NC-2, is fairly small, approximately 30 kDa, and it contains a segment with homology to the Kunitz protease inhibitor molecule (see **Fig. 2**A).[10,12]

Cloning of the human type VII collagen gene, *COL7A1*, revealed a complex structure consisting of a total of 118 separate exons (**Fig. 2**B).[9] However, the gene is fairly compact, and most of the intervening sequences (introns) are fairly small; consequently, the size of the human *COL7A1* gene is only approximately 32 kb, encoding a messenger RNA (mRNA) of approximately 8.9 kb. *COL7A1* has been mapped to the short arm of human chromosome 3, region 3p21.1.[13] At the time of the report of its structural organization, the type VII collagen gene was noted to be composed of more exons than any previously characterized gene.[9] Most of the *COL7A1* introns are small, including a 71-nucleotide intron that was the smallest intron yet reported in a collagen gene. The human type VII collagen gene structure and the encoded primary sequence of the protein are well conserved, and for example, the mouse gene shows 84.7% homology at the nucleotide and 90.4% identity at the protein level, attesting to the importance of type VII collagen as a structural protein.[14]

Type VII collagen gene expression displays a restricted, tissue-specific pattern. Specifically, type VII collagen has been localized by immunomapping to a select number of epithelia, including human skin, and the presence of type VII collagen correlated with the presence of ultrastructurally detected anchoring fibrils (**Table 2**).[5] The expression of the type VII collagen gene can be modulated by several cytokines, and in particular, transforming growth factor-β is a powerful upregulator of *COL7A1* in fibroblasts and keratinocytes, the regulation taking place primarily at the transcriptional level.[15,16]

TYPE VII COLLAGEN IS A MAJOR COMPONENT OF THE ANCHORING FIBRILS

Anchoring fibrils are specialized attachment complexes at the epithelium/mesenchyme interface in several tissues (see **Table 2**). In human skin, anchoring fibrils extend from the lower portion of the dermal-epidermal basement membrane to the underlying upper papillary dermis (**Fig. 3**). Initially, it was suggested that anchoring fibrils attach at one end to the lamina densa of the cutaneous basement membrane and at the other end to basement membrane-like structures, so-called anchoring plaques, that were thought to reside within the upper papillary dermis.[8] However, subsequent immunoelectron microscopic analyses indicated that

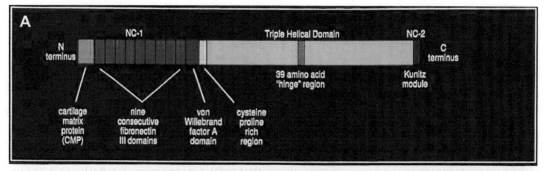

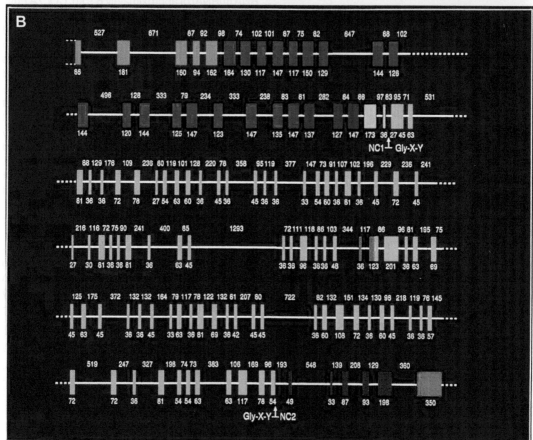

Fig. 2. Domain organization of type VII collagen polypeptides and the intron-exon organization of the corresponding gene, *COL7A1*. (*A*) The amino acid sequence of the pro-α1(VII) polypeptide, as deduced from cDNA sequences, indicates that type VII collagen consists of triple-helical central domain containing a 39-amino acid noncollagenous "hinge" region. The triple-helical domain is flanked by amino-terminal (NC-1) and carboxy-terminal (NC-2) noncollagenous domains. The NC-1 domain consists of submodules with homology to known adhesive proteins. The NC-2 domain contains a segment with homology to the Kunitz protease inhibitor molecule. (*B*) The intron-exon organization of *COL7A1* reveals that the gene consists of 118 distinct exons (*vertical colored blocks*) separated by fairly small introns (*horizontal white lines*). The sizes (in base pairs) of the exons and introns are indicated below and above the gene structure, respectively. The exons encoding distinct protein domains within the type VII collagen polypeptides, as shown in (*A*), are color-matched. (*Adapted from* Christiano AM, Uitto J. Impact of molecular genetic diagnosis on dystrophic epidermolysis bullosa. Curr Opin Dermatol 1996;3:225–32; with permission.[44])

Table 2
Correlation of the presence of type VII collagen as detected by immunofluorescence with anchoring fibrils detected ultrastructurally

	Immunofluorescence	Anchoring Fibrils
Skin	+	+
Chorioamnion	+	+
Placenta	−	−
Skeletal muscle	−	−
Cornea (Bowman membrane)	+	+
Oral mucosa	+	+
Cervix	+	+
Esophagus	+	+
Anal canal	+	+
Kidney cortex	−	−
Lung alvoli	−	−
Liver sinusoids	−	−
Stomach (fundus)	−	−
Large intestine	−	−
Elastic cartilage	−	−

Data from Sakai LY, Keene DR, Morris NP, et al. Type VII collagen is a major structural component of anchoring fibrils. J Cell Biol 1986;103:1577–86.

most, if not all, anchoring fibrils attach at both ends to the lamina densa, allowing entrapment of interstitial collagen fibers into the U-shaped structures (see **Fig. 3**).[17] In retrospect, the appearance of anchoring plaques in the upper papillary dermis may be an artifact resulting from preparation of skin samples for electron microscopy.

Type VII collagen is synthesized by epidermal keratinocytes and dermal fibroblasts in culture (**Fig. 4**).[18] Upon synthesis of complete pro-α1(VII) polypeptides, 3 polypeptides associate through their carboxy-terminal ends to a trimer molecule that in its collagenous portion folds into the triple-helical conformation (see **Fig. 3**). The triple-helical molecules are then secreted to the extra-cellular milieu where 2 type VII collagen molecules align into an antiparallel dimer with the amino-terminal domains present at both ends of the molecule (see Figs. 1B, C, and **3**).[5] This dimer assembly is accompanied by proteolytic removal of a portion of the carboxy-terminal end of both type VII collagen molecules and stabilization by intermolecular disulfide bond formation (see **Fig. 3**).[19] Subsequently, a large number of these antiparallel dimers aggregate laterally to form anchoring fibrils that can be recognized by trans-mission electron microscopy of the skin through their characteristic, centro-symmetric banding patterns.

Type VII collagen is a major component of the anchoring fibrils that provide stability to the dermal-epidermal adhesion on the dermal site at the lamina lucida/papillary dermis interface.[5] This stability has been attributed to the affinity of the NC-1(VII) domain to bind the principal components of the cutaneous basement membrane, laminin-332 (laminin-5), laminin-311 (laminin-6), and type IV collagen.[20,21] Kinetic assays of such associa-tions have demonstrated that the binding of the NC-1(VII) domain to laminin-332 and collagen IV are of high affinity, and the NC-1 domain uses the same region to bind both of these macromole-cules (**Fig. 5A, B**). In contrast, the NC-1(VII)-medi-ated binding to type I collagen is relatively weak (K_d value of approximately 10^{-6} M).[21] Thus, the high affinity binding of type VII collagen, particu-larly at the NC-1(VII) domains, seems to facilitate stabilization of the structure of the basement membrane zone (BMZ), and type VII collagen inter-actions with the interstitial collagen fibers in the dermis, consisting primarily of type I, III, and V collagens, may be due to physical entrapment of these fiber structures (see **Fig. 5**B; C).[21,22]

THE PATHOLOGIC CONSEQUENCES OF TYPE VII COLLAGEN GENE MUTATIONS

Considering the complexity of type VII collagen gene and protein structures and the critical

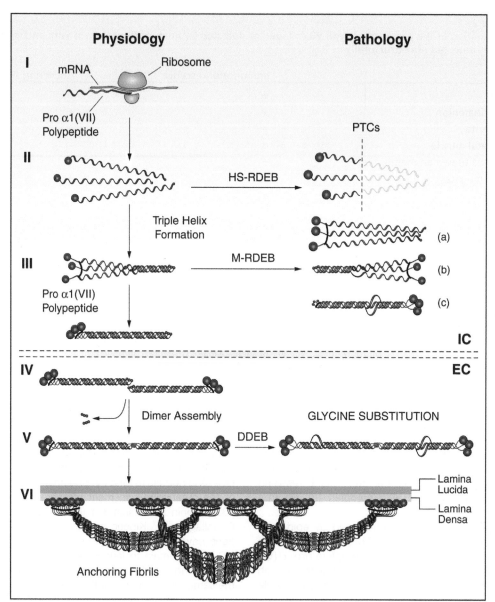

Fig. 3. Schematic presentation of the synthesis of pro-α1(VII) collagen polypeptides and their assembly into anchoring fibrils under physiologic conditions (*left side of the figure*) and perturbations in these processes leading to dystrophic epidermolysis bullosa (*right side*). Within the intracellular space (IC) of cells, such as keratinocytes and fibroblasts, pro-α1(VII) polypeptides are synthesized on ribosomes (*I*). Three polypeptides associate through their carboxy-terminal ends and their collagenous domains fold into a characteristic triple-helical conformation (*II*) and (*III*). After secretion into the extracellular space (EC), triple-helical type VII collagen molecules form antiparallel dimers (*IV*), and after proteolytic removal of a part of the carboxy-terminal end, the dimer assembly is stabilized by intermolecular disulfide bonds (*V*). Subsequently, a large number of dimer molecules laterally assemble in register to form cross- striated, centro-symmetric anchoring fibrils (*VI*). The amino-terminal noncollagenous globular domains (NC-1) attach to the extracellular macromolecules of the lamina densa, stabilizing the association of the lower part of the dermo-epidermal basement membrane to the underlying dermis. Mutations in the *COL7A1* gene can result in premature termination codons (PTCs), manifesting with the severe Hallopeau-Siemens (HS)-type recessive dystrophic epidermolysis bullosa (RDEB) when present in both alleles. Recessive missense mutations can interfere with chain assembly (*a*), triple helix formation (*b*), or stability of the triple-helix (*c*), resulting in mild (mitis, M) non-HS-RDEB. Glycine substitutions in the collagenous domain destabilize the triple helix and can result through dominant-negative interference in dominantly inherited DEB (DDEB). (*Adapted from* Varki R, Sadowski S, Uitto J, et al. Epidermolysis bullosa. II. Type VII collagen mutations and phenotype/genotype correlations in the dystrophic subtypes. J Med Genet 2007;44:181–92; with permission.)

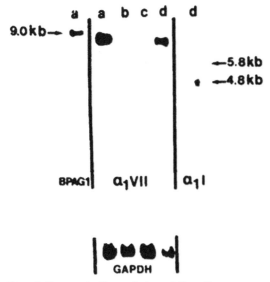

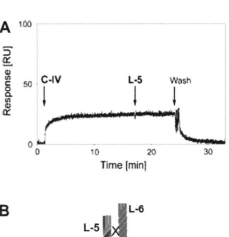

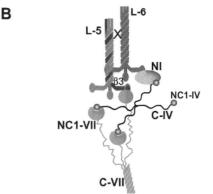

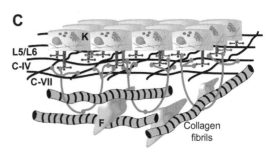

Fig. 4. Demonstration of type VII collagen gene expression in epidermal keratinocytes (*lane a*), Ras oncogene transformed human epidermal keratinocytes (RHK; *lane b*), human papilloma virus-transformed epidermal keratinocytes (HPK; *lane c*), and skin fibroblasts (*lane d*). Total mRNA was isolated from the cultured cells and subjected to Northern hybridization with a human type VII collagen cDNA probe (*middle panel*). Note the expression of human type VII collagen mRNA of approximately 8.9 kb in epidermal keratinocytes and dermal fibroblasts (a, d). For reference, hybridizations were performed with the 230-kDa bullous pemphigoid antigen (BPAG1) and type I collagen ($\alpha_1 I$) cDNAs. Rehybridization of the same filter with the *GAPDH* "housekeeping" gene served as an internal control for RNA loading. (*Adapted from* Ryynänen J, Sollberg S, Parente MG, et al. Type VII collagen gene expression by cultured human cells and in fetal skin. Abundant mRNA and protein levels in epidermal keratinocytes. J Clin Invest 1992;89:163–8; with permission.)

importance of its distinct domains in macromolecular interactions, one would have initially predicted that mutations in the *COL7A1* gene could have clinical consequences for integrity of the skin. The dystrophic forms of epidermolysis bullosa (DEB) emerged as candidate diseases for type VII collagen mutations when immunofluorescent staining of the skin of patients with the most severe recessive dystrophic EB (RDEB) demonstrated lack of type VII collagen epitopes.[23] Anchoring fibrils were shown by ultrastructural analysis to be morphologically altered, reduced in number, or completely absent in patients with different forms of DEB.[24,25] The cloning of human type VII collagen gene and cDNAs then provided the opportunity to assess the hypothesis that type VII collagen serves as the candidate gene/protein system for this group of blistering disorders.

Fig. 5. Demonstration of the binding of type VII collagen to type IV collagen and schematic representation of the dermal-epidermal junction with type VII collagen binding to basement membrane macromolecules. (*A*) Kinetic biosensor analysis demonstrates that recombinant NC-1 domain of human type VII collagen binds to type IV collagen (C-IV). After a wash, the NC-1/C-IV complex dissociates, indicating reversible nature of the binding. Addition of laminin-332 (laminin-5, L-5) did not result in additional binding, suggesting that the L-5 binding site corresponds to or is located close to that for binding of type IV collagen. (*B*) Binding of the NC-1-VII collagen domains to C-IV, L-5, and laminin-6 (L-6). (*C*) The anchoring fibrils entrap type VII collagen fibers, stabilizing the association of lamina densa of the dermo-epidermal basement membrane to underlying dermis. (*Adapted from* Brittingham R, Uitto J, Fertala A. High-affinity binding of the NC-1 domain of collagen VII to laminin 5 and collagen IV. Biochem Biophys Res Commun 2006;343:692–9; with permission.)

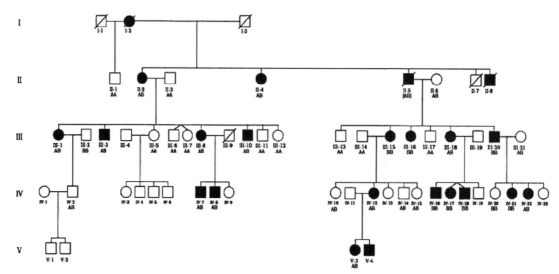

Fig. 6. Demonstration of genetic linkage between the dominant dystrophic epidermolysis bullosa phenotype and a type VII collagen allele in a family with 20 affected and 22 unaffected living individuals in 4 generations. The type VII collagen allele was tracked by inheritance of a *Pvu*II polymorphic marker. Note that the disease allele tracks with the B-allele of *COL7A1*. (*Adapted from* Ryynänen M, Knowlton RG, Parente MG, et al. Human type VII collagen: genetic linkage of the gene (COL7A1) on chromosome 3 to dominant dystrophic epidermolysis bullosa. Am J Hum Genet 1991;49:797–803; with permission.)

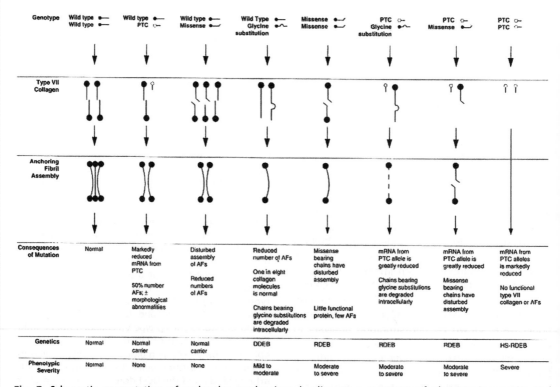

Fig. 7. Schematic presentation of molecular mechanisms leading to a spectrum of phenotypic severity and different types of inheritance in families with dystrophic forms of EB. (*Adapted from* Christiano AM, Uitto J. Molecular diagnosis of inherited skin diseases: the paradigm of dystrophic epidermolysis bullosa. Adv Dermatol 1996;11:199–214; with permission.[45])

Initial cloning of the *COL7A1* gene provided the tools to perform genetic linkage analyses in families with DEB and to explore the possibility that the inheritance of the disease in these families is linked to specific genetic markers, which allows tracking of the segregation of *COL7A1* alleles through the family pedigrees. One of the early markers was an intragenic *Pvu*II restriction fragment length polymorphism (RFLP), which was shown to reflect a single base-pair substitution within the type VII collagen gene in exon 21. This polymorphism occurs within the third nucleotide of a redundant proline codon, and, consequently, does not change the amino acid within the encoded polypeptide. The first genetic linkage analysis was performed with this marker in a large dominantly inherited DEB family (**Fig. 6**). In all cases within this family, there was complete cosegregation of the inheritance of one *COL7A1* allele and the DDEB phenotype.[26] The subsequent examination of 14 families with dominant DEB (DDEB) resulted in the combined logarithm of the odds favoring linkage (LOD) score of $\hat{Z} = 41.42$ at $\theta = 0$, establishing a robust linkage between the type VII collagen gene and the disease locus

causing skin fragility in DEB.[27] Similar genetic linkage studies were subsequently performed in families with RDEB, particularly with the most severe, Hallopeau-Siemens type.[28,29] Again, an unequivocal genetic linkage between *COL7A1* and the disease locus in RDEB was established. These early linkage studies were consistent with the notion that most, if not all, cases with DEB are the result of mutations in the *COL7A1* gene.

Subsequent development of streamlined mutation detection strategies[30,31] has allowed examination of a large number of cases with DEB with respect to type VII collagen mutations. In fact, more than 300 distinct mutations in the *COL7A1* gene have now been disclosed.[32,33] The types of mutations range from premature termination codon (PTC)-causing mutations as a result of nonsense mutations and small insertions or deletions or splice junction mutations resulting in frame shift of translation, to more subtle missense mutations. In fact, genotype/phenotype correlations in general terms have been established.[34] In recessively inherited forms of DEB, presence of PTC-causing mutations in both alleles results in complete absence of type VII collagen,

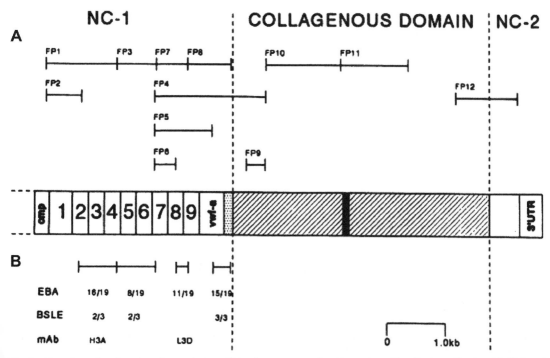

Fig. 8. Mapping of antigenic epitopes in type VII collagen recognized by autoantibodies in patients with EBA and bullous systemic lupus erythematosus (BSLE). (*A*) the positions of fusion proteins that correspond to the type VII collagen sequences are indicated by brackets. (*B*) The number of sera positive among the 19 EBA and 3 BSLE patients is indicated by the regions tested using recombinant fusion-proteins. Also, note the areas recognized by 2 monoclonal antibodies, H3A and L3D. (*Adapted from* Lapière JC, Woodley DT, Parente MG, et al. Epitope mapping of type VII collagen: identification of discrete peptide sequences recognized by sera from patients with acquired epidermolysis bullosa. J Clin Invest 1993;92:1831–9; with permission.)

manifesting with severe mutilating scarring and blistering (**Fig. 7**). Combinations of a PTC-causing mutation with a more subtle missense mutation can result in a milder autosomal recessive form of DEB. Most of the dominantly inherited cases of DEB result from glycine substitution mutations in the collagenous domain replacing one of the glycines in the Gly-X-Y repeat triplet sequence (see **Fig. 7**). Collectively, the precise degree of severity of DEB reflects the combinations of mutations in *COL7A1* and their consequences at the mRNA and protein levels combined with the effects of modifier genes on the individuals' genetic background and the exposure to environmental trauma.[34] For details on phenotypic presentations and genetic basis of different forms of DEB, see article by Leena Bruckner-Tuderman elsewhere in this issue.

involves pathology in type VII collagen. Specifically, circulating autoantibodies in patients with EBA recognize epitopes in type VII collagen molecules, and molecular cloning of the type VII collagen cDNAs again provided the tools to identify the most predominant immunoepitopes within the amino-terminal NC-1 domain of type VII collagen (**Fig. 8**).[35,36] The antigenic properties of the NC-1(VII) domain are further highlighted by monoclonal antibodies, such as H3A and L3D, which are in clinical use to map type VII collagen in the skin of patients with inherited forms of EB, also identifying epitopes in this portion of the protein (see **Fig. 8**).[36] In addition to circulating autoantibodies recognizing type VII collagen epitopes in EBA, bullous lesions in some patients with systemic lupus erythematosus have also been associated with anti-type VII collagen antibodies.[36,37]

CIRCULATING AUTOANTIBODIES TO TYPE VII COLLAGEN IN PATIENTS WITH EB ACQUISITA

In addition to inherited forms of EB, the acquired form of EB, epidermolysis bullosa acquisita (EBA),

THE ROLE OF TYPE VII COLLAGEN IN EPIDERMAL SQUAMOUS CELL CARCINOMA

The suggestion that type VII collagen is required for human epidermal tumorigenesis relates to the

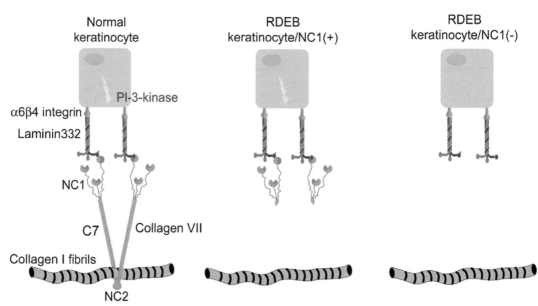

Fig. 9. Schematic representation of "anchorless" activation of α6β4 integrin-mediated signal transduction by NC-1(VII) in RDEB keratinocytes. In normal skin, type VII collagen is firmly anchored to the BMZ through interactions with other components of the extracellular matrix. Thus, activation of α6β4 integrin signaling is restricted to the appropriate tissue compartment within the epidermis (*left panel*). In contrast, expression of N-terminally truncated type VII collagen lacking the collagenous and the carboxy-terminal domains but depicting the presence of NC-1 may enable α6β4 integrin-dependent signal transduction in RDEB keratinocytes that are not firmly anchored in the BMZ, potentially supporting inappropriate cell survival during invasion and metastasis (*middle panel*). In the case of complete absence of NC-1 expression, activation of α6β4 integrin-dependent signal transduction will not occur (*right panel*). (*Adapted from* Rodeck U, Fertala A, Uitto J. Anchorless keratinocyte survival. An emerging pathogenic mechanism for squamous cell carcinoma in recessive dystrophic epidermolysis bullosa. Exp Dermatol 2007;16:465–7; with permission.)

observation that with extended life span of the affected individuals with RDEB, an increasing number of life-threatening complications related to development of squamous cell carcinomas (SCCs) has emerged.[38] The RDEB-associated SCCs usually manifest early in life, and they are distinguished by a particularly aggressive clinical course. These tumors have a high rate of metastatic spread, often leading to the early demise of the affected individual. The association of type VII collagen expression and development of SCCs in RDEB was derived from observations on tumorigenic conversion of keratinocytes cultured from these patients and xenotransplanted to immunodeficient mice.[39] Those keratinocytes expressing NC-1(VII) domain developed cancer, whereas those keratinocytes that did not express the same domain did not develop SCCs. A molecular mechanism potentially involving "anchorless" NC-1 activation of $\alpha6\beta4$ integrin-mediated signal transduction as a result of terminally truncated NC-1/laminin-332 interactions has also been proposed (**Fig. 9**).[40]

The notion that NC-1(VII) expression is required for SCC development in RDEB has been challenged by isolation of keratinocytes from RDEB patients with SCC, yet with complete absence of type VII collagen.[41] NC-1–dependent tumor formation has been described only in keratinocytes that were immortalized by co-expression of Ha-RasV12 and mutant IκBα to inhibit cellular nuclear factor (NF)-κB activity.[39] Nevertheless, the importance of the suggestion for the role of type VII collagen in SCC development in patients with RDEB is emphasized by the lack of information of the pathomechanistic features of SCC, precluding rational development of targeted therapies for this complication of DEB. Meanwhile, significant progress has been made toward development of molecular therapies to ameliorate and, eventually, to provide a cure for this, currently intractable, disease with significant morbidity and mortality.[42,43]

ACKNOWLEDGMENTS

GianPaolo Guercio assisted in preparation of this article. The authors' original research summarized in this article was supported by DHHS, NIH/NIAMS grants P01 AR38923 and R01 AR54876 and by the Dermatology Foundation.

REFERENCES

1. Uitto J, Chu ML, Gallo R, et al. Collagen, elastic fibers, and the extracellular matrix of the dermis. In: Wolff K, Goldsmith LA, Katz SI, et al, editors. Fitzpatrick's dermatology in general medicine. 7th edition. New York: McGraw-Hill; 2008. p. 517–42.

2. Myllyharju J, Kivirikko KI. Collagens, modifying enzymes and their mutations in humans, flies and worms. Trends Genet 2004;20:33–43.

3. Söderhäll C, Marenholz I, Kerscher T, et al. Variants in a novel epidermal collagen gene (COL29A1) are associated with atopic dermatitis. PLoS Biol 2007;5:e242.

4. Olsen BR. New insights into the function of collagens from genetic analysis. Curr Opin Cell Biol 1995;7:720–7.

5. Sakai LY, Keene DR, Morris NP, et al. Type VII collagen is a major structural component of anchoring fibrils. J Cell Biol 1986;103:1577–86.

6. Franzke CW, Tasanen K, Schäcke H, et al. Transmembrane collagen XVII, an epithelial adhesion protein, is shed from the cell surface by ADAMs. EMBO J 2002;21:5026–35.

7. de Pereda JM, Lillo MP, Sonnenberg A. Structural basis of the interaction between integrin alpha6-beta4 and plectin at the hemidesmosomes. EMBO J 2009;28:1180–90.

8. Burgeson RE. Type VII collagen, anchoring fibrils, and epidermolysis bullosa. J Invest Dermatol 1993; 101:252–5.

9. Christiano AM, Hoffman GG, Chung-Honet LC, et al. Structural organization of the human type VII collagen gene (COL7A1), comprised of more exons than any previously characterized gene. Genomics 1994;21:169–79.

10. Christiano AM, Greenspan DS, Lee S, et al. Cloning of human type VII collagen. Complete primary sequence of the α1(VII) chain and identification of intragenic polymorphisms. J Biol Chem 1994;269: 20256–62.

11. Christiano AM, Rosenbaum LM, Chung-Honet LC, et al. The large non-collagenous domain (NC-1) of type VII collagen is amino-terminal and chimeric. Homology to cartilage matrix protein, the type III domains of fibronectin and the A domains of von Willebrand factor. Hum Mol Genet 1992;1:475–81.

12. Greenspan DS. The carboxyl-terminal half of type VII collagen, including the non-collagenous NC-2 domain and intron/exon organization of the corresponding region of the COL7A1 gene. Hum Mol Genet 1993;2:273–8.

13. Parente MG, Chung LC, Ryynänen J, et al. Human type VII collagen: cDNA cloning and chromosomal mapping of the gene. Proc Natl Acad Sci U S A 1991;88:6931–5.

14. Kivirikko S, Li K, Christiano AM, et al. Cloning of mouse type VII collagen reveals evolutionary conservation of functional protein domains and genomic organization. J Invest Dermatol 1996;106: 1300–6.

15. Ryynänen J, Sollberg S, Olsen DR, et al. Transforming growth factor-beta up-regulates type VII

collagen gene expression in normal and transformed epidermal keratinocytes in culture. Biochem Biophys Res Commun 1991;180:673–80.

16. Vindevoghel L, Kon A, Lechleider RJ, et al. Smad-dependent transcriptional activation of human type VII collagen gene (COL7A1) promoter by transforming growth factor-β. J Biol Chem 1998;273: 13053–7.

17. Shimizu H, Ishiko A, Masunaga T, et al. Most anchoring fibrils in human skin originate and terminate in the lamina densa. Lab Invest 1997;76: 753–63.

18. Ryynänen J, Sollberg S, Parente MG, et al. Type VII collagen gene expression by cultured human cells and in fetal skin. Abundant mRNA and protein levels in epidermal keratinocytes. J Clin Invest 1992;89: 163–8.

19. Colombo M, Brittingham RJ, Klement JF, et al. Procollagen VII self-assembly depends on site-dpecific interactions and is promoted by cleavage of the NC-2 domain with procollagen C-proteinase. Biochemistry 2003;42:11434–42.

20. Chen M, Marinkovich MP, Veis A, et al. Interactions of the amino-terminal noncollagenous (NC-1) domain of type VII collagen with extracellular matrix components. A potential role in epidermal-dermal adherence in human skin. J Biol Chem 1997;272: 14516–22.

21. Brittingham R, Uitto J, Fertala A. High-affinity binding of the NC-1 domain of collagen VII to laminin 5 and collagen IV. Biochem Biophys Res Commun 2006;343:692–9.

22. Villone D, Fritsch A, Koch M, et al. Supramolecular interactions in the dermo-epidermal junction zone: anchoring fibril-collagen VII tightly binds to banded collagen fibrils. J Biol Chem 2008;283:24506–13.

23. Bruckner-Tuderman L, Mitsuhashi Y, Schnyder UW, et al. Anchoring fibrils and type VII collagen are absent from skin in severe recessive dystrophic epidermolysis bullosa. J Invest Dermatol 1989;93:3–9.

24. Tidman MJ, Eady RA. Evaluation of anchoring fibrils and other components of the dermal-epidermal junction in dystrophic epidermolysis bullosa by a quantitative ultrastructural technique. J Invest Dermatol 1985;84:374–7.

25. McGrath JA, Ishida-Yamamoto A, O'Grady A, et al. Structural variations in anchoring fibrils in dystrophic epidermolysis bullosa: correlation with type VII collagen expression. J Invest Dermatol 1993;100: 366–72.

26. Ryynänen M, Knowlton RG, Parente MG, et al. Human type VII collagen: genetic linkage of the gene (COL7A1) on chromosome 3 to dominant dystrophic epidermolysis bullosa. Am J Hum Genet 1991;49:797–803.

27. Uitto J, Christiano AM. Molecular basis for the dystrophic forms of epidermolysis bullosa: mutations in the type VII collagen gene. Arch Dermatol Res 1994;287: 16–22.

28. Hovnanian A, Duquesnoy P, Blanchet-Bardon C, et al. Genetic linkage of recessive dystrophic epidermolysis bullosa to the type VII collagen gene. J Clin Invest 1992;90:1032–6.

29. Dunnill MG, Richards AJ, Milana G, et al. Genetic linkage to the type VII collagen gene (COL7A1) in 26 families with generalised recessive dystrophic epidermolysis bullosa and anchoring fibril abnormalities. J Med Genet 1994;31:745–8.

30. Pulkkinen L, Uitto J. Mutation analysis and molecular genetics of epidermolysis bullosa. Matrix Biol 1999; 18:29–42.

31. Christiano AM, Hoffman GG, Zhang X, et al. Strategy for identification of sequence variants in COL7A1 and a novel 2-bp deletion mutation in recessive dystrophic epidermolysis bullosa. Hum Mutat 1997; 10:408–14.

32. Varki R, Sadowski S, Uitto J, et al. Epidermolysis bullosa. II. Type VII collagen mutations and phenotype/genotype correlations in the dystrophic subtypes. J Med Genet 2007;44:181–92.

33. Dang N, Murrell DF. Mutation analysis and characterization of COL7A1 mutations in dystrophic epidermolysis bullosa. Exp Dermatol 2008;17: 553–68.

34. Uitto J, Richard G. Progress in epidermolysis bullosa: from eponyms to molecular genetic classification. Clin Dermatol 2005;23:33–40.

35. Woodley DT, Briggaman RA, O'Keefe EJ, et al. Identification of the skin basement-membrane autoantigen in epidermolysis bullosa acquisita. N Engl J Med 1984;310:1007–13.

36. Lapière JC, Woodley DT, Parente MG, et al. Epitope mapping of type VII collagen: identification of discrete peptide sequences recognized by sera from patients with acquired epidermolysis bullosa. J Clin Invest 1993;92:1831–9.

37. Chan LS, Lapiere JC, Chen M, et al. Bullous systemic lupus erythematosus with autoantibodies recognizing multiple skin basement membrane components, bullous pemphigoid antigen 1, laminin-5, laminin-6, and type VII collagen. Arch Dermatol 1999;135:569–73.

38. Fine JD, Eady RA, Bauer EA, et al. The classification of inherited epidermolysis bullosa (EB): report of the Third International Consensus Meeting on Diagnosis and Classification of EB. J Am Acad Dermatol 2008; 58:931–50.

39. Ortiz-Urda S, Garcia J, Green CL, et al. Type VII collagen is required for Ras-driven human epidermal tumorigenesis. Science 2005;307: 1773–6.

40. Rodeck U, Fertala A, Uitto J. Anchorless keratinocyte survival. An emerging pathogenic mechanism for squamous cell carcinoma in recessive dystrophic

epidermolysis bullosa. Exp Dermatol 2007;16: 465–7.

41. Pourreyron C, Cox G, Mao X, et al. Patients with recessive dystrophic epidermolysis bullosa develop squamous-cell carcinoma regardless of type VII collagen expression. J Invest Dermatol 2007;127:2438–44.

42. Uitto J. Progress in heritable skin diseases: translational implications of mutation analysis and prospects of molecular therapies. Acta Derm Venereol 2009;89:228–35.

43. Tamai K, Yasufumi K, Uitto J. Molecular therapies for heritable blistering diseases. Trends Mol Med 2009; 15:285–92.

44. Christiano AM, Uitto J. Impact of molecular genetic diagnosis on dystrophic epidermolysis bullosa. Curr Opin Dermatol 1996;3:225–32.

45. Christiano AM, Uitto J. Molecular diagnosis of inherited skin diseases: the paradigm of dystrophic epidermolysis bullosa. Adv Dermatol 1996;11: 199–214.

Dystrophic Epidermolysis Bullosa: Pathogenesis and Clinical Features

Leena Bruckner-Tuderman, MD

KEYWORDS

- Blistering • Scarring • Dermal–epidermal junction
- Anchoring fibrils

Dystrophic epidermolysis bullosa (DEB) is an epidermolysis bullosa (EB) subtype with rather well understood pathogenesis. Its molecular basis— abnormalities of collagen VII—has been known for almost two decades,[1,2] and, so far, several hundred different mutations in the gene for collagen VII, COL7A1, have been disclosed in both recessive and dominant forms of DEB (human gene mutation database: www.hgmd.cf.ac.uk/ac/index.php). Several studies have addressed genotype–phenotype correlations and found the spectrum of biologic and clinical phenotypes to be much broader than initially anticipated.[3–5] Nevertheless, the cellular and molecular disease mechanisms are reasonably well known and reveal realistic perspectives for the development of biologically valid therapies for DEB in the future.[5,6]

The clinical hallmarks of DEB are trauma-induced blisters and healing with scarring. Dermal–epidermal separation occurs beneath the basement membrane in the uppermost papillary dermis. DEB occurs in all races worldwide and is equally common in boys and girls; its prevalence, however, is not known precisely. Data from the German EB-Network (www.netzwerk-eb.de) and the US national EB registry[7] indicate that about 40% of all patients in these databases have DEB. There is some variation in the frequency of the recessive and dominant DEB forms among different populations, however, reflecting each population's genetic pool.

MOLECULAR PATHOGENESIS OF DEB

Blistering in DEB results from structural and functional alterations of the anchoring fibrils (AF), polymers of collagen VII, which anchor the epidermal basement membrane with the dermis. Normal AF are visible in the electron microscope as centrosymmetrically cross-banded fibrils with frayed ends, which emanate from the lamina densa of the basement membrane into the dermal connective tissue.[8] Collagen VII polymerizes in a highly organized manner into the fibrils,[9] which are stabilized by tissue transglutaminase[10] and bind covalently to dermal collagen fibrils,[11] thus securing dermal–epidermal adherence. In DEB skin, collagen VII often is reduced or absent, and electron microscopy reveals paucity, rudimentary structure, or complete lack of the AF.

All DEB forms are caused by mutations in the collagen VII gene, COL7A1.[3] The spectrum of mutations is broad, and many families have their private mutations. In recessive DEB compound heterozygosity is common (ie, the patient has two different mutations, one inherited from the father and one from the mother). Different combinations of mutations generate a continuum of biologic phenotypes, which explains the varying clinical severity and overlap between different DEB forms.

In most patients with most severe recessive DEB, both COL7A1 mutations cause premature termination codons (PTC), which lead to nonsense

The author's work on dystrophic epidermolysis bullosa was supported by the EB-Network grant from the Federal Ministry for Education and Research 2003–2011 and by a grant from Debra International.
Department of Dermatology, University Medical Center Freiburg, Hauptstraße 7, 79104 Freiburg, Germany
E-mail address: bruckner-tuderman@uniklinik-freiburg.de

Dermatol Clin 28 (2010) 107–114
doi:10.1016/j.det.2009.10.020

derm.theclinics.com

mediated mRNA decay, or residual expression of truncated collagen VII polypeptides that are degraded within the cell. As a result, the AF are usually missing in the skin. The genetic background of other recessive DEB forms is heterogeneous, including missense or splice site mutations in COL7A1 in at least one allele. Frequently, the second mutation causes a PTC. These mutation combinations lead to synthesis of defective collagen VII and to structurally abnormal AF. In dominant DEB, heterozygous glycine substitution mutations interfere in a dominant–negative manner with collagen VII synthesis and impair its secretion or the fibrillogenesis of the AF.

Two different mouse models with complete or partial deficiency of collagen VII recapitulate the clinical and morphologic characteristics of recessive DEB in people and have been useful for understanding the molecular pathology of the disease. The collagen VII-knockout mouse[12] exhibits severe blistering that is lethal within about a week after birth. The collagen - hypomorphic mouse,[13] which has about 10% of normal collagen VII levels, lives into adulthood and develops a severe recessive DEB with scarring, nail dystrophy, and mutilating deformities of the paws. Molecular analysis of the extremities of this mouse has revealed that transforming growth factor-beta mediated fibroblast-to-myofibroblast transformation leads to contractile fibrosis, which underlies the mutilating deformities.[13] Both mouse models are also valuable for testing of molecular therapy strategies for DEB.

MAIN CLINICAL SUBTYPES OF DEB

Because all DEB subtypes are allelic variants (ie, caused by mutations in the COL7A1 gene), the most recent revised classification of EB[14] has simplified the division into subtypes and eliminated most eponyms. It is reasonable to define three major categories for easier clinical assessment, although the subtypes often overlap

(Table 1). The main clinical features of these are summarized.

Severe Generalized Recessive DEB

This is the most severe DEB form, and it was previously known as the Hallopeau-Siemens subtype. Blistering usually starts at birth. The skin is extremely fragile, forming large blisters both spontaneously and secondary to mechanical forces, typically on trauma-exposed sites or over bony prominences. The blisters heal with scarring and sometimes with hypo- or hyperpigmentation. Milia are very common (Fig. 1). The most devastating problem is the excessive scarring of the hands and feet, leading to mitten deformities. Initially, there are adhesions between the digits (webbing), and insidiously over time the individual digits fuse into a scarred mass (Fig. 2). Contractures of other joints also tend to develop. The nails may be absent or dystrophic. The hair is typically sparse with scarring alopecia. The oral, genital, anal and ocular mucous membranes can be affected with erosions and scarring. Perianal disease often leads to painful stools and, as a result, constipation. Dental abnormalities are common, including dystrophic teeth and severe caries. Opening of the mouth may become restricted and the tongue less mobile because of scarring. Additionally, esophageal strictures are common, further contributing to nutritional problems. Therefore, many affected individuals have reduced food intake, protein loss, bleeding, anemia, and impaired growth. The risk of squamous cell carcinoma is increased markedly . In the course of the disease, the patients become severely disabled and have a shortened life expectancy because of multiple secondary complications and increased risk of skin cancer.

Recessive DEB–other

These clinical forms, collectively called recessive DEB–other in the revised classification, are similar

---

Table 1
Characteristic features of the most common DEB subtypes

DEB Subtype	Clinical Severity	COL7A1 Mutations	Collagen VII Protein in the Skin
Recessive severe generalized	Very severe, mitten deformities	Mostly PTCs	Strongly reduced or negative
Recessive–other	Mild–moderate	Missense, nonsense, splice site mutations, deletions, insertions	Positive or reduced
Dominant	Mild–moderate	Glycine substitution mutations common	Positive or reduced

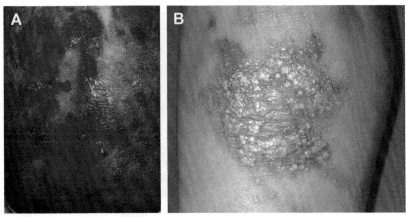

Fig. 1. Skin lesions in DEB. (A) Erosions and scarring on the back of an 11-year-old patient with DEB. (B) Milia.

to the severe generalized DEB, but the blistering is less severe. Mutilating deformities also do not develop (Fig. 3). Blisters are usually present at birth and continue to develop throughout the life. The clinical picture is highly variable. Some patients have widespread disease, while others have blisters limited primarily to the extremities. Blisters heal invariably with scars and milia (see Fig. 1). Oral, dental, nail, and hair problems are similar to severe generalized DEB, but less extensive. The localized forms tend to improve over time and overlap with dominant DEB. The risk of squamous cell carcinoma is elevated also in this form, and regular follow-up is needed.

Dominant DEB

Patients with dominant DEB generally have milder clinical phenotypes, which range from mainly acral involvement to disseminated blistering and scarring. Mucosal involvement, however, is rare, and the teeth are normal. Blistering usually starts at birth or soon thereafter, but the disease activity diminishes with advancing age. There is

a predilection for the extremities, but mechanical stress can induce blisters anywhere on the body. Scars, milia, and dystrophy or loss of nails are common (Fig. 4).

RARE SUBTYPES OF DEB

Several rather rare, localized subtypes of DEB have been described in the literature,[14–19] including inverse, pretibial, pruriginous, or nails only forms (Table 2, Fig. 5). Because all DEB forms are allelic and result from COL7A1 mutations, the prediction is that genetic or environmental modifiers contribute particularly strongly to these subtypes. Despite repeated trials, no distinct pathogenetic markers or modifying factors have been identified that would distinguish these forms from localized recessive or dominant DEB.[20,21] The subtype first described as transient bullous dermolysis of the newborn[22] has turned out not to be transient, but rather a form of recessive or dominant DEB.[17] Therefore, in this author's

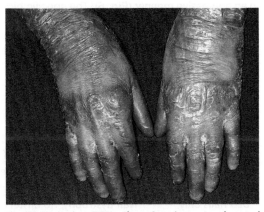

Fig. 2. Severe generalized recessive DEB. Mitten deformity of the left hand of a 12-year-old girl.

Fig. 3. Recessive DEB–other. Scarring, atrophy, and partial synechia in both hands of a 14 year-old boy.

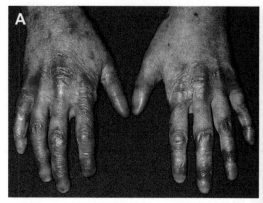
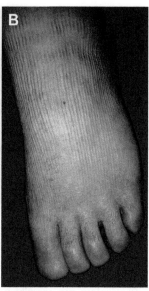

Fig. 4. Dominant DEB. (*A*) Moderate scarring and loss of all fingernails in a 25-year-old man. (*B*) Loss of toenails is associated with mild scarring.

opinion, the term is obsolete and should not be used any more.

DEB-ASSOCIATED SKIN CANCER

Individuals with DEB have a highly increased risk of squamous cell carcinoma (SCC) from early adulthood on, and aggressive SCC is the cause of death in a high percentage of patients with severe DEB. The tumors develop much earlier than in normal population, and the cumulative risk of developing SCC in severe DEB is more than 80% by age 45 and more than 90% by age 55.[23] The DEB-associated SCCs (DEB-SCC) typically develop on the limbs and over bony prominences, the areas that are most trauma-exposed. Despite their rather well differentiated morphology, DEB-SCCs behave in an aggressive manner (**Fig. 6**). The specific biologic and molecular mechanisms underlying DEB-SCC remain elusive. Tissue injury is known to play a substantial role in the pathogenesis of malignant lesions, with chronic inflammation and the contractile fibrosis in DEB being perhaps the most important factors perturbing epithelial–mesenchymal interactions, which are required for normal tissue homeostasis. Current treatments of DEB-SCC include surgery and, in some instances, radiotherapy or chemopreventive measures. Recently, successful application of epidermal growth factor receptor (EGFR) antagonists in treating EGFR-expressing DEB-SCC was reported.[24] Because the tumors are aggressive and therapeutic options limited, once- or twice-yearly skin cancer screening with clinical examination of the entire integument, biopsy of suspicious lesions, and patient education are pivotal preventive measures.

MOLECULAR DIAGNOSTICS OF DEB

For precise diagnosis and determination of the disease subtype, molecular diagnostics are recommended for all individuals with EB. The anxiety

Table 2
Rare phenotypes of DEB with special features

DEB Subtype	Clinical Hallmark	Inheritance	References
DEB inversa	Prominent involvement of inverse skin areas	AR	19
Pretibial DEB	Mainly pretibial involvement	AR, AD	14,15
DEB pruriginosa	Strongly pruritic blisters and nodules	AR, AD	16,20,21
DEB nails only	Nail dystrophy, no blisters	AD	17,18

Abbreviations: AR, autosomal recessive; AD, autosomal dominant.

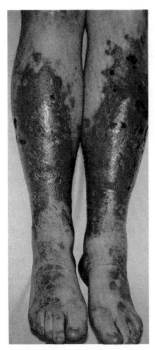

Fig. 5. Dominant DEB. Predominantly pretibial blistering and scarring in a 55-year-old man.

of patients and their families is reduced by precise diagnosis, because it allows prognostication, genetic counseling, prenatal diagnosis, and—in the future—design of individual molecular therapies. The basic diagnostic procedure is the same for all EB subtypes; a perilesional native skin biopsy is required for immunofluorescence mapping and determination of the candidate gene,[13,14] and a sample of EDTA blood is needed for mutation screening.

Immunofluorescence mapping of a skin biopsy using a panel of antibodies against molecular components of the dermal–epidermal junction zone is rapid and easy to perform,[4–6] although the interpretation of the results requires good knowledge of the molecular architecture of the skin. Most of the antibodies are commercially available. The immunofluorescence mapping indicates the level of skin split and alterations in the expression and distribution of the different proteins. As a general rule, the degree of the molecular defect correlates with the clinical severity (ie, complete absence of a protein is associated with a severe subtype). In DEB skin, the mapping reveals blister formation below the lamina densa, and, depending on the subtype, presence or absence of collagen VII. In severe recessive DEB, collagen VII is strongly reduced or absent (**Fig. 7**); in less severe recessive DEB–other and in dominant DEB subtypes, the collagen VII signal usually is reduced to variable degree.

Mutation analysis of the *COL7A1* gene is performed using PCR amplification of all 118 exons, subsequent direct automated DNA sequencing, and implementation of software tools. The efficiency of the screening can be increased with a priority strategy[25] that uses mutation detection based on prioritization of commonly occurring mutations. For example, in a cohort of 32 patients with dominant DEB investigated in the author's laboratory, 75% of the mutations were found in exons 73 to 75, a fact that clearly facilitates the screening.[6,25] Mutation analysis remains expensive, laborious, and time consuming, however, because of the complexity of the *COL7A1* gene and the large number of different mutations.

GENOTYPE–PHENOTYPE CORRELATIONS AND PROGNOSTICATION

The above knowledge is useful for prognostication of newly diagnosed DEB. In case of null mutations and complete absence of collagen VII, the phenotype is likely to become very severe, and mitten deformities are likely to develop. Missense mutations combined with positive, albeit attenuated collagen VII signals in immunofluorescence staining predict a milder

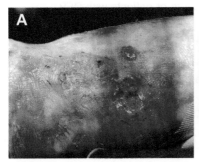
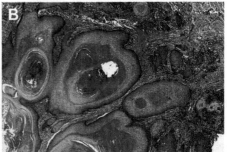

Fig. 6. DEB-associated squamous cell carcinoma. (*A*) Clinically, the tumor can appear as a nonhealing wound. (*B*) The histopathology of the tumor can appear well-differentiated, but the tumors behave in an aggressive manner.

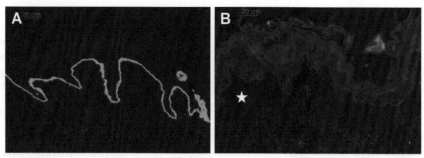

Fig. 7. Immunofluorescence mapping of a skin biopsy with antibodies to collagen VII. (*A*) Linear staining at the dermal–epidermal junction in normal control skin. (*B*) blister formation (star) and a negative collagen VII staining in the skin of a patient with severe generalized DEB.

phenotype. Different genetic and environmental phenotype modifying factors, however, exist. Yet neither their nature nor their effects are well understood yet; therefore, accurate prognostication of mild–moderate DEB phenotypes remains difficult.

THERAPEUTIC MANAGEMENT

The current therapy for DEB encompasses modern wound care and minimization of external factors, which induce blistering and complicate wound healing. Appropriate skin care includes a high standard of personal hygiene and intensive moisturizing care. Blisters without secondary trauma or infection usually heal well with everyday skin care and disinfection. Modern aqueous disinfectants are highly effective and pleasant to use. Adhesives and compressive dressings must be avoided, because they induce new blisters. Silicon-based, slightly adherent wound care products have proven very useful, in particular for difficult skin areas, such as elbows, shoulders, or the trunk. Usually, systemic therapy is not required for DEB. Sometimes, systemic antibiotics or corticosteroids can be indicated for short periods of time. Care of severely affected patients with extracutaneous involvement requires multidisciplinary management of secondary symptoms in different organs and collaboration of pediatricians, dermatologists, gastroenterologists, hand surgeons, dentists, nutritionists, physical therapists, psychologists, and other specialists.

PERSPECTIVES FOR MOLECULAR THERAPIES

Because the current treatment of EB is only symptomatic, development of curative molecular therapies is needed urgently. Although the clinical application of such treatments still may be years away, new technologies hold promise for individually designed, evidence-based treatments.[26] For recessive DEB, several such therapies, ranging from protein[27] therapy to nonviral gene transfer,[28] have been considered. Gene augmentation in an ex vivo approach comprises genetic correction of patient keratinocytes in vitro, and their cultivation into epithelial sheets for grafting onto the patient's skin. Treatment of canine DEB epidermal sheets of keratinocytes transduced with a retroviral vector containing the entire collagen VII cDNA delivered promising results (eg, enhanced expression and deposition of collagen VII at the dermal–epidermal junction).[29] Recent murine studies have shown that intradermal injections of recombinant human collagen VII[27] or allogenic fibroblasts[13,30] lead to type VII collagen deposition at the dermal–epidermal junction. A human pilot study with a few individuals with recessive DEB treated with a single intradermal injection of allogeneic fibroblasts indicated an increase of collagen VII expression in the skin.[31] The most recent therapeutic approach using transplantation of bone marrow-derived stem cells showed homing of a small number of stem cells into the skin and some improvement of DEB symptoms.[32] All of these approaches are currently at the stage of preclinical testing, however, and future research must show which of these promising experimental approaches will become suitable for effective and practical treatments of patients with DEB.

ACKNOWLEDGMENTS

The help by Dimitra Kiritsi, MD, with the figures is gratefully acknowledged.

REFERENCES

1. Bruckner-Tuderman L, Rüegger S, Odermatt B, et al. Lack of type VII collagen in unaffected skin of patients with severe recessive dystrophic epidermolysis bullosa. Dermatologica 1988;176:57–64.

2. Christiano AM, Greenspan DS, Hoffman GG, et al. A missense mutation in type VII collagen in two affected siblings with recessive dystrophic epidermolysis bullosa. Nat Genet 1993;4:62–6.

3. Dang N, Murrell DF. Mutation analysis and characterization of COL7A1 mutations in dystrophic epidermolysis bullosa. Exp Dermatol 2008;17:553–68.

4. Has C, Bruckner-Tuderman L. Molecular and clinical aspects of genetic skin fragility. J Dermatol Sci 2006;44:129–44.

5. Kern JS, Has C. Update on diagnosis and therapy of inherited epidermolysis bullosa. Expert Rev Dermatol 2008;3:721–33.

6. Aumailley M, Has C, Tunggal L, et al. Molecular basis of inherited skin blistering disorders and therapeutic implications. Expert Rev Mol Med 2006;8: 1–21.

7. Fine J-D, Bauer EA, McGuire J, et al. Epidermolysis bullosa. Clinical, epidemiologic, and laboratory advances, and the findings of the national epidermolysis bullosa registry. Baltimore (MD): The Johns Hopkins University Press; 1999.

8. Bruckner-Tuderman L, Stanley JR. Epidermal and epidermal/dermal cohesion. In: Wolff K, Goldsmith L, Katz SI, et al, editors. Fitzpatrick's dermatology in general medicine. 7th edition. New York: McGraw-Hill Medical; 2008. p. 736–52.

9. Bruckner-Tuderman L, Höpfner B, Hammami-Hauasli N. Biology of anchoring fibrils: lessons from dystrophic epidermolysis bullosa. Matrix Biol 1999;18:43–54.

10. Raghunath M, Höpfner B, Aeschlimann D, et al. Cross-linking of the dermo-epidermal junction of skin regenerating from keratinocyte autografts. Anchoring fibrils are a target for tissue transglutaminase. J Clin Invest 1996;98:1174–84.

11. Villone D, Fritsch A, Koch M, et al. Supramolecular interactions in the dermo-epidermal junction zone: anchoring fibril–collagen VII tightly binds to banded collagen fibrils. J Biol Chem 2008;283:24506–13.

12. Heinonen S, Männikkö M, Klement JF, et al. Targeted inactivation of the type VII collagen gene (Col7a1) in mice results in severe blistering phenotype: a model for recessive dystrophic epidermolysis bullosa. J Cell Sci 1999;112:3641–8.

13. Fritsch A, Loeckermann S, Kern JS, et al. A hypomorphic mouse model for dystrophic epidermolysis bullosa reveals disease mechanisms and responds to fibroblast therapy. J Clin Invest 2008;118: 1669–79.

14. Fine J-D, Eady RAJ, Bauer EA, et al. The classification of inherited epidermolysis bullosa (EB): report of the third international consensus meeting on diagnosis and classification of EB. J Am Acad Dermatol 2008;58:931–50.

15. Bruckner-Tuderman L. Epidermolysis bullosa. In: Burgdorf W, Plewig G, Wolff HH, et al, editors. Braun-Falco's dermatology. 3rd edition. Heidelberg (Germany): Springer Medizin Verlag; 2009. p. 628–40.

16. McGrath JA, Schofield OMV, Eady RAJ. Epidermolysis bullosa pruriginosa: dystrophic epidermolysis bullosa with distinctive clinicopathological features. Br J Dermatol 1994;130:617–25.

17. Hammami-Hauasli N, Raghunath M, Küster W, et al. Transient bullous dermolysis of the newborn associated with compound heterozygosity for recessive and dominant COL7A1 mutations. J Invest Dermatol 1998;111:1214–9.

18. Sato-Matsumura KC, Yasukawa K, Tomita Y, et al. Toenail dystrophy with COL7A1 glycine substitution mutations segregates as an autosomal dominant trait in 2 families with dystrophic epidermolysis bullosa. Arch Dermatol 2002;138:269–71.

19. Lin AN, Smith LT, Fine J-D. Dystrophic epidermolysis bullosa inversa: report of two cases with further correlation between electron microscopic and immunofluorescence studies. J Am Acad Dermatol 1995;33:361–5.

20. Schumann H, Has C, Kohlhase J, et al. Dystrophic epidermolysis bullosa pruriginosa is not associated with frequent FLG gene mutations. Br J Dermatol 2008;159:464–9.

21. Almaani N, Liu L, Harrison N, et al. New glycine substitution mutations in type VII collagen underlying epidermolysis bullosa pruriginosa, but the phenotype is not explained by a common polymorphism in the matrix metalloproteinase-1 gene promoter. Acta Derm Venereol 2009;89:6–11.

22. Hashimoto K, Matsumoto M, Iacobelli D. Transient bullous dermolysis of the newborn. Arch Dermatol 1985;121:1429–38.

23. Fine JD, Johnson LB, Weiner M, et al. Epidermolysis bullosa and the risk of life-threatening cancers: the National EB Registry experience, 1986–2006. J Am Acad Dermatol 2009;60:203–11.

24. Arnold AW, Bruckner-Tuderman L, Züger C, et al. Cetuximab therapy of metastasizing cutaneous squamous cell carcinoma in a patient with severe recessive dystrophic epidermolysis bullosa. Dermatology 2009;219:80–3.

25. Kern JS, Kohlhase J, Bruckner-Tuderman L, et al. Expanding the COL7A1 mutation database: novel and recurrent mutations and unusual genotype–phenotype constellations in 41 patients with dystrophic epidermolysis bullosa. J Invest Dermatol 2006;126:1006–12.

26. Uitto J. Epidermolysis bullosa: prospects for cell-based therapies. J Invest Dermatol 2008;128: 2140–2.

27. Remington J, Wang X, Hou Y, et al. Injection of recombinant human type VII collagen corrects the disease phenotype in a murine model of dystrophic epidermolysis bullosa. Mol Ther 2009;17:26–33.

28. Ortiz-Urda S, Thyagarajan B, Keene DR, et al. Stable nonviral genetic correction of inherited human skin disease. Nat Med 2002;8:1166–70 [erratum in: Nat Med 2003;9:237].

29. Baldeschi C, Gache Y, Rattenholl A, et al. Genetic correction of canine dystrophic epidermolysis bullosa mediated by retroviral vectors. Hum Mol Genet 2003; 12:1897–905.

30. Woodley DT, Remington J, Huang Y, et al. Intravenously injected human fibroblasts home to skin wounds, deliver type VII collagen, and promote wound healing. Mol Ther 2007;15:628–35.

31. Wong T, Gammon L, Liu L, et al. Potential of fibroblast cell therapy for recessive dystrophic epidermolysis bullosa. J Invest Dermatol 2008;128: 2179–89.

32. Tolar J, Ishida-Yamamoto A, Riddle M, et al. Amelioration of epidermolysis bullosa by transfer of wild-type bone marrow cells. Blood 2009;113: 1167–74.

Kindler Syndrome Pathogenesis and Fermitin Family Homologue 1 (Kindlin-1) Function

Maria-Anna M.A. D'Souza, BSc, MSc,
Roy M. Kimble, MBBS, MD, FRCS,
James R. McMillan, BSc, MSc, PhD*

KEYWORDS

- Genodermatosis • Keratinocyte adhesion
- Keratinocyte proliferation • Signaling
- Focal contact • Fermitin family homologue 1 (FFH1)
- Ultrastructure

KIND1 GENE PRODUCT BIOLOGY, STRUCTURE, AND FUNCTION

Kindler syndrome (KS) (OMIM173650) is a rare autosomal recessive skin disorder, first described in 1954.[1] The precise mechanism by which FERMT1 gene mutations (encoding fermitin family homolog 1 protein [FFH1]) result in KS symptoms, including blistering, epidermal atrophy, increased risk of cancer, and poor wound healing, remains unclear. Knowledge of some of the more basic FFH1 functions in skin and, in particular, keratinocytes, however, is steadily growing. Cell-matrix interactions are mediated by integrins, heterodimeric transmembrane proteins comprising α and β subunits, and are controlled through integrin activation and cytoskeletal organization.[2] Overall, studies suggest a critical role of FFH1 in cell-matrix interactions via integrin adhesion receptors. An important step in integrin activation is the binding of FERM (four point one protein, ezrin, radixin, and moesin) domain proteins, such as talin, to the cytoplasmic tail of β integrin subunits.[3] FFH1 (also a FERM or fermitin family homologue protein) can bind to several cytoplasmic motifs within the tail domains of β1 and β3 integrins, colocalizing with vinculin at focal adhesions in cultured keratinocytes.[4,5] In addition, FFH1 associates with FFH2 (a kindlin-1 homologue, formerly known as kindlin-2) and filamin-binding LIM protein[6] together with other focal adhesions components at sites of cell-matrix contact. Recent cell biologic mutational analysis demonstrated that the second conserved NXXY motif (Tyr795) and the threonine-containing region (Thr788 and Thr789) of the integrin β1A tail, together with the conserved tryptophan in the F3 subdomain of the FFH FERM domain (kindlin-1 Trp612 and kindlin-2 Trp615), are required for direct FFH-integrin interactions.[7] Tissue-specific expression of FFH protein regulates integrin activation, including FFH1 (in epithelia), FFH2 (expressed predominantly in the heart and other tissues), and FFH3 (where expression is restricted to hematopoietic lineages). FFH2/3 proteins are essential regulators of integrin activation, and deficiencies in these focal adhesions proteins leads to cardiac

This work was supported by the Royal Children's Hospital Foundation (JRM/RMK) and by A New Research Staff Startup Grant from The University of Queensland (JRM).
Children's Centre for Burns Research, The University of Queensland, Queensland Children's Medical Research Institute, L/4 RCH Foundation Building, Herston, Brisbane, Queensland 4029, Australia
* Corresponding author.
E-mail address: j.mcmillan@uq.edu.au (J.R. McMillan).

Dermatol Clin 28 (2010) 115–118
doi:10.1016/j.det.2009.10.012

malformation and platelet dysfunction, respectively.[8–12] These defects make knockout mouse work difficult or prohibitive due to poor survival.[8–12] From patients with KS disease, it is known that long-term FFH1 deficiency leads to an increased cancer risk; however, the precise mechanisms causing these effects are unknown. Focal adhesions are thought to have important roles in preventing disease by controlling cell survival, growth, signaling, and cell invasion, making them central to the study and treatment of cancer.[4] The role of FFH proteins is thought to be related to stem cell maintenance via its control of important cell cycle processes and also via the regulation of multiple growth factors that are associated with cancer progression and tumor cell survival[13] and, critically, are involved in wounding.[4] FFH1, -2, and -3 form part of a protein family that share a high degree of sequence homology in addition to a bipartite FERM domain interrupted by a pleckstrin homology domain that is important in cell signaling (**Fig. 1A**).[14] Nevertheless, the precise downstream roles of FFH proteins after integrin activation and their involvement in

precise signaling pathways controlling specific cell functions remain to be determined.

KIND1 GENE DISCOVERY

Since Theresa Kindler's discovery of a rare skin syndrome in 1954,[1] there has been some dispute as to the precise clinical entity of KS patients, as several cases with a clinical overlap to KS have been reported, including hereditary acrokeratotic poikiloderma and dystrophic epidermolysis bullosa.[15] It took a long time before the precise defects in the protein FFH1 encoded by the gene FERMT1 (also known as C20ORF42 or KIND1) were identified that underlie this disease.[16,17] Mutations in the FERMT1-encoding FFH1 protein have been identified in the majority of patients with KS.[16–24] In-depth examination of FERMT1 in a small proportion of patients, however, has failed to identify the underlying genetic defects, suggesting that KS may be caused by more the one gene.

KS can also affect other organs, including urethral, anal, esophageal and genital mucosa[25–27] and gastrointestinal involvement,[28] manifesting as

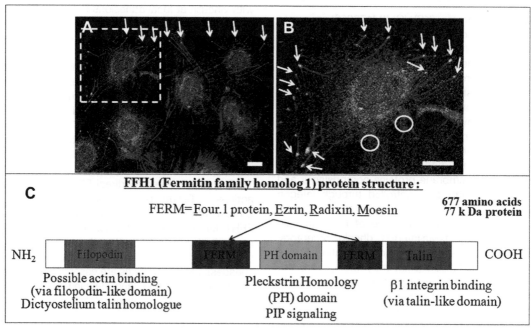

Fig. 1. (A) Indirect immunofluorescent staining using a rabbit polyclonal anti-FFH1 (*green punctate* staining highlighted by *white arrows*) in a mouse RAC-11P cell line demonstrating the localization of FFH1 at the ends of actin bundles (highlighted by tetramethyl rhodamine iso-thiocyanate (TRITC)–phalloidin staining, *red*) where they terminate at focal contacts at the edge of the cell. (B) At higher power, view of the area highlighted by the *dashed box* in (A) shows the discrete localization of FFH1 in greater detail at focal adhesion structures but not at sites of cell-cell adhesion (highlighted by two *white circles*). Scale bars 2 μm. (C) Schematic representation of FFH1 structure highlighting the two FERM domains (*blue*) separated by a pleckstrin homologous (PH) domain. Towards the C terminus of FFH1 domains is a talin-like β1 integrin-binding domain (*red box*) and at the N terminus is a filopodin-like putative actin binding domain (*orange box*).

ulcerative colitis.[5] Apart from esophageal or anal stenosis, gastrointestinal tract participation is rare in KS.[5,27]

ULTRASTRUCTURAL FINDINGS IN KINDLER SYNDROME

The first reported ultrastructural changes in KS skin were published in 1989 and highlighted epidermal atrophy, poikiloderma with hyperkeratosis, telangiectasia, and hyper- and hypopigmentation.[29] Depending on a patient's skin type, other features included disruptions in melanosome transport (manifesting as melanosome leakage from melanocytes or keratinocytes) and the presence of multiple melanophages.[15] This loss of normal melanosome distribution protecting basal keratinocytes may play some role in the increased risk of skin cancer observed in KS patients. Together with keratinocyte integrin dysadhesion, these combined effects may serve to allow DNA damage resulting from the reductions in the normally abundant melanosomes/melanin capping the keratinocyte basal cell nuclei while simultaneously increasing tumour promotion activity after the release of cytokine/growth factors resulting from the loss of cell adhesion and integrity after FFH1 depletion. Other ultrastructural changes in KS patient skin include the disruption of the normal collagen and elastic fiber organization in the papillary dermis.[15] Classically, ultrastructural examination of KS skin reveals a distinct disorganization within the epidermal basement membrane exhibiting as lamina densa reduplication with branching, folding, and formation of loops and circles. Inconsistent multiple levels of cleavage within the dermal-epidermal junction were also seen.[15,17,20,24,30] In 2002, using electron microscopy, Yasukawa and colleagues reported multiple levels of epidermal separation, including minor disruption to the keratin intermediate filament-hemidesmosome linkage but no decrease in hemidesmosome size or number.[15] In 2006, Has and colleagues[19] reported the clinical features of Italian patients with suspected KS. Acral poikiloderma with skin atrophy and dyschromia were the prominent features of adults. Only recently, however, has the distinctive skin atrophy on the dorsal aspects of the hands and feet and the digital webbing provided any diagnostic clues to the underlying causes of this disease.

Although basal lamina reduplication is not absolutely specific to KS, it remains useful in distinguishing this disorder from dystrophic epidermolysis bullosa.[15] In dystrophic epidermolysis bullosa, the typical plane of cleavage through the basement membrane zone occurs beneath the lamina densa with morphologic abnormalities of the anchoring fibril comprising collagen VII. In KS skin, however, apart from extensive reduplication in the lamina densa, patients often exhibit multiple planes of separation within epidermal basement membrane zone, including within the basal keratinocytes and separation between the lamina lucida and sublamina densa.[23] Although a prominent feature, the mechanism behind the thickening and reduplication of the lamina densa remains unclear. It may be related, however, to repeated episodes of keratinocyte dysadhesion and overcompensation for this by excessive matrix production. Accordingly, it has been suggested that this characteristic is not a primary, but a secondary, change brought about by constant remodeling of the matrix beneath the basement membrane.[24,31]

REFERENCES

1. Kindler T. Congenital poikiloderma with traumatic bulla formation and progressive cutaneous atrophy. Br J Dermatol 1954;66(3):104–11.
2. Larjava H, Plow EF, Wu C. Kindlins: essential regulators of integrin signalling and cell-matrix adhesion. EMBO Rep 2008;9(12):1203–8.
3. Calderwood DA. Talin controls integrin activation. Biochem Soc Trans 2004;32(Pt3):434–7.
4. Kloeker S, Major MB, Calderwood DA, et al. The Kindler syndrome protein is regulated by transforming growth factor-beta and involved in integrin-mediated adhesion. J Biol Chem 2004;279(8):6824–33.
5. Ussar S, Moser M, Widmaier M, et al. Loss of kindlin-1 causes skin atrophy and lethal neonatal intestinal epithelial dysfunction. PLoS Genet 2008;4(12):e1000289.
6. Lai-Cheong JE, Ussar S, Arita K, et al. Colocalization of kindlin-1 kindlin-2, and migfilin at keratinocyte focal adhesion and relevance to the pathophysiology of Kindler syndrome. J Invest Dermatol 2008;128(9):2156–65.
7. Harburger DS, Bouaouina M, Calderwood DA. Kindlin-1 and -2 directly bind the C-terminal region of beta integrin cytoplasmic tails and exert integrin-specific activation effects. J Biol Chem 2009;284(17):11485–97.
8. Dowling JJ, Gibbs E, Russell M, et al. Kindlin-2 is an essential component of intercalated discs and is required for vertebrate cardiac structure and function. Circ Res 2008;102(4):423–31.
9. Kruger M, Moser M, Ussar S, et al. SILAC mouse for quantitative proteomics uncovers kindlin-3 as an essential factor for red blood cell function. Cell 2008;134(2):353–64.

10. Montanez E, Ussar S, Schifferer M, et al. Kindlin-2 controls bidirectional signaling of integrins. Genes Dev 2008;22(10):1325–30.

11. Mory A, Feigelson SW, Yarali N, et al. Kindlin-3: a new gene involved in the pathogenesis of LAD-III. Blood 2008;112(6):2591.

12. Moser M, Nieswandt B, Ussar S, et al. Kindlin-3 is essential for integrin activation and platelet aggregation. Nat Med 2008;14(3):325–30.

13. Lahn M, Kloeker S, Berry BS. TGF-beta inhibitors for the treatment of cancer. Expert Opin Investig Drugs 2005;14(6):629–43.

14. Ussar S, Wang HV, Linder S, et al. The Kindlins: subcellular localization and expression during murine development. Exp Cell Res 2006;312(16): 3142–51.

15. Yasukawa K, Sato-Matsumura KC, McMillan JR, et al. Exclusion of COL7A1 mutation in Kindler syndrome. J Am Acad Dermatol 2002;46(3): 447–50.

16. Jobard F, Bouadjar B, Caux F, et al. Identification of mutations in a new gene encoding a FERM family protein with a pleckstrin homology domain in Kindler syndrome. Hum Mol Genet 2003;12(8): 925–35.

17. Siegel DH, Ashton GH, Penagos HG, et al. Loss of kindlin-1, a human homolog of the caenorhabditis elegans actin-extracellular-matrix linker protein UNC-112, causes Kindler syndrome. Am J Hum Genet 2003;73(1):174–87.

18. Burch JM, Fassihi H, Jones CA, et al. Kindler syndrome: a new mutation and new diagnostic possibilities. Arch Dermatol 2006;142(5):620–4.

19. Has C, Wessagowit V, Pascucci M, et al. Molecular basis of Kindler syndrome in Italy: novel and recurrent Alu/Alu recombination, splice site, nonsense, and frameshift mutations in the KIND1 gene. J Invest Dermatol 2006;126(8):1776–83.

20. White SJ, McLean WH. Kindler surprise: mutations in a novel actin-associated protein cause Kindler syndrome. J Dermatol Sci 2005;38(3): 169–75.

21. Sethuraman G, Fassihi H, Ashton GH, et al. An Indian child with Kindler syndrome resulting from a new homozygous nonsense mutation (C468X) in the KIND1 gene. Clin Exp Dermatol 2005;30(3):286–8.

22. Ashton GH, McLean WH, South AP, et al. Recurrent mutations in kindlin-1, a novel keratinocyte focal contact protein, in the autosomal recessive skin fragility and photosensitivity disorder, Kindler syndrome. J Invest Dermatol 2004;122(1):78–83.

23. Ashton GH. Kindler syndrome. Clin Exp Dermatol 2004;29(2):116–21.

24. Lanschuetzer CM, Muss WH, Emberger M, et al. Characteristic immunohistochemical and ultrastructural findings indicate that Kindler's syndrome is an apoptotic skin disorder. J Cutan Pathol 2003;30(9): 553–60.

25. Periodontal disease linked with Kindler syndrome. J Am Dent Assoc 2003;134(4):424–8.

26. Szczerba SM, Yokoo KM, Bauer BS. Release of acquired syndactylies in Kindler syndrome. Ann Plast Surg 1994;33(4):434–8.

27. Forman AB, Prendiville JS, Esterly NB, et al. Kindler syndrome: report of two cases and review of the literature. Pediatr Dermatol 1989;6(2):91–101.

28. Sadler E, Klausegger A, Muss W, et al. Novel KIND1 gene mutation in Kindler syndrome with severe gastrointestinal tract involvement. Arch Dermatol 2006;142(12):1619–24.

29. Hovnanian A, Blanchet Bardon C, de Prost Y. Poikiloderma of Theresa Kindler: report of a case with ultrastructural study, and review of the literature. Pediatr Dermatol 2008;6(2):82–90.

30. Ghaninejad H, Balighi K, Ehsani A, et al. Kindler's syndrome: the first report of four siblings with new findings. Acta Med Iran 2004;42(2):146–8.

31. Nofal E, Assaf M, Elmosalamy K. Kindler syndrome: a study of five Egyptian cases with evaluation of severity. Int J Dermatol 2008;47:658–62.

Kindler Syndrome

Joey E. Lai-Cheong, MBBS, MRCP (UK),
John A. McGrath, MD, FRCP*

KEYWORDS

- *FERMT1*, Fermitin family homolog 1 • Actin
- Blistering • Skin atrophy • Poikiloderma

Understanding of blistering skin disorders involving the dermal-epidermal junction (DEJ) has improved considerably over the past 2 decades. This has been possible with the discovery of pathogenic mutations in genes encoding several structural components of cell–extracellular matrix (ECM) junctions in conjunction with the identification of autoantibodies targeting specific ECM proteins.[1] Epidermolysis bullosa (EB) is the term used for the spectrum of inherited mechanobullous skin disorders that result from mutations in at least 13 different proteins' involvement in epithelial or basement membrane integrity. Until the publication of the revised classification of EB in 2008, the molecular pathology of this condition was restricted to disorders that result from disruption of keratin intermediate filament-ECM anchorage.[2] These skin fragility disorders include clinical subtypes of EB simplex, junctional EB, and dystrophic EB. In the latest classification of EB, however, Kindler syndrome (KS) (MIM173650) has been added as a further, specific form of EB.[2] Trauma-induced blistering is common to KS and EB but individuals with KS soon develop progressive skin atrophy and poikiloderma. In addition, from a molecular viewpoint, KS differs from the other types of EB in that it results from disruption of the actin cytoskeleton-ECM anchorage network.[3] The gene implicated in KS is *FERMT1*, which encodes fermitin family homolog 1 (FFH1) protein, a focal adhesion protein that links the actin cytoskeleton with the underlying ECM.[3] In the skin, FFH1 is predominantly expressed in the basal keratinocyte layer close to the DEJ.[3–6] In cultured keratinocytes, it is present at focal adhesions where it mediates integrin-dependent ECM interactions.[5] This article reviews the clinical and pathologic features of KS and provides an overview on patient management.

BACKGROUND TO KINDLER SYNDROME

In 1954, Theresa Kindler reported the case of a 14-year old white girl who had congenital acral trauma-induced blistering and mottled pigmentation on her cheeks. This individual also burned easily in the sun and developed progressive skin atrophy.[7] These features were suggestive of a subtype of EB and a form of inherited poikiloderma, but the precise nature of the disorder and the inheritance pattern, was unclear. In 1971, Weary and colleagues[8] reported a family with overlapping clinical features. The pattern of inheritance was autosomal dominant but the clinical features were variable (vesicopustules, eczema, poikiloderma, and acral keratotic papules). The partial similarities between the Weary pedigree and the Kindler case report led to the introduction of the term, *Weary-Kindler syndrome*, and a further similar autosomal dominant pedigree was reported by Larregue and colleagues[9] in 1981. Evidence for a distinct recessive disease, however, that more closely resembled the original Kindler case was published in 1985 and several other cases of unequivocal autosomal recessive inheritance followed.[10] In recent years, characterization of the molecular basis of

The authors' original studies on Kindler syndrome have received funding from The Wellcome Trust, the British Association of Dermatologists, and the British Skin Foundation. The authors also acknowledge financial support from the Department of Health via the National Institute for Health Research comprehensive Biomedical Research Centre award to Guy's and St Thomas' NHS Foundation Trust in partnership with King's College London and King's College Hospital NHS Foundation Trust.

Division of Genetics and Molecular Medicine, St John's Institute of Dermatology, King's College London, Floor 9 Tower Wing, Guy's Hospital, Great Maze Pond, London SE1 9RT, UK

* Corresponding author.

E-mail address: john.mcgrath@kcl.ac.uk (J.A. McGrath).

Dermatol Clin 28 (2010) 119–124

doi:10.1016/j.det.2009.10.013

several genodermatoses that partly resemble KS has provided further evidence that it is a distinct disorder. The mechanobullous disease, dystrophic EB, has been shown to result from mutations in the type VII collagen gene, *COL7A1*.[11] Likewise, KS does not map to the Rothmund-Thomson syndrome gene, *RECQL4,* on 8q24.3 or other known DNA helicase genes.[12] Another genodermatosis that overlaps with KS, EB simplex with mottled pigmentation, has been found to result from a specific mutation, p.Pro25Leu, in the cytokeratin 5 gene (*KRT5*),[13] thus also distinguishing this genodermatosis from true KS.

CLINICAL FEATURES OF KINDLER SYNDROME

The main clinical features of KS are trauma-induced skin blistering predominantly involving acral sites and progressive poikiloderma and mucosal inflammation (**Fig. 1**). Some individuals with KS suffer with varying degrees of photosensitivity, which often lessens with age.[14] The skin blistering also has a tendency to subside with age

although this is not a universal finding. Marked skin atrophy develops early in life (under the age of 5) especially on the dorsal aspects of the hands and feet and, in most cases, becomes generalized by adolescence.[15] Gingivitis and periodontitis are also prominent features.[16] Mucosal stenoses involving the esophagus, vagina, anus, and urethra have been reported. Gastrointestinal symptoms, including constipation and severe colitis, can also occur in KS.[17,18] Other features may include pseudosyndactyly, conjunctivitis, mandibular abnormalities and orogenital leukokeratosis, although the diagnosis of KS in many reports detailing these clinical findings has not been substantiated by molecular analysis.[19,20] There is also an increased of nonmelanoma skin cancer in KS with squamous cell carcinomas reported in acral skin or the mouth.[18,21–25]

SKIN BIOPSY FINDINGS IN KINDLER SYNDROME

Light microscopy of KS skin may show hyperkeratosis, epidermal atrophy, loss of the rete ridges,

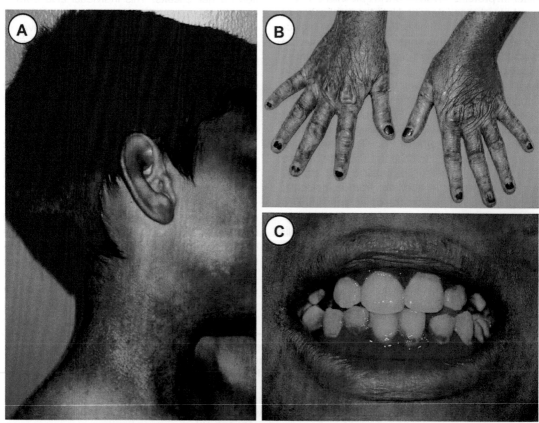

Fig. 1. Clinical features of KS. (*A*) Poikiloderma involving the neck of this 10-year-old boy with KS harboring a homozygous *FERMT1* nonsense mutation, p.S14X/p.S14X. (*B*) Marked skin atrophy present on dorsal aspects of the hands in this 16-year-old girl with a homozygous *FERMT1* nonsense mutation, p. E168X/p.E168X. (*C*) Gingival inflammation and dental caries present in the same female patient with KS.

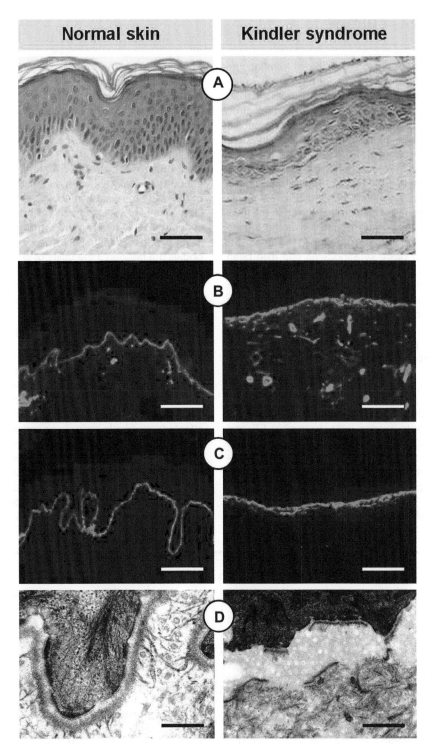

Fig. 2. Histologic abnormalities in KS skin. (*A*) Hematoxylin and eosin staining of normal human skin shows the presence of rete ridges whereas in KS skin, there is marked skin atrophy associated with complete loss of the rete ridges. In the pigmented KS skin illustrated (Fitzpatrick skin type V), pigmentary incontinence and melanophages are observed in the dermis (bar = 50 μm). Immunofluorescence microscopy labeling for type IV collagen (*B*) and type VII collagen (*C*) in normal human skin shows linear labeling at the DEJ whereas in KS skin there is extensive reduplication and basement membrane interruptions (bar = 50 μm). (*D*) Transmission electron microscopy of normal skin shows an intact basement membrane zone consisting of an electron dense hemidesmosomal complex, lamina lucida, and lamina densa from which anchoring fibrils project into the dermis (bar = 0.1 μm). In KS skin, there are variable planes of cleavage: the lamina densa is fragmented and appears in the roof and base of the blistered skin (bar = 0.5 μm).

and focal vacuolization of the basal keratinocyte layer, consistent with poikiloderma (**Fig. 2**). In the papillary dermis, melanophages and colloid bodies may be found.[15] Transmission electron microscopy findings in KS are variable. In nonblistered skin there is reduplication of the lamina densa, focal interruptions of the lamina densa at the DEJ, and areas of collagen lysis and disrupted elastic tissue in the dermis. The ultrastructural abnormalities in blistered skin in KS reveal single or multiple planes of cleavage at the DEJ: the level of blister formation can occur below the lamina densa, although tissue separation in the lamina lucida or within basal keratinocytes has also been documented.[26] Duplication of the lamina densa is a useful clue to the diagnosis of KS, and skin immunohistochemistry with an anti–type IV or –type VII collagen antibody may illustrate the features of basement membrane reduplication with broad patchy staining at the DEJ.[15] This finding is not diagnostic for KS but is a helpful clue.

DIAGNOSIS OF KINDLER SYNDROME

KS can be difficult to diagnose at birth because of its considerable overlap with dystrophic EB and EB simplex with mottled pigmentation. The combination of progressive skin atrophy and poikiloderma (both of which tend to be generalized), acral blistering, mucosal inflammation, and varying degrees of photosensitivity, however, is more suggestive of KS. Identification of loss-of-function

mutations in the *FERMT1* gene by gene sequencing confirms the diagnosis of KS.[3,4,18] Since the identification of the *FERMT1* gene in 2003, 37 different pathogenic *FERMT1* mutations have been reported.[18,27,28] These comprise 14 nonsense, 13 frameshift, 7 splice site, and 3 large deletion mutations (**Fig. 3**). Skin immunofluorescence microscopy using a C-terminal anti-FFH1 antibody typically shows reduced immunolabeling of FFH1 in the basal keratinocyte layer and at the DEJ. This is not a universal finding, however, and variable FFH1 labeling has been observed in several patients with KS.[5] New anti-FFH1 antibodies are needed if the utility of skin immunolabeling as a diagnostic probe is to be fully realized, as is typically the case for skin immunohistochemistry in other autosomal recessive forms of EB.

MANAGEMENT OF KINDLER SYNDROME

The management of KS is largely symptomatic. The skin in KS is often dry and pruritic and may require frequent topical application of emollients. Photoprotection is advocated because of the development of photosensitivity in KS; many affected individuals typically go red within minutes of sun exposure.[29] There is an increased risk of squamous cell carcinomas and, therefore, repeated screening checks for premalignant keratoses and early malignancy are indicated. Regular dental care is advised because of erosive gingivitis and aggressive periodontitis in KS. Esophageal

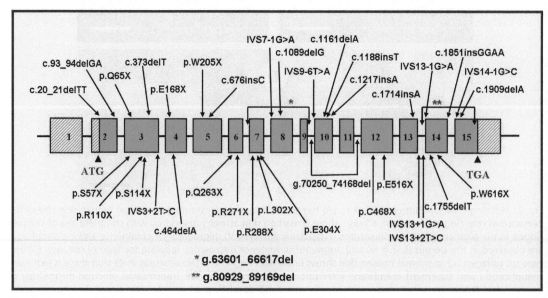

Fig. 3. A total of 37 different loss-of-function *FERMT1* mutations have been reported. These comprise 14 nonsense, 13 frameshift, 7 splice site, and 3 large deletion mutations. Single/double asterisks indicate sites of large intragenic deletions. (*Adapted from* Lai-Cheong JE, Tanaka A, Hawche G, et al. Kindler syndrome: a focal adhesion genodermatosis. Br J Dermatol 2009;160:233–42.)

dilatation may be indicated in patients with dysphagia.[30,31] In cases of severe esophageal dysfunction, temporary parenteral nutrition may be necessary.[30] Affected individuals with colitis-like symptoms may develop iron-deficiency anemia. In some cases, surgical bowel resection may be required for severe colitis.[17] Urethral strictures may also require stenting or surgical intervention. In pregnant women with KS, careful obstetric planning, such as consideration of an elective cesarean section, should be considered because vaginal stenosis may occur in KS.[32]

SUMMARY

Since the first clinical description of KS more than 50 years ago, the syndrome has come to represent a distinct autosomal recessive genodermatosis that is characterized as a subtype of EB. In contrast to other forms of EB, however, KS results from disruption of the attachment of the actin cytoskeleton to focal adhesion junctions at the DEJ and the consequences of impaired epithelial mesenchymal signaling via these complexes. KS results from loss-of-function mutations in the *FERMT1* gene, which encodes FFH1. Identification of KS as a discrete clinical entity with a specific molecular basis provides an opportunity to establish an accurate diagnosis in patients with this disorder, notably in distinguishing it from other forms of EB or poikilodermatous syndromes. Clinical management involves monitoring for specific complications, including scarring, strictures, and anemia. Practically, a major problem is gingivitis, which requires regular and careful dental assessment. It is also important to remember that patients with KS maybe prone to develop squamous cell carcinomas, in sun-exposed sites or in chronically inflamed mucosae.

REFERENCES

1. Mellerio JE. Molecular pathology of the cutaneous basement membrane zone. Clin Exp Dermatol 1999;24:25–32.
2. Fine JD, Eady RA, Bauer EA, et al. The classification of inherited epidermolysis bullosa (EB): report of the third international consensus meeting on diagnosis and classification of EB. J Am Acad Dermatol 2008;58:931–50.
3. Siegel DH, Ashton GH, Penagos HG, et al. Loss of kindlin-1, a human homolog of the *Caenorhabditis elegans* actin-extracellular-matrix linker protein UNC-112, causes Kindler syndrome. Am J Hum Genet 2003;73:174–87.
4. Jobard F, Bouadjar B, Caux F, et al. Identification of mutations in a new gene encoding a FERM family protein with a pleckstrin homology domain in Kindler syndrome. Hum Mol Genet 2003;12:925–35.
5. Lai-Cheong JE, Ussar S, Arita K, et al. Colocalization of kindlin-1, kindlin-2, and migfilin at keratinocyte focal adhesion and relevance to the pathophysiology of Kindler syndrome. J Invest Dermatol 2008;128:2156–65.
6. Ussar S, Wang HV, Linder S, et al. The Kindlins: subcellular localization and expression during murine development. Exp Cell Res 2006;312:3142–51.
7. Kindler T. Congenital poikiloderma with traumatic bulla formation and progressive cutaneous atrophy. Br J Dermatol 1954;66:104–11.
8. Weary PE, Manley WF Jr, Graham GF. Hereditary acrokeratotic poikiloderma. Arch Dermatol 1971;103:409–22.
9. Larregue M, Prigent F, Lorette G, et al. [Bullous and hereditary Weary-Kindler's acrokeratotic poikiloderma]. Ann Dermatol Venereol 1981;108:69–76 [in French].
10. Hacham-Zadeh S, Garfunkel AA. Kindler syndrome in two related Kurdish families. Am J Med Genet 1985;20:43–8.
11. Hilal L, Rochat A, Duquesnoy P, et al. A homozygous insertion-deletion in the type VII collagen gene (COL7A1) in Hallopeau-Siemens dystrophic epidermolysis bullosa. Nat Genet 1993;5:287–93.
12. Kitao S, Lindor NM, Shiratori M, et al. Rothmund-Thomson syndrome responsible gene, RECQL4: genomic structure and products. Genomics 1999;61:268–76.
13. Uttam J, Hutton E, Coulombe PA, et al. The genetic basis of epidermolysis bullosa simplex with mottled pigmentation. Proc Natl Acad Sci U S A 1996;93:9079–84.
14. Lai-Cheong JE, Liu L, Sethuraman G, et al. Five new homozygous mutations in the KIND1 gene in Kindler syndrome. J Invest Dermatol 2007;127:2268–70.
15. Ashton GH. Kindler syndrome. Clin Exp Dermatol 2004;29:116–21.
16. Wiebe CB, Petricca G, Hakkinen L, et al. Kindler syndrome and periodontal disease: review of the literature and a 12-year follow-up case. J Periodontol 2008;79:961–6.
17. Kern JS, Herz C, Haan E, et al. Chronic colitis due to an epithelial barrier defect: the role of kindlin-1 isoforms. J Pathol 2007;213:462–70.
18. Lai-Cheong JE, Tanaka A, Hawche G, et al. Kindler syndrome: a focal adhesion genodermatosis. Br J Dermatol 2009;160:233–42.
19. Ezzine Sebai N, Trojjet S, Khaled A, et al. Kindler syndrome: three cases reports in three siblings. Ann Dermatol Venereol 2007;134:774–8.
20. Sharma RC, Mahajan V, Sharma NL, et al. Kindler syndrome. Int J Dermatol 2003;42:727–32.

21. Arita K, Wessagowit V, Inamadar AC, et al. Unusual molecular findings in Kindler syndrome. Br J Dermatol 2007;157:1252–6.

22. Ashton GH, McLean WH, South AP, et al. Recurrent mutations in kindlin-1, a novel keratinocyte focal contact protein, in the autosomal recessive skin fragility and photosensitivity disorder, Kindler syndrome. J Invest Dermatol 2004;122:78–83.

23. Emanuel PO, Rudikoff D, Phelps RG. Aggressive squamous cell carcinoma in Kindler syndrome. Skinmed 2006;5:305–7.

24. Has C, Wessagowit V, Pascucci M, et al. Molecular basis of Kindler syndrome in Italy: novel and recurrent Alu/Alu recombination, splice site, nonsense, and frameshift mutations in the KIND1 gene. J Invest Dermatol 2006;126:1776–83.

25. Lotem M, Raben M, Zeltser R, et al. Kindler syndrome complicated by squamous cell carcinoma of the hard palate: successful treatment with high-dose radiation therapy and granulocyte-macrophage colony-stimulating factor. Br J Dermatol 2001;144:1284–6.

26. Hovnanian A, Blanchet-Bardon C, de Prost Y. Poikiloderma of Theresa Kindler: report of a case with ultrastructural study, and review of the literature. Pediatr Dermatol 1989;6:82–90.

27. Zhou C, Song S, Zhang J. A novel 3017-bp deletion mutation in the FERMT1 (KIND1) gene in a Chinese family with Kindler syndrome. Br J Dermatol 2009;160:1119–22.

28. Has C, Yordanova I, Balabanova M, et al. A novel large FERMT1 (KIND1) gene deletion in Kindler syndrome. J Dermatol Sci 2008;52:209–12.

29. Thomson MA, Ashton GH, McGrath JA, et al. Retrospective diagnosis of Kindler syndrome in a 37-year-old man. Clin Exp Dermatol 2006;31:45–7.

30. Mansur AT, Elcioglu NH, Aydingoz IE, et al. Novel and recurrent KIND1 mutations in two patients with Kindler syndrome and severe mucosal involvement. Acta Derm Venereol 2007;87:563–5.

31. Martignago BC, Lai-Cheong JE, Liu L, et al. Recurrent KIND1 (C20orf42) gene mutation, c.676insC, in a Brazilian pedigree with Kindler syndrome. Br J Dermatol 2007;157:1281–4.

32. Hayashi S, Shimoya K, Itami S, et al. Pregnancy and delivery with Kindler syndrome. Gynecol Obstet Invest 2007;64:72–4.

Ectodermal Dysplasia-Skin Fragility Syndrome

John A. McGrath, MD, FRCP[a],*,
Jemima E. Mellerio, MD, FRCP[b]

KEYWORDS

- Desmosome • Cell adhesion • Blister
- Keratinocyte • Genodermatosis

In 1997, details were published of a child with a clinical combination of skin fragility (erosions, fissures, scale-crust, and keratoderma) and abnormalities of ectodermal development (growth delay, hypotrichosis, and nail dystrophy).[1] Skin biopsy showed acantholysis and loss of expression of the desmosomal protein plakophilin 1 (PKP1) and subsequently loss-of-function mutations were identified on both alleles of *PKP1*, the PKP1 gene. The case was termed *ectodermal dysplasia–skin fragility (ED-SF) syndrome* and represented the first inherited disorder of desmosomes (MIM604536). The syndrome is now classified as a specific suprabasal form of epidermolysis bullosa simplex.[2] Desmosomes are intricate intercellular structures that mediate adhesion between cells by anchoring intermediate filaments to the cell membrane.[3,4] Structurally, desmosomes are present in certain simple, stratified, and complex epithelia, but several "desmosomal" proteins are also expressed in the nuclei of cells that do not have desmosomes.[3,4] These findings indicate that desmosomal proteins may play key structural and signaling roles in several aspects of cell biology and tissue homeostasis. PKP1 is expressed throughout the epidermis, particularly in suprabasal cells, where it is required for stabilization of

desmosomes.[5] The two principal isoforms of PKP1, designated 1a and 1b, are generated through alternative splicing of exon 7.[6] PKP1a is expressed in both desmosomes and nuclei whereas PKP1b is only expressed in nuclei. The specific biologic significance of the two isoforms, however, is unknown. The carboxyl terminus of PKP1 is required for its localization to the plasma membrane and the amino terminus is involved in the recruitment of desmoplakin to the cell membrane and desmosome assembly.[7] PKP1 is also relevant to calcium stability of desmosomes.[5] Following the initial report of ED-SF syndrome, nine other cases have been reported. These have established the disorder as a specific autosomal recessive genodermatosis.[8–15] Pathogenic mutations in nine other desmosomal components (plakophilin 2; desmoplakin; plakoglobin; desmoglein 1, 2, and 4; desmocollin 2, and 3; and corneodesmosin) have also been reported.[16] These mutations may cause skin, hair, or cardiac abnormalities, alone or in combination. Some inherited desmosomal disorders, notably those arising from mutations in desmoplakin or plakoglobin, may be associated with cardiomyopathy, although this is not a feature in ED-SF syndrome since PKP1 is not expressed in the heart.

Funding: The authors acknowledge financial support from the Department of Health via the National Institute for Health Research (NIHR) comprehensive Biomedical Research Centre award to Guy's & St Thomas' NHS Foundation Trust in partnership with King's College London and King's College Hospital NHS Foundation Trust.
[a] St John's Institute of Dermatology, Floor 9 Tower Wing, Guy's Campus, Great Maze Pond, London SE1 9RT, UK
[b] St John's Institute of Dermatology, The Guy's and St Thomas's NHS Foundation Trust, Lambeth Palace Road, London SE1 7EH, UK
* Corresponding author.
E-mail address: john.mcgrath@kcl.ac.uk (J.A. McGrath).

Dermatol Clin 28 (2010) 125–129
doi:10.1016/j.det.2009.10.014

CLINICAL FEATURES OF ECTODERMAL DYSPLASIA–SKIN FRAGILITY SYNDROME

All cases of ED-SF syndrome have some degree of skin fragility, which is partly related to trauma, but which mostly occurs as spontaneous erosions and fissures. A useful clinical clue to diagnosing the syndrome is chronic cheilitis and perioral scale and cracking (**Fig. 1**). Nearly all cases also have palmoplantar keratoderma with painful fissures that are often disabling; indeed, many affected individuals find it difficult to walk or bear weight. All cases have abnormal hair. Usually this abnormality is expressed as hypotrichosis or complete alopecia. Occasionally, depending on the consequences of the particular *PKP1* mutations, the hair may be woolly rather than reduced. These hair abnormalities appear to persist over time.

Nail dystrophy is a further universal clinical finding. Typically, there are growth abnormalities. Affected children are small for age, usually below the third centile for height and weight, although data regarding growth parameters into adulthood are lacking. The first case of ED-SF syndrome reported was noted to have reduced sweating, astigmatism, and dental caries.[1] However, these do not appear to be present in most other affected individuals. Other variable clinical features include scattered scale-crust on the trunk and limbs, pruritus, recurrent systemic infections, follicular hyperkeratosis, inflammatory scaly plaques in the flexures, perianal erythema and erosions, and chronic diarrhea. One case was reported to have a patent foramen ovale,[11] but no other cardiac pathology has been noted.

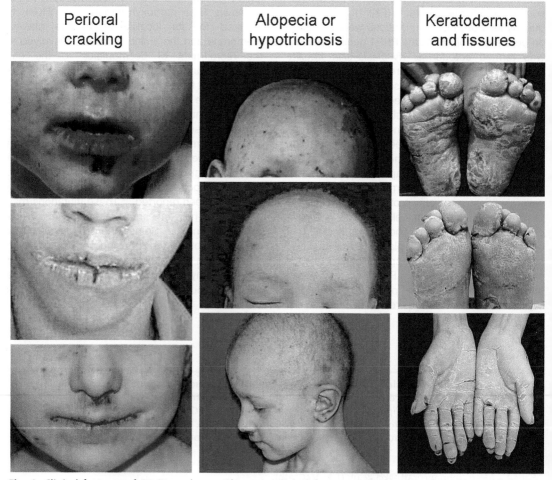

Fig. 1. Clinical features of ED-SF syndrome. The main clinical features include perioral cracking and cheilitis, hypotrichosis or alopecia, and palmoplantar keratoderma, typically with painful fissuring.

SKIN PATHOLOGY OF ECTODERMAL DYSPLASIA–SKIN FRAGILITY SYNDROME

Light microscopy of skin in ED-SF syndrome typically shows hyperkeratosis and acanthosis with widening of spaces between adjacent keratinocytes, particularly throughout the spinous layer (**Fig. 2**). Ultrastructurally, there is a reduced number of small, poorly formed desmosomes. Although there appears to be acantholysis, the actual plane of cleavage/weakness is within the desmosomal plaque (ie, inside the keratinocyte). This leads to desmosomal detachment from the keratinocyte and subsequent cell-cell separation. Immunofluorescence microscopy typically shows markedly reduced or completely absent labeling for PKP1, although the nature of the mutations in some cases may lead to some residual staining. Expression of other desmosomal proteins is usually of normal intensity, but some redistribution of staining patterns can be seen. Notably, labeling for desmoplakin tends to show more cytoplasmic staining and less membranous labeling. Likewise, keratin immunolabeling is often compacted in a perinuclear pattern with less staining at the cell periphery close to desmosomes.

MOLECULAR PATHOLOGY OF ECTODERMAL DYSPLASIA–SKIN FRAGILITY SYNDROME

The first individual with *PKP1* mutations was a compound heterozygote for a nonsense/frameshift combination of mutations. Subsequently, 10 other *PKP1* mutations have been published. These include 2 nonsense, 1 frameshift, and 7 splice-site mutations (**Fig. 3**). The mutations have been located within the amino terminus as well as the second, third, fourth, seventh, eighth, and ninth armadillo-repeat domains of PKP1. In 7 of the 10 published cases the mutations have been homozygous. With respect to genotype-phenotype correlation, nearly all cases involve loss of expression of PKP1, but in 1 case there was a slightly milder clinical variant of the syndrome, which was possibly accounted for by the presence of at least one in-frame transcript arising from

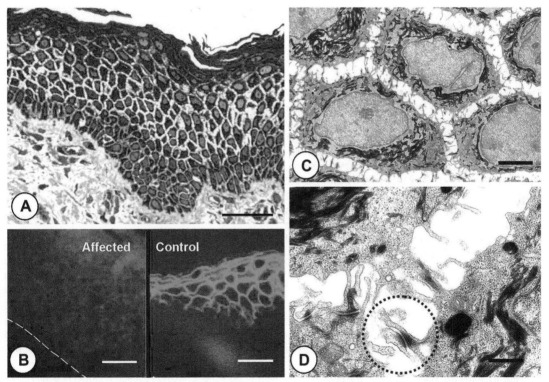

Fig. 2. Skin biopsy abnormalities in ED-SF syndrome. (*A*) Light microscopy shows acanthosis and widening of spaces between adjacent keratinocytes throughout the spinous layer. Note that the basal keratinocyte layer appears intact (bar = 50 μm). (*B*) Immunofluorescence microscopy using an anti-PKP1 antibody shows a complete absence of epidermal labeling in patient skin (*left*) in contrast to the bright peripheral cell staining in normal control skin (*right*) (bar = 50 μm). (*C*) Transmission electron microscopy of the epidermis in an affected individual shows keratinocyte separation and retraction of keratin filaments in a compacted perinuclear distribution (bar = 1 μm). (*D*) At higher magnification, desmosomes appear small and the plane of separation (within *dotted circle*) is occurring just within the intracellular side of the cell in the desmosomal plaque (bar = 0.1 μm).

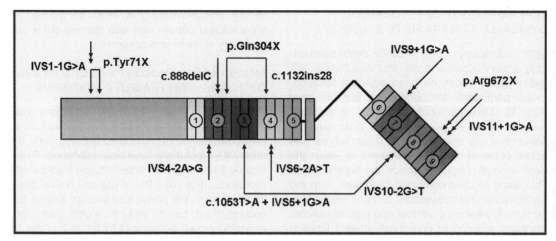

Fig. 3. Database of mutations in *PKP1* in ED-SF syndrome. *Double arrows* indicate homozygous mutations. Joined *arrows* depict compound heterozygous mutations. Colored circled numbers 1 through 9 refer to the armadillo-domains of the PKP1 protein.

a homozygous splice-site mutation (IVS9+1 G>A).[12] Individuals who have haploinsufficiency for PKP1 (eg, parents of affected children who are carriers of one *PKP1* mutation) appear to show no phenotypic abnormalities.

SUMMARY

The autosomal recessive disorder ED-SF syndrome represents the first inherited disorder of desmosomes to be described. It is caused by loss-of-function mutations in *PKP1*, the PKP1 gene. Ten cases of this syndrome have been reported. The clinical features of skin erosions, skin crusting and keratoderma with painful fissures as well as the ultrastructural findings of poorly formed desmosomes with acantholysis collectively underscore the clinicopathologic significance of PKP1 in maintaining desmosomal and epidermal integrity.

REFERENCES

1. McGrath JA, McMillan JR, Shemanko CS, et al. Mutations in the plakophilin 1 gene result in ecto-dermal dysplasia/skin fragility syndrome. Nat Genet 1997;17:241–4.
2. Fine JD, Eady RA, Bauer EA, et al. The classification of inherited epidermolysis bullosa (EB): report of the third International Consensus Meeting on diagnosis and classification of EB. J Am Acad Dermatol 2008;58:931–50.
3. Green KJ, Simpson CL. Desmosomes: new perspectives on a classic. J Invest Dermatol 2007; 127:2499–515.
4. Hoethofer B, Windoffer R, Troyanovsky S, et al. Structure and function of desmosomes. Int Rev Cytol 2007;264:65–163.
5. South AP. Plakophilin 1: an important stabilizer of desmosomes. Clin Exp Dermatol 1997;108:139–46.
6. Schmidt A, Langbein L, Rode M, et al. Plakophi-lins 1a and 1b: widespread nuclear proteins re-cruited in specific epithelial cells as desmosomal plaque components. Cell Tissue Res 1997;290: 481–99.
7. Sobolik-Delmaire T, Katafiasz D, Wahl JK 3rd. Carboxyl terminus of plakophilin 1 recruits to its plasma membrane, whereas amino terminus recruits desmoplakin and promotes desmosome assembly. J Biol Chem 2006;281:16962–70.
8. McGrath JA, Hoeger PH, Christiano AM, et al. Skin fragility and hypohidrotic ectodermal dysplasia re-sulting from ablation of plakophilin 1. Br J Dermatol 1999;140:297–307.
9. Whittock NV, Haftek M, Angoulvant N, et al. Genomic amplification of the human plakophilin 1 gene and detection of a new mutation in ectodermal dysplasia/skin fragility syndrome. J Invest Dermatol 2000;15:368–74.
10. Hamada T, South AP, Mitsuhashi Y, et al. Genotype-phenotype correlation in skin fragility-ectodermal dysplasia syndrome resulting from mutations in pla-kophilin 1. Exp Dermatol 2002;11:107–14.
11. Sprecher E, Molho-Pessach V, Ingber A, et al. Homo-zygous splice site mutations in PKP1 result in loss of epidermal plakophilin 1 expression and underlie ectodermal dysplasia/skin fragility syndrome in two consanguineous families. J Invest Dermatol 2004; 122:647–51.
12. Steijlen PM, van Steensel MA, Jansen BJ, et al. Cryptic splicing at a non-consensus splice-donor

in a patient with a novel mutation in the plakophilin 1 gene. J Invest Dermatol 2004;122:1321–4.

13. Zheng R, Bu DF, Zhu XJ. Compound heterozygosity for new splice site mutations in the plakophilin 1 gene (PKP1) in a Chinese case of ectodermal dysplasia–skin fragility syndrome. Acta Derm Venereol 2005;85:394–9.

14. Ersoy-Evans S, Erkin G, Fassihi H, et al. Ectodermal dysplasia–skin fragility syndrome resulting from a new homozygous mutation, 888 delC, in the desmosomal protein plakophilin 1. J Am Acad Dermatol 2006;55:157–61.

15. Tanaka A, Lai-Cheong JE, Café ME, et al. Novel truncating mutations in PKP1 and DSP cause similar skin phenotypes in two Brazilian families. Br J Dermatol 2009;160:692–7.

16. Lai-Cheong JE, Arita K, McGrath JA. Genetic diseases of junctions. J Invest Dermatol 2007;127:2713–25.

Lethal Acantholytic Epidermolysis Bullosa

John A. McGrath, MD, FRCP[a],*, Maria C. Bolling, MD[b],
Marcel F. Jonkman, MD, PhD[b]

KEYWORDS

- Desmoplakin • Keratin • Keratinocyte • Skin fragility
- Desmosome • Genodermatosis

A single case of lethal acantholytic epidermolysis bullosa (LAEB) was born to nonconsanguineous parents and presented with rapidly progressive generalized epidermolysis, which started at the time of the vaginal delivery.[1] Within 24 hours, more than two thirds of the infant's skin was denuded, with a positive Nikolsky's sign. There were no intact blisters or vesicles. Instead, there were areas of large sheets of detached skin with superficial red wound surfaces (**Fig. 1**A). The skin on the hands and feet had detached in a glove and stocking pattern (**Fig. 1**B). No excessive granulation tissue was noted and some sites resembled aplasia cutis. Clinical assessment also revealed complete absence of scalp hair, eyebrows, and eyelashes, although there were some discrete follicular openings on the scalp. All finger- and toenails had shed. Three triangular natal teeth were noted along with extensive erosions affecting the oral cavity. Erosions were also present on the glans penis. Over the first few days of life the skin erosions extended to more than 90% of the surface area, which led to loss of profuse amounts of fluid from the eroded skin. Ten days postpartum the child died. Autopsy revealed extensive suprabasal acantholytic separation within several epithelia, including the mouth, epiglottis, larynx, lung, gastrointestinal tract, and bladder. Cardiac dilatation was noted, but the changes in the heart were attributed to the large amounts of intravenous fluid given to compensate for the cutaneous fluid loss. The cause of death was considered to be multiorgan failure

precipitated by heart failure, but there was no evidence of infection, either cutaneous or systemic. Neither parent of this infant had any cutaneous, hair, or cardiac abnormalities.

SKIN PATHOLOGY OF LETHAL ACANTHOLYTIC EPIDERMOLYSIS BULLOSA

Light microscopy of skin revealed extensive suprabasal clefting with some spongiosis and acantholysis (**Fig. 1**C). These changes extended into hair follicles and eccrine ducts. Ultrastructurally, there was evidence for detachment of keratin intermediate filaments from the inner plaques of desmosomes in all layers of the epidermis (**Fig. 2**). The number and size of the desmosomes appeared normal and both inner and outer plaques were clearly discernible. In contrast to many other autosomal-recessive blistering genodermatoses, however, immunolabeling of skin with antibodies to a panel of desmosomal and hemidesmosomal proteins was not helpful in establishing a candidate gene for mutations. Notably, all antibodies showed normal intensity staining although the pattern of staining for several desmosomal proteins was more punctate: This was the case for desmoplakin (DSP), plakoglobin, plakophilins, desmogleins, and desmocollins. In addition, labeling with keratin antibodies showed a condensed perinuclear staining, rather than a diffuse cytoplasmic pattern. The skin biopsy clue that led to the DSP gene (DSP) as the candidate gene was the ultrastructural observation that keratin filaments failed to connect

[a] St John's Institute of Dermatology, King's College London, Guy's Campus, London, UK
[b] Department of Dermatology, University Medical Centre Groningen, PO Box 30.001, 9700 RB, Groningen, The Netherlands
* Corresponding author.
E-mail address: john.mcgrath@kcl.ac.uk (J.A. McGrath).

Dermatol Clin 28 (2010) 131–135
doi:10.1016/j.det.2009.10.015

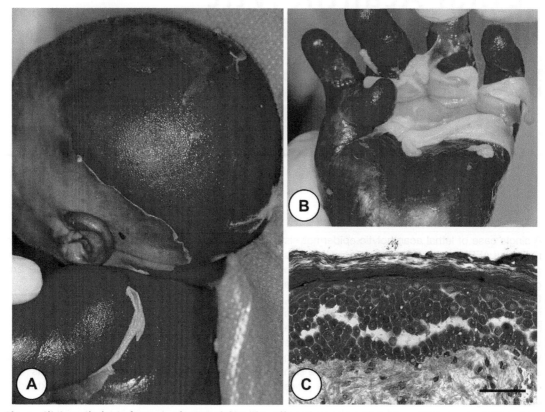

Fig. 1. Clinicopathologic features of LAEB. (*A*) In the affected neonate, there are widespread erosions, here shown on the head, upper trunk, and arm. (*B*) Degloving of the epidermis is present on the hand. (*C*) Light microscopy reveals hyperkeratosis and keratinocyte cell-cell separation with suprabasal clefting (bar = 50 μm).

properly to the inner dense plaques of desmosomes, a finding that had been observed previously in *DSP* knockout mice and in patients with nonsense/missense combinations of mutations in *DSP*, resulting in skin fragility–woolly hair syndrome (MIM607655).[2,3]

MOLECULAR PATHOLOGY OF LETHAL ACANTHOLYTIC EPIDERMOLYSIS BULLOSA

Molecular screening of *DSP* revealed two heterozygous mutations in the last exon (exon 24). The patient was a compound heterozygote for the mutations p.Arg1934X and a 2–base pair deletion, c.6370delTT, which led to a premature termination-codon 27 amino acids downstream (**Fig. 3**). Nevertheless, reverse transcription–polymerase chain reaction showed that both mutant transcripts were detectable in the proband's keratinocyte complementary DNA, indicating that neither mutation resulted in DSP haploinsufficiency by nonsense-mediated messenger RNA decay. Instead, the transcripts encoded for truncated DSP proteins (detectable by immunoblotting) that lacked the C-terminal tail. The nonsense mutation led to truncation at the end of the rod domain and thus lacked all three intermediate filament-binding subdomains (see **Fig. 3**), whereas the frameshift mutation truncated the protein shortly after the start of subdomain A and therefore lacked subdomains B and C within the keratin filament association region.[4,5] These transcripts were translated into truncated proteins, confirming that the pathology of LAEB involved truncation of the DSP tail, and that the clinicopathologic abnormalities were a direct consequence of failure of intermediate filament attachment to the desmosomal inner plaques.

DIFFERENTIAL DIAGNOSIS OF LETHAL ACANTHOLYTIC EPIDERMOLYSIS BULLOSA

Although LAEB is a distinct subtype of suprabasal epidermolysis bullosa simplex resulting from loss of the DSP tail, the clinicopathologic findings initially had a differential diagnosis. The first impression of the clinical phenotype was reminiscent of neonatal pemphigus, although the mother was not affected by pemphigus and no antidesmoglein antibodies were detected in the patient's

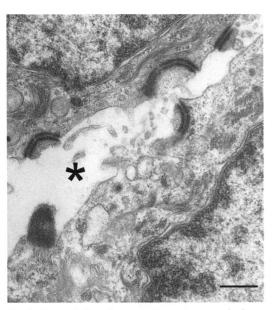

Fig. 2. Transmission electron microscopy reveals cleavage (*asterisk*) between two suprabasal keratinocytes. The plane of cleavage is within the keratinocyte at sites where keratin filaments normally insert in to desmosomes. The desmosomes appear normal in size and number but there is complete detachment from the intermediate filament network within the desmosomal plaques in each of the four desmosomes illustrated (bar = 0.1 μm).

skin or serum. Likewise, a possible diagnosis of mucosal dominant pemphigus vulgaris associated with anti-DSP auto-antibodies was excluded. Netherton's syndrome (MIM256500) was also considered to be a putative diagnosis. The differential diagnosis of the histopathology with acantholysis included Hailey-Hailey disease (benign familial pemphigus, MIM169600), although, atypically for this disorder, the adnexae were involved in the LAEB case. There was also some clinicopathologic overlap with ectodermal dysplasia–skin fragility syndrome (MIM604536), an autosomal recessive disorder of the desmosomal plaque protein plakophilin 1,[6] although the latter disorder tends to have less severe erosions and the histologic acantholysis typically involves the mid- and upper spinous layer in contrast to LAEB, in which acantholysis is most prominent in the lower epidermis.

SPECTRUM OF *DSP* MUTATIONS

Pathogenic mutations in the *DSP* gene may result in a number of distinct autosomal-dominant and autosomal-recessive disorders (see **Fig. 3**).[7,8] The first mutation reported in *DSP* was in 1999 in an autosomal-dominant pedigree

with striate palmoplantar keratoderma (MIM148700).[9] Affected individuals were shown to have DSP haploinsufficiency. In 2000, the first recessive *DSP* mutation was reported in siblings from Ecuador who had Carvajal-Huerta syndrome (MIM605676) with clinical features of striate palmoplantar keratoderma, woolly hair, and severe cardiomyopathy.[10] Subsequently, a number of other mutations in the DSP gene, both dominant and recessive, have been reported.[8] In these cases, there have been variable abnormalities in skin, hair, and heart, although some cases only have skin and hair involvement, while others just have cardiac disease and no skin phenotype. Two important issues have emerged from *DSP* mutation screening reports. First, the clinicopathologic consequences of loss-of-function mutations in the DSP gene can be variable: they may lead to nonsense-mediated RNA decay and haploinsufficiency or, alternatively, synthesis of a truncated peptide.[11] Although some *DSP* mutations have clearly been shown to result in haploinsufficiency, both mutations in the LAEB case led to the translation of truncated DSP proteins that lacked the keratin binding tail.[1] Secondly, there is the issue of which *DSP* mutations are associated with cardiomyopathy. In the LAEB case, although some cardiac abnormalities were observed, there was no histologic evidence of myocyte loss, subepicardial fibrosis, or mediomural fibrofatty replacement. However, in other individuals with desmosomal cardiomyopathy, these pathologic changes typically only tend to occur in patients over 7 years of age and therefore may be absent in the neonate. As such, it remains to be determined if cardiac dilation in LAEB is a primary consequence of the underlying desmosome anomaly (no immunohistochemistry was performed on cardiac tissue) or secondary to overfilling. DSP has two alternative splice variants: a cardiac expressed isoform (DSP1) and a more widely expressed isoform (DSP2),[12] and the expanding *DSP* mutation database indicates that the site and nature of the pathogenic mutations in the DSP isoforms can have important prognostic implications for the presence, severity, and age of onset of cardiac disease, or lack thereof.[13–17] In genodermatoses arising from *DSP* mutations, the clinical phenotype can resemble other genetic or acquired dermatoses and a comprehensive understanding of the molecular pathology and its effects on different transcripts of *DSP* and their expression in various tissues is fundamental in determining an accurate clinical

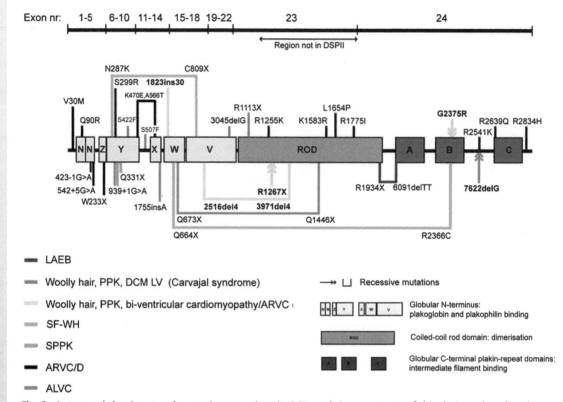

Fig. 3. Autosomal-dominant and -recessive mutations in *DSP* result in a spectrum of skin, hair, and cardiac disease phenotypes. The LAEB mutations are highlighted in red. These mutations lead to truncation of the DSP protein, which lacks the keratin-binding region (domains A, B, and C). The assorted phenotypes are illustrated in different colors. The single lines represent dominant mutations. The double arrowheads represent homozygous, recessive mutations. Joined lines represent compound heterozygosity (recessive). ALVC, arrthymogenic left ventricular cardiomyopathy; ARVC/D, arrhthymogenic right ventricular cardiomyopathy/dysplasia; DCM, dilated cardiomyopathy; LV, left ventricle; PPK, palmoplantar keratoderma; SF-WH, skin fragility–woolly hair; SPPK, striate palmoplantar keratoderma. (*From* Bolling MC, Jonkman MF. Skin and heart: une liaison dangereuse. Exp Dermatol 2009;18:658–68; with permission.)

diagnosis and, most importantly, a likely prognosis for the patient.

SUMMARY

DSP mutations result in a spectrum of autosomal-dominant and autosomal-recessive disorders that have variable skin, hair, and heart anomalies. Within this group of diseases a specific subtype is LAEB, an autosomal-recessive disorder resulting from loss-of-function mutations that lead to truncation of the DSP protein rather than messenger RNA decay. The lack of a DSP tail results in impaired attachment between the keratin intermediate filaments and the desmosomal inner plaque. This leads to profound fragility with acantholysis in several epithelial tissues. Although only a single case of LAEB has been described, the clinicopathologic abnormalities clearly attest to the key role of certain

subdomains of DSP in keratinocyte biology and human disease.

REFERENCES

1. Jonkman MF, Pasmooij AM, Pasmans SG, et al. Loss of desmoplakin tail causes lethal acantholytic epidermolysis bullosa. Am J Hum Genet 2005;77:653–60.
2. Gallicano GI, Kouklis P, Bauer C, et al. Desmoplakin is required early in development for assembly of desmosomes and cystoskeletal linkage. J Cell Biol 1998;143:2009–22.
3. Whittock NV, Wan H, Morley SM, et al. Compound heterozygosity for nonsense and missense mutations in desmoplakin underlies skin fragility/woolly hair syndrome. J Invest Dermatol 2002;118:232–8.
4. Choi HJ, Park-Snyder S, Pascoe LT, et al. Structures of two intermediate filament-binding fragments of

desmoplakin reveal a unique repeat motif structure. Nat Struct Biol 2002;9:612–20.

5. Fontao L, Favre B, Riou S, et al. Interaction of the bullous pemphigoid antigen 1 (BP230) and desmoplakin with intermediate filaments is mediated by distinct sequences within their COOH terminus. Mol Biol Cell 2003;14:1977–92.

6. McGrath JA, McMillan JR, Shemanko CS, et al. Mutations in the plakophilin 1 gene result in ectodermal dysplasia/skin fragility syndrome. Nat Genet 1997;17:240–4.

7. Lai-Cheong, Wessagowit V, McGrath JA. Molecular abnormalities of the desmosomal protein desmoplakin in human disease. Clin Exp Dermatol 2005;30: 261–6.

8. Lai-Cheong JE, Arita K, McGrath JA. Genetic diseases of junctions. J Invest Dermatol 2007;127: 2713–25.

9. Armstrong DK, McKenna KE, Purkis PE, et al. Haploinsufficiency of desmoplakin causes a striate subtype of palmoplantar keratoderma. Hum Mol Genet 1999;8:143–8.

10. Norgett EE, Hatsell SJ, Carvajal-Huerta L, et al. Recessive mutation in desmoplakin disrupts desmoplakin-intermediate filament interactions and causes dilated cardiomyopathy, woolly hair and keratoderma. Hum Mol Genet 2000;9:2761–6.

11. Nagy E, Maquat LE. A rule for termination-codon position within intron-containing genes: when nonsense affects RNA abundance. Trends Biochem Sci 1998;23:198–9.

12. Green KJ, Goldman RD, Chisholm RL. Isolation of cDNAs encoding desmosomal plaque proteins: evidence that bovine desmoplakins I and II are derived from two mRNAs and a single gene. Proc Natl Acad Sci U S A 1998;85:2613–7.

13. Alcalai R, Metzger S, Rosenheck S, et al. A recessive mutation in desmoplakin causes arrhythmogenic right ventricular dysplasia, skin disorder and woolly hair. J Am Coll Cardiol 2003;42:319–27.

14. Uzumcu A, Norgett EE, Dindar A, et al. Loss of desmoplakin isoform I causes early onset cardiomyopathy and heart failure in a Naxos-like syndrome. J Med Genet 2006;43:e5.

15. Tanaka A, Lai-Cheong JE, Café ME, et al. Novel truncating mutations in PKP1 and DSP cause similar skin phenotypes in two Brazilian families. Br J Dermatol 2009;160:692–7.

16. Van Tintelen JP, Hofstra RM, Wiesfeld AC, et al. Molecular genetics of arrhythmogenic right ventricular cardiomyopathy: emerging horizon? Curr Opin Cardiol 2007;22:185–92.

17. Bolling MC, Jonkman MF. Skin and heart: une liaison dangereuse. Exp Dermatol 2009;18:658–68.

Animal Models of Epidermolysis Bullosa

Ken Natsuga, MD*, Satoru Shinkuma, MD,
Wataru Nishie, MD, PhD, Hiroshi Shimizu, MD, PhD

KEYWORDS

- Epidermolysis bullosa • Transgenic mice
- Knock-out mice • Knock-in mice

For more than 2 decades, animal models have been used to clarify the pathogenic mechanisms of human diseases and develop new therapeutics for these diseases. Several therapies for human diseases have become available through trials using animal models.

Epidermolysis bullosa (EB) is one of the most severe inherited skin disorders, whose effective treatments have not been fully available. EB is characterized by abnormalities of the proteins that consist of the dermoepidermal junction (DEJ). EB has been classified into three major subtypes according to the level of skin cleavage: EB simplex (EBS), junctional EB (JEB), and dystrophic EB (DEB). To date, 13 genes have been shown to cause EB phenotype.[1,2] After the discovery of the causative genes responsible for each EB subtype, many researchers have tried to develop EB animal models by genetically manipulating the corresponding genes.[3]

CHARACTERIZATION OF ANIMAL MODELS OF EPIDERMOLYSIS BULLOSA, AND THERAPEUTIC EXPERIMENTS USING THESE MODELS

Table 1 summarizes previously described EB animal models whose genetic abnormalities are clarified. The characteristics of each EB animal model and therapeutic experiments using the models are described in this section.

Junctional Epidermolysis Bullosa

Six genes, COL17A1, LAMA3, LAMB3, LAMC2, ITGA6, and ITGB4, have been identified as responsible for the JEB phenotype. Twelve JEB animal models have been developed, although most of the models die perinatally. Recently, the authors' group developed a Col17a1 knock-out (KO) mice that can survive for approximately 12 months.[15]

Defective type XVII collagen (COL17) encoded by mutated COL17A1 causes non-Herlitz JEB (nH-JEB).[27,28] The authors recently developed Col17a1 KO mice whose blistering phenotype is similar to that of human nH-JEB.[15] Notably, 20% of the Col17a1 KO mice exhibited long survival, allowing for the therapeutic experiments, including bone marrow transplantation, cell therapy, protein therapy, and gene therapy.[15] The authors described transgenic rescue experiments for Col17a1 KO mice using human COL17A1 cDNA transgenic mice driven under the keratin-14 promoter, and the rescued mice were born without any skin defects and were able to reacquire reproductive ability.[15] In addition, the tooth abnormalities seen in Col17a1 KO mice were also correctable after incorporation of human COL17A1 cDNA.[29]

Herlitz JEB (H-JEB) is a severe form of EB with short-term survival expectancy. H-JEB is caused by mutations in the genes encoding laminin 332, which consists of the laminin $\alpha 3$, $\beta 3$, and $\gamma 2$ chains (LAMA3/LAMB3/LAMC2).[28,30–35] Lama3 and Lamc2 KO mouse models have been generated.[17,19] Furthermore, spontaneous mutant dog,[16] horse,[20,21] and mouse[18] models whose laminin genes are inactivated have also been described. Those animal models exhibited severe skin detachment with perinatal lethality. Among

---

Department of Dermatology, Hokkaido University Graduate School of Medicine, North 15 West 7, Sapporo 060-8638, Japan
* Corresponding author.
E-mail address: natsuga@med.hokudai.ac.jp (K. Natsuga).

Dermatol Clin 28 (2010) 137–142
doi:10.1016/j.det.2009.10.016

Table 1
Animal models of epidermolysis bullosa

Disease	Causative Gene	Species	Type	Survival	References
EBS	KRT5	Mouse	KO	Neonatal death	4
EBS	KRT14	Mouse	Tg	Neonatal death	5
EBS	KRT14	Mouse	KO	Neonatal death	6
EBS	KRT14	Mouse	KI	Neonatal death	7
EBS	KRT14	Mouse	KI (an inducible model)	Not mentioned	7
EBS-MD/EBS-PA	PLEC1	Mouse	KO	Neonatal death	8
EBS-MD/EBS-PA	PLEC1	Mouse	Conditional KO	Neonatal death	9
JEB-PA	ITGA6	Mouse	KO	Neonatal death	10
JEB-PA	ITGB4	Mouse	KO	Neonatal death	11
JEB-PA	ITGB4	Mouse	KO	Neonatal death	12
JEB-PA	ITGB4	Mouse	Partial ablation (expressing ectodomain of $\beta4$ integrin)	Neonatal death	13
JEB-PA	ITGB4	Mouse	Conditional KO	Not mentioned	14
nH-JEB	COL17A1	Mouse	KO	Prolonged survival in 20% of mice	15
nH-JEB	LAMA3	Dog	Naturally occurring	Not mentioned	16
H-JEB	LAMA3	Mouse	KO	Neonatal death	17
H-JEB	LAMB3	Mouse	Naturally occurring	Neonatal death	18
H-JEB	LAMC2	Mouse	KO	Neonatal death	19
H-JEB	LAMC2	Horse	Naturally occurring	Not mentioned	20
H-JEB	LAMC2	Horse	Naturally occurring	Not mentioned	21
RDEB-sev gen	COL7A1	Mouse	KO	Neonatal death	22
RDEB-O	COL7A1	Dog	Naturally occurring	Not mentioned	23
RDEB-O	COL7A1	Mouse	Hypomorphic	Prolonged survival	24
RDEB-O	COL7A1	Mouse	KO with transgenic rescue using mutated human cDNA	Prolonged survival	25
Kindler syndrome	FERMT1	Mouse	KO	Neonatal death	26

Abbreviations: EBS, epidermolysis bullosa simplex; EBS-MD, epidermolysis bullosa simplex with muscular dystrophy; EBS-PA, epidermolysis bullosa simplex with pyloric atresia; H-JEB, Herlitz junctional epidermolysis bullosa; JEB, junctional epidermolysis bullosa; JEB-PA, junctional epidermolysis bullosa with pyloric atresia; KI, knock-in; KO, knock-out; nH-JEB, non-Herlitz JEB; RDEB, recessive dystrophic epidermolysis bullosa; RDEB-O, generalized other recessive dystrophic epidermolysis bullosa; RDEB-sev gen, severe generalized recessive dystrophic epidermolysis bullosa; Tg, transgenic.

them, Swiatek and colleagues[18] reported spontaneous mutant mice in which the defective $\beta3$ chain of laminin-332 resulted from insertion of an intracisternal-A particle between the exon/intron junction of *Lamb3* (Lamb3[IAP] mutant).[18]

Schneider and colleagues[36] described prenatal intra-amniotic human *LAMB3* cDNA delivery into LamB3[IAP] mutant mice using adenovirus and adeno-associated virus vectors.[36] They showed that the defective $\beta3$ chain of laminin-332 was expressed in the skin of treated mice, although they found only a minor increase of the lifespan of these mice.[36]

JEB with pyloric atresia (JEB-PA) is caused by mutations in the genes encoding $\alpha6$ integrin or $\beta4$ integrin (*ITGA6/ITGB4*).[28,37,38] $\alpha6$ or $\beta4$ integrin null mice exhibited severe skin detachment with perinatal lethality.[10–12] Sonnenberg and colleagues[39] generated human *ITGB4* cDNA transgenic mice driven under keratin-5 promoter and then tried transgenic rescue for *Itgb4* KO mice using those transgenic mice, although the rescued mice still exhibited skin fragility and high mortality.[39]

The same group generated *Itgb4* conditional knock-out mice, in which *Itgb4* was inactivated only in a small area of the skin. Those mice did not have obvious skin defects, although microscopy showed a small number of blisters in which β4 integrin had been deleted.[14] Giancotti and colleagues[13] generated mice carrying targeted deletion of the β4 integrin cytoplasmic domain.[13] Although those mice expressed truncated extracellular domain β4 integrin protein, their phenotypes were almost the same as mice with complete loss of β4 integrin.[13]

Dystrophic Epidermolysis Bullosa

Mutations in the gene encoding type VII collagen (*COL7A1*) are responsible for dystrophic EB (DEB).[40–42] *Col7a1* KO mice were developed as a severe generalized recessive DEB (RDEB) model by Uitto and colleagues.[22] *Col7a1* KO mice exhibited severe skin detachment with perinatal lethality.[22] Chen and colleagues[43] injected recombinant human type VII collagen (COL7) protein into *Col7a1* KO mice and found that the injected human COL7 was incorporated into the DEJ and that the treated mice exhibited longer survival rates than the controls.[43]

Tamai and colleagues[44] reported that embryonic transplantation with bone marrow cells derived from green fluorescent protein (GFP) transgenic mice through vitelline vein–alleviated skin phenotypes of *Col7a1* KO mice.[44] Tolar and colleagues[45] also showed that administration of hematopoietic stem-cell–enriched bone marrow cells derived from GFP transgenic mice ameliorated skin fragility and reduced lethality of newborn *Col7a1* KO mice.[45] However, the short survival time in which the treatment can show a significant effect in *Col7a1* KO mice is still an obstacle to new therapeutics for RDEB.

Bruckner-Tuderman and colleagues[24] developed a DEB hypomorphic mouse model in which the amount of mouse COL7 in skin was approximately 10% of that of wild-type mice and those mice had a prolonged survival.[24] Using this hypomorphic mouse model, they showed that injection of cultured fibroblasts derived from wild-type mice increased the expression of mouse COL7 at the DEJ above the treated area in the hypomorphic mouse skin.[24,46]

The authors' group showed transgenic rescue of the previously described *Col7a1* KO mouse using two transgenic mouse models comprising human *COL7A1* cDNA under keratin-14 promoter or type I collagen promoter.[22,25] They also used novel methods to develop a milder blistering phenotype in humanized RDEB model mice. They generated human *COL7A1* transgenic mice with a premature termination codon (PTC) expressing truncated human COL7 protein.[25] Then, transgenic rescue of *Col7a1* KO mice using PTC-causing human *COL7A1* transgenic mice resulted in a significantly milder clinical skin blistering manifestation resembling generalized other RDEB and prolonged survival.[25]

Epidermolysis Bullosa Simplex

Mutations in genes encoding keratin 5 and 14 (*KRT5/KRT14*) have been known to cause EBS, where an abnormal keratin network leads to blister formation.[47,48] Magin and colleagues[4] developed *Krt5* KO mice in which severe skin detachment and perinatal death were noted.[4] Fuchs and colleagues[5] generated transgenic mice expressing a truncated human keratin 14 protein.[5] Those mice exhibited severe skin detachment from the dominant negative effects of aberrantly expressed protein.[5] The same group generated *Krt14* KO mice that exhibited a milder phenotype than *Krt5* KO mice.[6] Although keratin-null mice showed skin fragility,[4,6] their mechanism of blister formation is different from that of human patients who have EBS, in which aberrant keratin protein from *KRT5/14* missense mutations interferes with the structural assembly of keratin filaments. Roop and colleagues[7] adopted a knock-in strategy to represent the dominant negative effects of abnormal protein encoded by *Krt14* harboring a missense mutation in the knock-in mice.[7] They showed that one amino acid substitution is enough to cause an EBS disease phenotype in the knock-in mice.[7] Furthermore, they generated an inducible animal model of EBS, in which topical application of a chemical inducer allows focal activation of a mutant keratin 14 protein in the epidermis of the treated area.[7]

Mutations in the gene encoding plectin (*PLEC1*) are responsible for EBS with muscular dystrophy[49–51] and EBS with pyloric atresia.[52,53] Wiche and colleagues[8] reported that mice with targeted inactivation of *Plec1* exhibited severe skin fragility and perinatal death.[8] They also succeeded in obtaining mice with conditional ablation of *Plec1* in the stratified epithelia,[9] although those mice also showed markedly short survival.[9]

Kindler Syndrome

The Third International Consensus Meeting on Diagnosis and Classification of EB proposed to include Kindler syndrome within the category of EB.[2] Kindler syndrome is caused by mutations in the gene encoding Kindlin-1 or fermitin family homolog protein 1 (FFH1, *FERMT1, KIND1*).[54] Targeted ablation of *Fermt1* failed to show any skin fragility phenotype in mice, although skin specimens from those mice showed skin atrophy.[26]

FUTURE DIRECTIONS

Most EB subtypes already have been represented as animal models. Although perinatal death was a major obstacle in using genetically engineered EB animal models to develop new therapeutic strategies, several methods have been successful at overcoming the problem of short survival, and longer surviving animal models are suitable to observe the efficacy of therapeutic interventions. Several transgenic rescue trials have shown that successfully delivered human transgenes are able to function in vivo. In addition, cell therapy and protein replenishment used in many animal models have potential as future therapeutic options for patients who have EB.

RNA interference is a promising way to treat the dominant negative effects of mutated keratin genes in EBS and considerable work is underway in this field. In the future, safe, and efficient gene delivery systems will be developed for EB gene therapy to benefit patients. Researchers and clinicians should continue to explore new therapeutic options using animal models and test their efficacy for application to human diseases.

ACKNOWLEDGMENTS

We thank Dr James R. McMillan for reviewing and commenting on this manuscript and Mr Michael O'Connell for his proofreading.

REFERENCES

1. Fine JD, Eady RA, Bauer EA, et al. Revised classification system for inherited epidermolysis bullosa: report of the Second International Consensus Meeting on diagnosis and classification of epidermolysis bullosa. J Am Acad Dermatol 2000;42(6):1051–66.
2. Fine JD, Eady RA, Bauer EA, et al. The classification of inherited epidermolysis bullosa (EB): report of the Third International Consensus Meeting on diagnosis and classification of EB. J Am Acad Dermatol 2008;58(6):931–50.
3. Jiang QJ, Uitto J. Animal models of epidermolysis bullosa–targets for gene therapy. J Invest Dermatol 2005;124(3):xi–xiii.
4. Peters B, Kirfel J, Bussow H, et al. Complete cytolysis and neonatal lethality in keratin 5 knockout mice reveal its fundamental role in skin integrity and in epidermolysis bullosa simplex. Mol Biol Cell 2001;12(6):1775–89.
5. Vassar R, Coulombe PA, Degenstein L, et al. Mutant keratin expression in transgenic mice causes marked abnormalities resembling a human genetic skin disease. Cell 1991;64(2):365–80.
6. Lloyd C, Yu QC, Cheng J, et al. The basal keratin network of stratified squamous epithelia: defining K15 function in the absence of K14. J Cell Biol 1995;129(5):1329–44.
7. Cao T, Longley MA, Wang XJ, et al. An inducible mouse model for epidermolysis bullosa simplex: implications for gene therapy. J Cell Biol 2001;152(3):651–6.
8. Andra K, Lassmann H, Bittner R, et al. Targeted inactivation of plectin reveals essential function in maintaining the integrity of skin, muscle, and heart cytoarchitecture. Genes Dev 1997;11(23):3143–56.
9. Ackerl R, Walko G, Fuchs P, et al. Conditional targeting of plectin in prenatal and adult mouse stratified epithelia causes keratinocyte fragility and lesional epidermal barrier defects. J Cell Sci 2007;120(Pt 14):2435–43.
10. Georges-Labouesse E, Messaddeq N, Yehia G, et al. Absence of integrin alpha 6 leads to epidermolysis bullosa and neonatal death in mice. Nat Genet 1996;13(3):370–3.
11. Dowling J, Yu QC, Fuchs E. Beta4 integrin is required for hemidesmosome formation, cell adhesion and cell survival. J Cell Biol 1996;134(2):559–72.
12. van der Neut R, Krimpenfort P, Calafat J, et al. Epithelial detachment due to absence of hemidesmosomes in integrin beta 4 null mice. Nat Genet 1996;13(3):366–9.
13. Murgia C, Blaikie P, Kim N, et al. Cell cycle and adhesion defects in mice carrying a targeted deletion of the integrin beta4 cytoplasmic domain. EMBO J 1998;17(14):3940–51.
14. Raymond K, Kreft M, Janssen H, et al. Keratinocytes display normal proliferation, survival and differentiation in conditional beta4-integrin knockout mice. J Cell Sci 2005;118(Pt 5):1045–60.
15. Nishie W, Sawamura D, Goto M, et al. Humanization of autoantigen. Nat Med 2007;13(3):378–83.
16. Capt A, Spirito F, Guaguere E, et al. Inherited junctional epidermolysis bullosa in the German Pointer: establishment of a large animal model. J Invest Dermatol 2005;124(3):530–5.
17. Ryan MC, Lee K, Miyashita Y, et al. Targeted disruption of the LAMA3 gene in mice reveals abnormalities in survival and late stage differentiation of epithelial cells. J Cell Biol 1999;145(6):1309–23.
18. Kuster JE, Guarnieri MH, Ault JG, et al. IAP insertion in the murine LamB3 gene results in junctional epidermolysis bullosa. Mamm Genome 1997;8(9):673–81.

19. Meng X, Klement JF, Leperi DA, et al. Targeted inactivation of murine laminin gamma2-chain gene recapitulates human junctional epidermolysis bullosa. J Invest Dermatol 2003;121(4):720–31.

20. Spirito F, Charlesworth A, Linder K, et al. Animal models for skin blistering conditions: absence of laminin 5 causes hereditary junctional mechanobullous disease in the Belgian horse. J Invest Dermatol 2002;119(3):684–91.

21. Milenkovic D, Chaffaux S, Taourit S, et al. A mutation in the LAMC2 gene causes the Herlitz junctional epidermolysis bullosa (H-JEB) in two French draft horse breeds. Genet Sel Evol 2003;35(2):249–56.

22. Heinonen S, Mannikko M, Klement JF, et al. Targeted inactivation of the type VII collagen gene (Col7a1) in mice results in severe blistering phenotype: a model for recessive dystrophic epidermolysis bullosa. J Cell Sci 1999;112(Pt 21):3641–8.

23. Baldeschi C, Gache Y, Rattenholl A, et al. Genetic correction of canine dystrophic epidermolysis bullosa mediated by retroviral vectors. Hum Mol Genet 2003;12(15):1897–905.

24. Fritsch A, Loeckermann S, Kern JS, et al. A hypomorphic mouse model of dystrophic epidermolysis bullosa reveals mechanisms of disease and response to fibroblast therapy. J Clin Invest 2008; 118(5):1669–79.

25. Ito K, Sawamura D, Nishie W, et al. Keratinocyte-/fibroblast-targeted rescue of Col7a1 disrupted mice and generation of an exact dystrophic epidermolysis bullosa model using a human COL7A1 mutation. Am J Pathol, in press.

26. Ussar S, Moser M, Widmaier M, et al. Loss of Kindlin-1 causes skin atrophy and lethal neonatal intestinal epithelial dysfunction. PLoS Genet 2008;4(12): e1000289.

27. McGrath JA, Gatalica B, Christiano AM, et al. Mutations in the 180-kD bullous pemphigoid antigen (BPAG2), a hemidesmosomal transmembrane collagen (COL17A1), in generalized atrophic benign epidermolysis bullosa. Nat Genet 1995;11(1):83–6.

28. Varki R, Sadowski S, Pfendner E, et al. Epidermolysis bullosa. I. Molecular genetics of the junctional and hemidesmosomal variants. J Med Genet 2006; 43(8):641–52.

29. Asaka T, Akiyama M, Domon T, et al. Type XVII collagen is a key player in tooth enamel formation. Am J Pathol 2009;174(1):91–100.

30. Kivirikko S, McGrath JA, Baudoin C, et al. A homozygous nonsense mutation in the alpha 3 chain gene of laminin 5 (LAMA3) in lethal (Herlitz) junctional epidermolysis bullosa. Hum Mol Genet 1995;4(5):959–62.

31. McGrath JA, Kivirikko S, Ciatti S, et al. A homozygous nonsense mutation in the alpha 3 chain gene of laminin 5 (LAMA3) in Herlitz junctional epidermolysis bullosa: prenatal exclusion in a fetus at risk. Genomics 1995;29(1):282–4.

32. Vidal F, Baudoin C, Miquel C, et al. Cloning of the laminin alpha 3 chain gene (LAMA3) and identification of a homozygous deletion in a patient with Herlitz junctional epidermolysis bullosa. Genomics 1995;30(2):273–80.

33. Pulkkinen L, Christiano AM, Gerecke D, et al. A homozygous nonsense mutation in the beta 3 chain gene of laminin 5 (LAMB3) in Herlitz junctional epidermolysis bullosa. Genomics 1994;24(2):357–60.

34. Aberdam D, Galliano MF, Vailly J, et al. Herlitz's junctional epidermolysis bullosa is linked to mutations in the gene (LAMC2) for the gamma 2 subunit of nicein/kalinin (LAMININ-5). Nat Genet 1994;6(3): 299–304.

35. Pulkkinen L, Christiano AM, Airenne T, et al. Mutations in the gamma 2 chain gene (LAMC2) of kalinin/laminin 5 in the junctional forms of epidermolysis bullosa. Nat Genet 1994;6(3):293–7.

36. Muhle C, Neuner A, Park J, et al. Evaluation of prenatal intra-amniotic LAMB3 gene delivery in a mouse model of Herlitz disease. Gene Ther 2006;13(23):1665–76.

37. Ruzzi L, Gagnoux-Palacios L, Pinola M, et al. A homozygous mutation in the integrin alpha6 gene in junctional epidermolysis bullosa with pyloric atresia. J Clin Invest 1997;99(12):2826–31.

38. Vidal F, Aberdam D, Miquel C, et al. Integrin beta 4 mutations associated with junctional epidermolysis bullosa with pyloric atresia. Nat Genet 1995;10(2): 229–34.

39. van der Neut R, Cachaco AS, Thorsteinsdottir S, et al. Partial rescue of epithelial phenotype in integrin beta4 null mice by a keratin-5 promoter driven human integrin beta4 transgene. J Cell Sci 1999; 112(Pt 22):3911–22.

40. Christiano AM, Greenspan DS, Hoffman GG, et al. A missense mutation in type VII collagen in two affected siblings with recessive dystrophic epidermolysis bullosa. Nat Genet 1993;4(1):62–6.

41. Hilal L, Rochat A, Duquesnoy P, et al. A homozygous insertion-deletion in the type VII collagen gene (COL7A1) in Hallopeau-Siemens dystrophic epidermolysis bullosa. Nat Genet 1993;5(3):287–93.

42. Varki R, Sadowski S, Uitto J, et al. Epidermolysis bullosa. II. Type VII collagen mutations and phenotype-genotype correlations in the dystrophic subtypes. J Med Genet 2007;44(3):181–92.

43. Remington J, Wang X, Hou Y, et al. Injection of recombinant human type VII collagen corrects the disease phenotype in a murine model of dystrophic epidermolysis bullosa. Mol Ther 2009;17(1): 26–33.

44. Chino T, Tamai K, Yamazaki T, et al. Bone marrow cell transfer into fetal circulation can ameliorate genetic skin diseases by providing fibroblasts to the skin and inducing immune tolerance. Am J Pathol 2008; 173(3):803–14.

45. Tolar J, Ishida-Yamamoto A, Riddle M, et al. Amelioration of epidermolysis bullosa by transfer of wild-type bone marrow cells. Blood 2009;113(5): 1167–74.

46. Kern JS, Loeckermann S, Fritsch A, et al. Mechanisms of fibroblast cell therapy for dystrophic epidermolysis bullosa: high stability of collagen VII favors long-term skin integrity. Mol Ther 2009;17:1605–15.

47. Lane EB, Rugg EL, Navsaria H, et al. A mutation in the conserved helix termination peptide of keratin 5 in hereditary skin blistering. Nature 1992; 356(6366):244–6.

48. Coulombe PA, Hutton ME, Letai A, et al. Point mutations in human keratin 14 genes of epidermolysis bullosa simplex patients: genetic and functional analyses. Cell 1991;66(6):1301–11.

49. Gache Y, Chavanas S, Lacour JP, et al. Defective expression of plectin/HD1 in epidermolysis bullosa simplex with muscular dystrophy. J Clin Invest 1996;97(10):2289–98.

50. McLean WH, Pulkkinen L, Smith FJ, et al. Loss of plectin causes epidermolysis bullosa with muscular dystrophy: cDNA cloning and genomic organization. Genes Dev 1996;10(14):1724–35.

51. Smith FJ, Eady RA, Leigh IM, et al. Plectin deficiency results in muscular dystrophy with epidermolysis bullosa. Nat Genet 1996;13(4):450–7.

52. Nakamura H, Sawamura D, Goto M, et al. Epidermolysis bullosa simplex associated with pyloric atresia is a novel clinical subtype caused by mutations in the plectin gene (PLEC1). J Mol Diagn 2005;7(1):28–35.

53. Pfendner E, Uitto J. Plectin gene mutations can cause epidermolysis bullosa with pyloric atresia. J Invest Dermatol 2005;124(1):111–5.

54. Siegel DH, Ashton GH, Penagos HG, et al. Loss of kindlin-1, a human homolog of the Caenorhabditis elegans actin-extracellular-matrix linker protein UNC-112, causes Kindler syndrome. Am J Hum Genet 2003;73(1):174–87.

Ophthalmic Involvement in Inherited Epidermolysis Bullosa

Edwin C. Figueira, MBBS, MS (Ophth)[a],*,
Dédée F. Murrell, MA, BMBCh, FAAD, MD[b],
Minas T. Coroneo, MS, FRANZCO[a,c]

KEYWORDS

• Epidermolysis bullosa • Amblyopia • Cornea

Eye involvement in inherited epidermolysis bullosa (EB) can occur as a spectrum of symptoms and signs, ranging from mild conjunctival irritation to severe cicatrisation of the eyelids, cornea, and the conjunctiva as reviewed in published case reports and case series.[1,2] The ocular surface formed by the conjunctiva and the cornea and covered by the protective eyelids is derived embryonically from the surface ectoderm like the skin. There are various biochemical and ultrastructural similarities common to the skin and cornea, particularly the plasma membrane and the epidermal–dermal basement membrane zone of the two stratified epithelia.[3] Careful ophthalmologic examination should become an integral part of the management of all patients with inherited EB. Ocular and adnexal abnormalities may be acute or chronic, symptomatic or asymptomatic, and they can be of variable clinical severity. Ocular involvement in EB can occur at any age (even as early as 1 month of age).[4] Common ocular symptoms and signs in EB described are red watery eyes,[5] photophobia,[3,6] ocular pain,[3,4,6] conjunctival injection,[7] conjunctival edema,[5] blepharoconjunctivitis,[1,6,8] exposure keratopathy,[9–11] corneal erosions, or abrasions.[1,6,8,10–14] Ophthalmologists have a major role in the multidisciplinary approach in treating EB by preventing and controlling complications that occur in the eye.

SUMMARY OF REPORTS AND STUDIES REPORTING ON THE FREQUENCY OF OCULAR INVOLVEMENT

Common ocular involvement described in inherited EB includes corneal abrasions, corneal scars, corneal pannus, eyelid blisters or ectropion, conjunctival blisters, and symblephara.[11,13,15] Other ocular associations reported in EB include cataracts, cornea plana, sclerocornea, refractive errors, amblyopia, lacrimal duct obstruction, strabismus, lens subluxation, posterior vitreous detachment.

The first publication report of ocular involvement in inherited EB was in 1904.[16] Later, there were limited case reports[4,6,7,9,10,12,14,17–23] and case series[1,5,8,11,13] suggesting that various forms of involvement of the ocular surface and its adnexa can occur in some subtypes of inherited EB. Very few large series of EB patients have been studied. One of the largest involved 181 consecutive patients who were seen and given full ophthalmologic examination at London's Great Ormond Street Children's Hospital from 1980 to 1996.[11] The overall frequency of ocular complications was 12%, 40%, 4%, and 51% in their children with EBs, junctional epidermolysis bullosa (JEB), dominant dystrophic EB (DDEB), and recessive dystrophic EB (RDEB), respectively. The only

---

[a] Department of Ophthalmology, Prince Of Wales Hospital, Randwick, NSW 2031, Australia
[b] Department of Dermatology, St George Hospital, University of NSW, Gray Street, Kogarah, Sydney, NSW 2217, Australia
[c] University of New South Wales, Randwick, Sydney, NSW 2031, Australia
* Corresponding author.
E-mail address: e_c_figueira@hotmail.com (E.C. Figueira).

Dermatol Clin 28 (2010) 143–152
doi:10.1016/j.det.2009.10.021

derm.theclinics.com

finding seen in a single patient with DDEB was conjunctival blistering. The only findings in EBs were present in those having the usually clinically severe Dowling-Meara subtype. Of these, 12% had peripheral corneal vascularization; eyelid blistering and corneal abrasions also were noted. In contrast, 14% of RDEB patients had a history of recurrent ocular erosions; 68% had some type of corneal complication (eg, abrasions, scarring, or pannus formation). Eight percent had exposure keratitis with ectropions of both upper and lower lids; 24% had conjunctival involvement, and 14% had eyelid blisters. The most common findings in their JEB patients were corneal scarring (20%) and exposure keratopathy (33%). Miscellaneous ocular findings in rare patients included amblyopia, squints, lacrimal punctal occlusion, punctal papilloma of the eyelid, subconjunctival hemorrhage, pseudopterygia, microophthalmos, and anterior polar cataract with astigmatism. Lin and colleagues[13] reported findings in 204 patients with EB seen at Rockefeller University (New York) from 1986 to 1993. Findings were similar in type and frequency to those reported by Tong and associates.[11] Gans reported the findings in 78 EB patients studied in nonlongitudinal fashion at Washington University (St Louis) from 1979 to 1986.[1] The most common finding was the presence of corneal erosions in 55.5% of patients with junctional epidermolysis bullosa-Herlitz type (JEB-H) and 52.9% of patients with RDEB. About 25% of the RDEB patients had evidence of corneal scarring; blepharitis and eyelid blistering each occurred in about 20% of patients.

Before the reports of the National EB Registry (NEBR) database, the case series reported and published indicated the frequencies of ocular involvement in inherited EB as depicted in **Table 1**.

The 3280 consecutively enrolled patients in the NEBR comprise the largest cohort of EB patients ever assembled in the world and reflect up to 16 years of methodical clinical follow-up. Although the primary study was a cross-sectional one, most patients had some longitudinal data collection also. About one eighth of the entire study population also was selected randomly for formal prospective evaluation every 2 years. The only significant longitudinal data reported of ocular involvement in inherited EB have been the data that are extrapolated from the NEBR, an epidemiologic project established in 1986 by the National Institutes of Health (NIH).[24] This registry contains both cross-sectional and longitudinal data of 3280 EB patients that are aimed at determining the risk of selected extracutaneous affection in inherited EB. The demographics of the study population included in the database closely resembled

the general American population.[25] The data reported by the NEBR database were significant, as the distribution of patients defined by major EB types and subtypes were observed to closely mimic data of reported cohorts of EB patients elsewhere in the world. Therefore, the NEBR data results are applicable to EB patients universally. Fine and colleagues were able to perform a rigorous analysis of the NEBR's database, thereby enabling them to precisely measure the impact of ocular disease, by accurately estimating cumulative lifetime risk of corneal blistering, erosion, and scarring, for each of the major types and subtypes of inherited EB (**Table 2**).

The distribution of patients by major EB type and subtype also was shown to closely mimic that seen within much smaller cohorts of EB patients elsewhere in the world, suggesting that these data are applicable to EB patients everywhere. Rigorous analysis of the NEBR registry's database has allowed for more precise measurement of the impact of ocular disease, to include accurate estimation of the cumulative lifetime risk of corneal blistering, erosion, and scarring, for each of the major types and subtypes of inherited EB. The NEBR registry reported the ocular abnormalities secondary to EB as described in **Table 3**.

OCULAR TISSUE-WISE COMPLICATIONS

The most common ocular finding in EB patients as reported by the NEBR study group was corneal blisters in the form of intact vesicles or secondary erosions. These blisters or erosions most often were seen in the severe forms of EB, that is JEB and recessive DEB. The corneal blisters were seen more commonly in the more severe JEB subset, Herlitz subset of severe JEB disease with 50% of these patients involved. Around 25% of all non-Herlitz JEB patients had findings suggestive of corneal blistering. Around 66% of the recessive dystrophic epidermolysis bullosa-Hallopeau-Siemens type (RDEB-HS) patients and 33% each of the recessive dystrophic epidermolysis bullosa-non Hallopeau-Siemens type (RDEB-nHS), and RDEB-I patients were reported to have experienced at least one episode of corneal blisters or erosions. Corneal blistering was reported to be low in other forms of EB, with values ranging from 0.92% (in the mildest EB subtype, Weber-Cockayne EBs) to 6.19% (in the most severe EBs subtype, Dowling-Meara disease). Corneal scarring rates were lower than those of corneal blisters and erosions across all major EB types and subtypes, which may be due to the fact that blistering may have occurred only once or infrequently or if it was self-limited in its duration. Corneal

Table 1
Eye involvement in EB reports before the National EB Registry data

Form of EB	Study Gans et al 1988[1]	Study Lin et al 1994[13]	Study Tong et al 1999[11]
Simplex EB	Ocular involvement Weber Cockayne 8%, Dowling Meara 22%, Koebner 0%	Ocular involvement 3%	Ocular involvement 12%
	Weber Cockayne (localized) 8% blepharitis Dowling-Meara 22% corneal scarring; 11% had eyelid blistering	No description of type 3%	Dowling subtype – 12% peripheral corneal vascularization
Junctional EB	55% 55% corneal erosions, 22% corneal scarring, 11% blepharitis, 22% eyelid blistering	39% 39%	40% 20% corneal involvement; no eyelid or conjunctival involvement
Recessive dystrophic EB	52% 52% corneal erosions 26% corneal scarring 20% eyelid blistering 20% blepharitis.	51% No description 51%	51% 68% cornea involved 35% corneal scarring 24% corneal pannus 8% exposure keratitis, eyelid scarring 24% conjunctival involvement 14% eyelid involvement
Dominant dystrophic EB	10% 10% corneal erosions	17.6% No description 51%	4% 4% conjunctival blistering

Data from Fine JD, Johnson LB, Suchindran CM. The National Epidermolysis Bullosa Registry. J Invest Dermatol 1994;102: 54S–6S; Fine J-D, Johnson LB, Weiner M, et al. Eye involvement in inherited epidermolysis bullosa: experience of the National Epidermolysis Bullosa Registry. Am J Ophthalmol 2004;138:254–62.

scarring was seen most frequently in RDEB-HS (50%), RDEB-I (29.4%), and JEB-H (26.8%) patients. Other ocular associations reported in EB include cataracts, cornea plana and sclerocornea, refractive errors, amblyopia, lacrimal duct obstruction, strabismus, lens subluxation, posterior vitreous detachment, and Graves' disease.[13]

EYELIDS

Blepharitis is reported uncommonly in EB, with highest frequencies reported in the RDEB-HS and RDEB-I (18% in each form) and JEB (6% to 7% in both subtypes). Ectropion formation most often occurs in JEB-H, and it is reported in approximately 14% of JEB cases. Eyelid retraction, scarring, and eversion of the lower eyelids are compatible with the presence of chronic exuberant granulation tissue in adjacent skin. About half as many patients with RDEB-HS were reported to have had some evidence of ectropion formation. In the authors' experience, those ectropions were much milder than those seen in patients with JEB-H. Exuberant granulation tissue

Table 2
Ocular involvement in EB—anatomic wise (correlation with the data from the multicenter, national study using the data from the National Epidermolysis Bullosa Registry (NEBR), 1995)

Tissue Involved	Recessive DEB	Dominant DEB	JEB	EBs
Eyelid	Bullae, ulcers, crusted lesions, cicatrisation[25] Blepharitis–8.9% Ectropion–1.4% Lacrimal duct obstruction–5.7%	Bullae, ulcers, crusted lesions, cicatrisation[25] Blepharitis–0.4% Ectropion–0.4% Lacrimal duct obstruction–nil	Not frequent involvement Blepharitis–3.0% Ectropion–4.2% Lacrimal duct obstruction–3.6%	Occasional involvement[25] Blepharitis–0.3% Ectropion–nil Lacrimal duct obstruction–1.3%
Conjunctiva	Conjunctivitis, keratoconjunctivitis, cicatrisation[25] Symblepharon–3.6%	Conjunctivitis, keratoconjunctivitis, cicatrisation[25] Symblepharon–nil	Not frequent involvement[25] Symblepharon–1.2%	Occasional involvement[25] Symblepharon–nil
Cornea	Keratitis, ulcers, opacities, perforation, pitting[25] Corneal erosion–31.9% scarring–18.2%	Keratitis, ulcers, opacities, perforation, pitting[25] Corneal erosion–0.4% scarring–0.4%	Keratitis, ulcers, opacities, perforation, pitting[25] Corneal erosion–19.9% scarring–8.4%	Keratitis, ulcers, opacities, perforation, pitting[25] Corneal erosion–0.9% scarring–0.2%
Lens			Involved	
Retina			Occasionally retinal detachment, cysts, pigmentary changes.	

Abbreviation: DEB, dystrophic epidermolysis bullosa.

Data from Fine JD, Johnson LB, Suchindran C, et al. The epidemiology of inherited EB: findings within American, Canadian, and European study populations. In: Fine JD, Bauer EA, McGuire J, et al, editors. Epidermolysis bullosa: clinical, epidemiologic, and laboratory advances, and the findings of the National Epidermolysis Bullosa Registry. Baltimore (MD): Johns Hopkins University Press; 1999:101–13; Fine J-D, Johnson LB, Weiner M, et al. Eye involvement in inherited epidermolysis bullosa: experience of the National Epidermolysis Bullosa Registry. Am J Ophthalmol 2004;138:254–62.

Table 3
Frequency of occurrence (%) as indicated in the NEBR—an observational cross-sectional longitudinal study

	EB Simplex				Junctional EB		Dystrophic EB			
	Weber-Cockayne	Dowling-Meara	Koebner	EBS-O	Herlitz	Non-Herlitz	DDEB	RDEB-HS	RDEB-nHS	RDEB Inversa
Ocular abnormalities (case numbers)	1092	113	96	379	40	190	424	139	265	17
Corneal erosions or blisters	0.92	6.19	3.13	2.64	47.50	25.26	2.12	74.10	32.45	35.29
Corneal scarring	0.27	0.00	3.16	0.53	26.83	13.37	0.95	50.00	16.92	29.41
Symblepharon	0.00	0.00	0.00	0.00	4.76	2.11	0.00	10.07	1.89	11.76
Blepharitis	0.37	0.88	2.08	0.26	7.14	6.32	0.71	17.52	6.46	17.65
Ectropion	0.00	0.00	0.00	0.00	14.29	2.11	0.00	7.19	1.90	0.00
Lacrimal duct obstruction	1.19	2.65	1.04	1.85	2.38	4.23	1.65	5.80	5.30	11.76
Impaired vision	13.17	13.27	15.63	16.14	16.67	13.68	17.18	38.13	21.89	41.18
Blindness	0.82	1.77	0.00	0.53	0.00	1.58	0.94	6.47	1.14	0.00

Abbreviations: EBS-O, all other forms of EBs; HS, Hallopeau-Siemens; EB nHS, non-Hallopeau-Siemens; RDEB, recessive dystrophic EB.
Data from Fine J-D, Johnson LB, Weiner M, et al. Eye involvement in inherited epidermolysis bullosa: experience of the National Epidermolysis Bullosa Registry. Am J Ophthalmol 2004;138:254–62.

has been seen on the face of a boy with the Herlitz subtype of generalized junctional EB.

LACRIMAL SYSTEM

Lacrimal duct obstruction was reported rarely in each major EB subtype. Higher levels were noted only in RDEB, especially in those patients with inversa disease (nearly 12%). The fact that RDEB-I patients have the highest frequency of this finding may be compatible with this EB subtype's marked prevalence for epithelial blistering within other mucosal tissues to include the oral cavity, esophagus, urethra, and introitus. Lacrimal duct obstruction has been reported.[18] Reduced tear break-up time has been reported.

CONJUNCTIVAL

Symblepharon formation was confined to JEB and RDEB patients (**Fig. 1**). The highest frequencies were seen in RDEB-HS (10%), RDEB-I (12%), and JEB-H (5%). This is consistent with the severity of other external eye involvement noted in these three major EB types. Other involvement reported included red watering eyes,[5] photophobia,[3,6] ocular pain,[3,6,14] conjunctival injection,[7] conjunctival edema,[5] and blepharoconjunctivitis.[1,6,8] Symblepharon formation was confined to JEB and RDEB patients. The highest frequencies were seen in RDEB-HS (10%), RDEB-I (12%), and JEB-H (5%). This is consistent with the severity of other external eye involvement noted in these three major EB types (**Fig. 2**).

CORNEA

Exposure keratitis, corneal ulcerations,[3] corneal bullae,[5] corneal opacities,[5,8] corneal scarring,[1,5,10,11,13] limbal broadening,[5,8] pannus

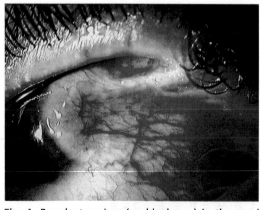

Fig. 1. Pseudopterygium (symblepharon) in the nasal conjunctiva of right eye in DEB (dystrophic epidermolysis bullosa).

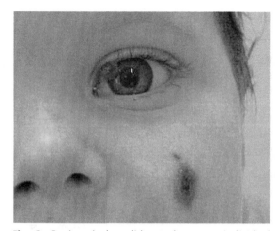

Fig. 2. Conjunctival eyelid papule on an individual with laryngo-onycho-cutaneous (LOC) syndrome.

formation,[5,11,13] symblephara,[8,22] and ectropions have been described in epidermolysis bullosa patients.[11,13] The cumulative risk of corneal blistering or erosions was estimated for the NEBR group. It is reported that for each major EB subtype, by 1 year of age, the cumulative risk of corneal lesions was 27.12%, 18.64%, 10.43%, and 8.79% in JEB-H, RDEB-HS, RDEB-nHS, and JEB-nH, respectively. These risk values reached a plateau of 83.18% in JEB-H by age 5. Ocular involvement of 79% in RDEB-HS, by age 35 years has been described in medical literature. Between 63.53% and 71.15% of all patients were predicted to have experienced corneal blisters or erosions by ages 10 and 20, respectively. The cumulative risk of corneal blistering or erosions in JEB-nH reached 46.5% by age 40, roughly half of that seen in JEB-H patients. Similarly, the maximum cumulative risk in RDEB-nHS achieved a level approximately half (35.11%) of the maximum level in RDEB-HS by age 30. An almost identical curve was observed for RDEB-I. Among EBS patients, only those with generalized Dowling-Meara disease were at significant risk for this outcome, with a cumulative risk of 7.73% predicted by age 20. The most common ocular finding in EB patients as reported by the NEBR study group was corneal blisters in the form of intact vesicles or secondary erosions. These blisters or erosions most often were seen in the severe forms of EB, that is JEB and recessive DEB. The corneal blisters were seen more commonly in the more severe JEB subset, Herlitz subset of severe JEB disease, with 50% of these patients having involvement. Around 25% of all non-Herlitz JEB patients had findings suggestive of corneal blistering. Around 66% of the RDEB-HS patients and 33% each of the RDEB-nHS and RDEB-I patients were reported to have experienced at least one episode of corneal blisters or erosions. Corneal blistering was reported to be low in other forms of EB, with values ranging from 0.92% (in the mildest EB subtype, Weber-Cockayne EBs) to 6.19% (in the most severe EBs subtype, Dowling-Meara disease). Corneal scarring rates were lower than those of corneal blisters and erosions across all major EB types and subtypes, which may be due to the fact that blistering may have occurred only once or infrequently or if it was self-limited in its duration. Corneal scarring was seen most frequently in RDEB-HS (50%), RDEB-I (29.4%), and JEB-H (26.8%) patients.

Other ocular associations reported in EB include cataracts, cornea plana and sclerocornea, refractive errors, amblyopia, lacrimal duct obstruction, strabismus, lens subluxation, posterior vitreous detachment, and Graves' disease.[13]

The only disadvantage of the NEBR study was that the frequencies of occurrence were determined for only the eight variables (corneal erosions or blistering, corneal scarring, symblepharons, blepharitis, ectropions, lacrimal duct obstruction, impaired vision, blindness).

LIFETIME RISK OF OCULAR COMPLICATIONS IN EB—DATA FROM THE NEBR

Using the life table analysis techniques, Fine and colleagues[15] estimated the cumulative risk of corneal blistering or erosions for each major EB subtype, particularly the four clinically severe EB subtypes (JEB-H and the three major subtypes of RDEB) is the highest cumulative risk for developing corneal blisters, erosions, and scarring. By 1 year of age, the cumulative risks of corneal blisters are 27.12%, 18.64%, 10.43%, and 8.79% in JEB-H, RDEB-HS, RDEB-nHS, and JEB-nH, respectively. The cumulative risk reached a plateau of 83.18% in JEB-H, 79.35% in RDEB-HS by age 5 years. Between 63.53% and 71.15% of all patients are predicted to experience corneal blisters or erosions by first and second decades of life respectively. The cumulative risk of corneal blistering or erosions in JEB-nH is reported to be 46.5% by the fourth decade (roughly half of that reported in JEB-H). The maximum cumulative risk in RDEB-nHS reaches 35.11% by age 30 years. Similar cumulated risks were reported in RDEB-I patients. EBs patients with generalized Dowling-Meara disease were reported to have the only EBs subtype with a predictable cumulative risk for corneal blisters of 7.73% by the second decade of life. Life tables for corneal scarring parallel those calculated for corneal blistering or erosions, although the absolute values for the former were lower. Cumulative risks for corneal scarring were predicted to occur in 3.45%, 5.93%, and 3.51% of all patients with JEB-H, RDEB-HS, and RDEB-I, respectively, during infancy. The highest cumulative risk (72.22%) was seen in JEB-H, reported by age 20 years. The predicted cumulative risks for corneal scarring in RDEB-HS, RDEB-nHS, and RDEB-I were 51.23%, 16.82%, and 21.21%, respectively, by the second decade of life. The cumulative risks were reported to plateau at 60.34% by age 35 in RDEB-HS, 23.55% by age 50 in RDEB-nHS, 29.97% by age 35 in RDEB-I, and 5.18% by age 40 in epidermolysis bullosa-Dowling-Meara (EBS-DM).[15]

MANAGEMENT OF OPHTHALMIC INVOLVEMENT IN EB PATIENTS

Management of the ocular complications in EB should part of a multidisciplinary team approach. EB patients should be managed based on the type and severity of ocular complication that presents. The method of treatment in most patients is usually conservative with regular ocular surface lubricants. Care needs to be taken not to hold the eyelids firmly when applying the drops in children, as this may result in damage to the skin and may trigger the blistering phenomenon.

Patients with mild forms of EB (eg, simplex EB, except the Dowling–Meara subtype) do not need regular ophthalmologic review, as long as the parents are adequately advised to watch for symptoms that are suspicious of ocular surface involvement (grittiness, pain, photophobia, persistent redness) and to seek the advice of an ophthalmologist urgently when these happen. After the initial ophthalmic evaluation and advice on ocular surface lubricants by the physician, all symptomatic patients should be referred to a specialist in ophthalmic care for an appropriate management and follow-up. The main therapy that must be initiated is the provision of supplementary moisture for the irritated ocular surface in states of deficiency of the tear film and poor eyelid function. Artificial tear drops are manufactured by different pharmaceutical companies, and these may be instilled at different frequencies matched to the degree of discomfort. Some patients prefer thicker more viscous preparations, while others prefer hypotonic preparations that serve to dilute the concentrated tears, ideal in situations of poor lid function or reduced tear secretion. Unpreserved formulations may be helpful for patients sensitive to preservatives. Drying of the ocular surface is typically more severe during the winter months, when indoor humidity is very low. An ultrasonic humidifier placed strategically close to the bedside, in the playroom, or in the workplace environment may mitigate the problem substantially. Dry eye syndrome is treated with lanolin-free ocular lubricants without preservatives. Soft contact lenses appear to protect the eyes from corneal erosions and also appear to reduce mild scarring and pannus formation, preventing possible blindness. Acute management of corneal erosions consists of supportive treatment with application of nontoxic antibiotic ointments, as long as no stromal infiltrates are seen. Gram's stains and culture samples should be obtained otherwise. Patients who fail these approaches sometimes are treated with limbal and corneal transplants. These patients require systemic immunosuppressants to remain the integrity of transplants. A novel technique for corneal reconstruction uses tissue-engineered cell sheets derived from autologous oral mucosal epithelium. Another technique is to cover the cornea with amniotic membranes; this facilitates re-epithelialization of the cornea within a 4-week period. Chronic blepharitis can result in cicatricial ectropion and exposure keratitis. Moisture chambers and ocular lubricants are used commonly for such management. Full-thickness skin grafting to the upper eyelid can be considered in these scarring conditions; however, complete correction is difficult to obtain.[26]

During sleep, the cornea is protected by the Bells phenomenon, in which the eyeballs spontaneously rotate upwards under the upper eyelids, even in the absence of eyelid closure. In the absence of Bells phenomenon, bland ophthalmic ointments may be useful at night, particularly in patients with a severe grade of lagophthalmic complications that are associated with inadequate bells.

Patching using a soft secured ocular patch or spectacle wear is not contraindicated if unavoidable. The clinician needs to monitor EB patients carefully for secondary cutaneous complications (triggering of epidermal blistering) resulting from these ophthalmic treatment options. Empirically preservative-free ocular lubricants should be used to minimize the risk of ocular surface problems associated with scarring and infection. Patients with resultant exposure keratitis are most difficult to manage and require the most frequent follow-up. Both eyelid cicatricial ectropion and severe symblepharon sequelae can result in exposure keratitis or lagophthalmos. Some patients with cutaneous blistering and induration of the upper eyelids tend to have a mild nocturnal lagophthalmos. Once a dense corneal scar is formed, little improvement can be obtained with ocular lubricants, and a lamellar keratoplasty can be considered, although its role has not been proved here. Management should be aimed to prevent the development of surface scarring complications. Tarsorrhaphy and ectropion surgery may have to be considered to prevent this. Patients with squints and problems with extraocular muscle motility should be assessed, and surgery may be performed with the usual indications to prevent strabismic amblyopia. Spectacle-dispensing opticians should be made aware of the problems (eg, friction-triggered blistering). The opticians should be advised to use large padded arms for the spectacle frames where necessary. Ideally an optician experienced in dealing with types of problems described previously would be involved. Amblyopia therapy such as ocular penalization can be considered in the case of corneal scarring and where there is potentially a risk of complicated lower visual outcome.

Recurrent corneal abrasions are a problem for many EB patients. Preverbal patients frequently may cry and tear, often inconsolably. The eye with the abraded cornea eye will be injected. It is important for the parents to recognize the problem and obtain definitive treatment promptly after each such episode to prevent progressive corneal scarring or infection. The initial examination always is facilitated by instillation of a topical anesthetic in the eye. The corneal abrasion can be highlighted by instillation of fluorescein; the abraded area will be bright yellow under blue light illumination. In cases with corneal abrasion, prophylactic antibiotic is instilled. If the abrasion is large, healing is facilitated by a pressure patch dressing. This is achieved using a wrapped head roll bandage, as taping eye pads to the skin is contraindicated in EB patients to avoid blisters. If the child is photophobic, a cycloplegic eye drop also is instilled in the injured eye to relieve the associated discomfort. In severe cases, a vascularized pannus will destroy the optical clarity of the cornea. This membrane frequently can be removed by careful lamellar dissection with substantial visual improvement.

Refractive errors require special attention in these patients. Small refractive error patients do not require treatment. Large errors should be corrected, generally with spectacles. A close alliance with a concerned optician is mandatory to provide large baring surfaces and an accurate fit, so as to not unduly stress the skin of the nose, temple or ears. Hard contact lenses are likely to cause frequent corneal abrasions in EB patients and are therefore contraindicated.

In the milder forms of EB, it may be possible to fit a patient with soft contact lenses provided the patient retains sufficient dexterity to manipulate the lenses. In the most severe cases (eg, dystrophic epidermolysis bullosa), corneal scars may reduce visual function to bare light perception. In desperate cases, it may be reasonable to consider corneal transplantation, particularly if lid function and tear secretion are relatively intact. Experience in such cases is limited, and the prognosis remains guarded.

Cicatricial damage to the eyelids is treated with ocular lubricants for as long as possible. In cases of chronic severe exposure, chronic epithelial defects of the corneal surface will be observed, more prominent in the form of a horizontal band corresponding to the palpebral fissure. When ocular discomfort or visual compromise becomes intolerable, it becomes necessary to attempt to restore the normal relationship of the eyelids to the globe surgically. Eyelid corrective procedures are performed best by experienced ophthalmic plastic surgeons. Generally, contractures of the eyelid skin are corrected best by release and autograft transplants using uninvolved skin. If no skin is available near the eyes, retroauricular skin can be the donor site, but this area also is affected frequently in EB patients. The autografts generally survive well, but genuine improvement in eyelid function and motility are achieved inconsistently.[27]

Adhesions between the eyelid and surface of the globe (symblepharon) are frequently well tolerated if they are small and do not substantially limit motility of the lid and globe. If the restriction becomes severe, surgical lysis may enhance visual or cosmetic function greatly. The procedure can be performed using retrobulbar or a general anesthetic. In order to prevent reformation of adhesions, it may be helpful to place a conformer in the conjunctival sac along with the liberal use of an ocular steroid ointment. If the anatomy of the adhesion is very simple, it may be adequate to simply approximate the cut edges of the conjunctiva with interrupted absorbable sutures to provide an intact epithelial surface as a guard against recurrence of the adhesions.

Given the clinical impact of external eye involvement in patients with EB, thorough semiannual to annual ophthalmologic evaluations should be considered and are an essential component of overall clinical management.

REFERENCES

1. Gans LA. Eye lesions of epidermolysis bullosa: clinical features, management, and prognosis. Arch Dermatol 1988;124:762–4.

2. Hochman MA, Mayers M. Stevens-Johnson syndrome, epidermolysis bullosa, staphylococcal scalded skin syndrome, and dermatitis herpetiformis. Int Ophthalmol Clin 1997;37:77–92.

3. Destro M, Wallow IH, Brightbill FS. Recessive dystrophic epidermolysis bullosa. Arch Ophthalmol 1987; 105:1248–52.

4. Silverberg M, Fan-Paul N, Kane S, et al. Junctional EB in the neonate: a case report. J Pediatr Ophthalmol Strabismus 1999;36:219–20.

5. McDonnell PJ, Schofield OMV, Spalton DJ, et al. Eye involvement in junctional epidermolysis bullosa. Arch Ophthalmol 1989;107:1635–7.

6. Granek H, Baden HP. Corneal involvement in epidermolysis bullosa simplex. Arch Dermatol 1980;98: 469–72.

7. Lechner S, Pleyer U, Hartmann C. Konjunktivale gemischte Injektion mit beginnender Symblepharonbildung. Ophthalmologe 2002;99:960–1.

8. McDonnell PJ, Spalton DJ. The ocular signs and complications of epidermolysis bullosa. J R Soc Med 1988;81:576–8.

9. Breit R. Epidermolysis bullosa dystrophica inversa, a review and case report. Hautarzt 1979;30:471–7.

10. Irak I, Soll SM, Camacho JM. Junctional epidermolysis bullosa in a young patient. J Pediatr Ophthalmol Strabismus 2003;40:168–9.

11. Tong L, Hodgkins PR, Denyer J, et al. The eye in epidermolysis bullosa. Br J Ophthalmol 1999;83: 323–6.

12. Hammerton ME, Turner TW, Pyne RJ. A case of junctional epidermolysis bullosa (Herlitz-Pearson) with corneal bullae. Aust J Ophthalmol 1984;12:45–8.

13. Lin AN, Murphy F, Brodie SE, et al. Review of ophthalmic findings in 204 patients with epidermolysis bullosa. Am J Ophthalmol 1994;118:384–90.

14. Steuhl KP, Anton-Lamprecht I, Arnold M-L, et al. Recurrent bilateral corneal erosions due to an association of epidermolysis bullosa simplex Kobner and X-linked ichthyosis with steroid sulfatase deficiency. Graefes Arch Clin Exp Ophthalmol 1988;226: 216–23.

15. Fine J-D, Johnson LB, Weiner M, et al. Eye involvement in inherited epidermolysis bullosa: experience of the National Epidermolysis Bullosa Registry. Am J Ophthalmol 2004;138:254–62.

16. Pernet G. Involvement of the eyes in a case of epidermolysis bullosa. Ophthalmoscope 1904;2: 308–9.

17. Aurora AL, Madhavan M, Rao S. Ocular changes in epidermolysis bullosa letalis. Am J Ophthalmol 1975;79:464–70.

18. Cohen M, Sulzberger MB. Essential shrinking of the conjunctiva in a case of probable epidermolysis bullosa dystrophica. Arch Ophthalmol 1935;13:374–90.

19. Iwanmoto M, Haik BG, Iwanmoto T, et al. The ultrastructural defect in conjunctiva from a case of

recessive dystrophic epidermolysis bullosa. Arch Ophthalmol 1991;109:1382–6.

20. Jay B. Genetic implications of oculocutaneous disorders. Proc R Soc Med 1969;62:7–8.

21. Le Jamtel MF. Epidermolyse bulleuse dystrophique a heredite recessive. Bul Soc Ophtalmol Fr 1958; 46:58–66.

22. Schreck E. Cutaneous muco-oculoepithelial syndromes. Arch Klin Exp Dermatol 1954;198:221–57.

23. Sorsby A, Fraser Roberts JA, Brain RT. Essential shrinking of the conjunctiva in a hereditary affection allied to epidermolysis bullosa. Doc Ophthalmol 1951;5:118–50.

24. Fine JD, Johnson LB, Suchindran CM. The National Epidermolysis Bullosa Registry. J Invest Dermatol 1994;102:54S–6S.

25. Fine JD, Johnson LB, Suchindran C, et al. The epidemiology of inherited EB: findings within American, Canadian, and European study populations. In: Fine JD, Bauer EA, McGuire J, et al, editors. Epidermolysis bullosa: clinical, epidemiologic, and laboratory advances, and the findings of the National Epidermolysis Bullosa Registry. Baltimore (MD): Johns Hopkins University Press; 1999. p. 101–13.

26. Uitto J, Eady R, Fine JD, et al. The DEBRA International Visioning/Consensus Meeting on Epidermolysis Bullosa; summary and recommendations. J Invest Dermatol 2000;114:734–7.

27. Hill JC, Rodrigue D. Cicatirical ectropion in epidermolysis bullosa and in congenital icthyosis: its plastic repair. Can J Ophthalmol 1971;6:89–97.

Nail Involvement in Epidermolysis Bullosa

Antonella Tosti, MD[a],*, Débora Cadore de Farias, MD[b],
Dédée F. Murrell, MA, BMBCh, FAAD, MD[c]

KEYWORDS

- Nail diseases • Epidermolysis bullosa • Pachyonychia
- Anonychia • Periungual granulomas • Onychogryphosis

Although the anatomy of the nail apparatus is different from that of the skin, the antigenic expression of basement membrane zone (BMZ) components in the normal matrix, nail bed, proximal nail fold, and hyponychium is similar to that of normal skin. In addition, there are no differences in the antigenic composition of the BMZ between the different portions of the nail matrix.[1,2] Nail expression of all the target antigens found in the normal nonappendage basement membrane explains why nail involvement is a feature of most epidermolysis bullosa (EB) subtypes.

Even though the absence or presence of nail changes at birth should not be used as absolute criteria for differential diagnosis between different subtypes of EB, nail involvement recently has been included among the criteria for scoring EB severity, as early nail dystrophy and loss are correlated with disease severity and progression, particularly in junctional epidermolysis bullosa (JEB) and recessive dystrophic epidermolysis bullosa (RDEB).[3]

Trauma undoubtedly contributes to the development of nail dystrophy, and for this reason, the great toenails more often are affected severely.

The nail abnormalities may be the first or the only symptom of EB. In fact they may precede the development of skin blistering as in the late-onset JEB (Fig. 1) and pretibial DEB, or be an isolated finding as reported in some families with dominant dystrophic EB (DDEB) (Figs. 2 and 3).[4–8]

Nail involvement is uncommon in localized EB simplex (EBS) and is not a feature of EBS migratory circinate or EBS with pyloric atresia (Table 1).[9]

NAIL CHANGES IN EBS

In most patients with localized EBS, the nails usually are not affected. In severe EBS subtypes, however, blistering may cause onycholysis and onychomadesis with regrowth of thickened dystrophic toenails, with or without onychogryphosis.

Horn in 2000 reported the clinical features of 130 EBS patients (seven patients with Dowling Meara subtype, 69 with Koebner subtype, and 54 with Weber Cockayne subtype). In the Dowling Meara EBS group, all subjects had nail involvement. The infants had periodic shedding of finger and toenails, and the adults had thickened great toenails. In the Koebner EBS group, nowadays classified by Fine and colleagues[9] as generalized EBS–other, 14% of the patients had thickened great toenails. In the Weber Cockayne EBS group, classified by Fine and colleagues[9] as localized EBS, thickened toenails were present in seven individuals (12%), including three children younger than 4 years.[10]

In EBS-Ogna, which is a dominant variant of EBS caused by plectin gene abnormalities, the skin involvement is usually similar to localized EBS, but the blisters are often blood stained, additionally, the nails may have blistering with bleeding underneath, leading to nail dystrophy.[11]

NAIL CHANGES IN JEB

Most JEB subtypes are associated with severe nail dystrophy. Subungual blistering causes onycholysis

[a] Department of Dermatology, Bologna University, Via Massarenti, 1, Bologna 40138, Italy
[b] Department of Dermatology, Santa Casa de São Paulo Hospital, João Moura Street, 975 (164), Jardim América, São Paulo, SP 05412-002, Brazil
[c] Department of Dermatology, St George Hospital, University of New South Wales, Sydney, NSW 2217, Australia
* Corresponding author.
E-mail address: antonella.tosti@unibo.it (A. Tosti).

Dermatol Clin 28 (2010) 153–157
doi:10.1016/j.det.2009.10.017

derm.theclinics.com

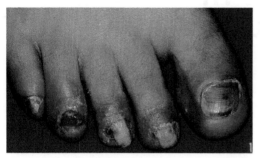

Fig. 1. Late-onset JEB: thickened toenails; in the fourth right toe there is loss of the nail and granulomatous tissue.

with loss of the nails. With time, the nails become thickened, abnormally shaped and sometimes onychogryphotic.

In most patients with Herlitz EB, nail involvement occurs soon after birth, with very typical paronychia-like lesions and nail loss with nail bed erosions due to extensive blistering. Development of subungual and periungual granulation tissue is typical and may cover the entire digit (**Fig. 4**). Patients with JEB caused by defects in lam332 often may have significant nail involvement leading to anonychia, while their systemic involvement can be mild.

The new subtype of JEB included in the most recent classification, laryngo-onycho-cutaneous syndrome (LOC), is characterized by early involvement of blistering under the nails. Eventually the nails may be lost.[12,13] This syndrome may occur in overlap with classical forms of JEB caused by LAMA3a mutations, and both result in exuberant granulation tissue.[11]

NAIL CHANGES IN DEB

Nail abnormalities in DEB range from a minor nail dystrophy to complete nail loss and mitten deformities. Nail loss is a constant feature of patients

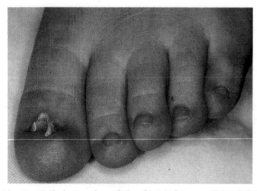

Fig. 2. Nail dystrophy of the first left toenail in child with dominant dystrophic EB nails only.

with severe subtypes who usually develop nail changes early in life. Repeated and extensive sub-basement membrane blistering followed by scarring leads to nail bed and matrix destruction with permanent anonychia.

In localized DEB, only few nails can be affected. Nails-only DDEB is a newly recognized subtype of DEB, in which nail dystrophy is the only clinical feature; the deformity, often limited to the toenails, can be mild and easily overlooked. This diagnosis should be considered in families with AD toenail dystrophy, even when there is no history of blistering (see **Figs. 2** and **3**).[6-8]

In 2001, Dharma described a family with AD nail dystrophy without blistering for four generations. The diagnosis was confirmed by genomic DNA studies, which showed glycine substitutions in COL7A1. The patient, a 7-month-old boy, had recurrent blisters affecting the hands and feet since birth; at 1 year, he had no more blisters but groups of milia on erythematous plaques over the hands, feet, knees, and thighs, and pachyonychia of the great toes and thumbnails. There was no family history of blisters, but there was a history of nail dystrophy in his mother, maternal uncle, maternal grandmother, maternal great uncle, and maternal great grandfather, who had thickened and dystrophic toenails.[6]

In 2002, Sato-Matsumura reported on two families with glycine substitutions in COL7A1 associated with dominant familial dystrophic toenail changes. The genetic study of their families showed that the G1815R and G1595R mutations resulted in familial dominant toenail deformities. The toenails of the affected members were thickened and shortened (pachyonychia).[7]

In the authors' experience, the nail dystrophy is seen first in childhood when the great toenail is affected by onycholysis associated with subungual hemorrhages and mild nail bed hyperkeratosis. With time, the nail becomes thickened and dystrophic (pachyonychia) because of nail bed scarring and hyperkeratosis.

In pretibial DEB, the nail dystrophy develops in childhood before the onset of skin lesions that typically occur after the age of 10 years. Nail dystrophy may occur in the absence of skin lesions in family members.[5]

Clinical Features

Nail abnormalities observed in EB are not specific or pathognomonic, as they result from nail bed and matrix scarring. In the same way, there are nail changes characteristic of specific EB subtypes. The severity of the nail changes, however, usually is related to the severity of the skin lesions.

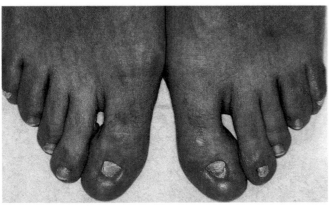

Fig. 3. Toenail dystrophy in the mother of the child from **Fig. 2.**

Pachyonychia (nail thickening)
The nail plate is shortened, thickened, and yellow-brown in color. Onycholysis and nail bed hemorrhages frequently are associated. The nail abnormalities may affect several nails or be limited to the great toenail. In fingernails, pachyonychia often is associated with pincer nail deformity. Pachyonychia usually is reported in the literature as thickened dystrophic nails, and it is the most common nail finding in EB (EBS, DEB, and JEB).

Onychogryphosis
The nail is thickened, opaque, and yellow with an oyster-like appearance caused by excessive growth in the upward and lateral directions. The dystrophy usually is limited to the great toenails. It may be observed in EBS and JEB.

Nail blistering
Periungual or subungual bullae produce hemorrhagic onycholysis and hemorrhagic paronychia with onychomadesis. Nail shedding may be followed by regrowth of normal or dystrophic nails (EBS, JEB) or produce loss of the nails (JEB, DEB).

Nail erosions with granular tissue
The nail plate is absent, and the distal digit is covered by granulation tissue producing a drumstick appearance (JEB) (**Fig. 5**). This feature is characteristic of Herlitz EB, where patients usually have dystrophic or absent nails with periungual granulation tissue. Periungual hypergranulation tissue occasionally may be present at birth before the development of widespread skin and mucosal blistering, but most patients develop this feature during the first year of life.[14]

Nail atrophy
The nail plate is very thin, brittle, and short. Nail changes result from nail matrix damage caused by repetitive blistering (JEB, DEB).

Anonychia
Nail loss caused by scarring is common in RDEB. Fusion of the digits by scar tissue leads to mitten-like appearance of hands and feet (pseudosyndactyly), which is typical of children with severe generalized RDEB, who usually develop the deformity by the age of 6 to 8 years. The collagen 7 hypomorphic mouse that serves as an immunocompetent animal model for DEB also develops mitten deformities in the extremities that closely resemble severe human RDEB. In this mouse model, mitten deformities result from aberrant wound healing with myofibroblast-mediated excessive contraction and extracellular matrix deposition.[15]

Anonychia is also a feature of Herlitz JEB and LOC syndrome,[14,16] where it may be associated with thickening and occasionally periungual inflammation with granulation tissue of other nails.[17]

Parrot beak nail deformity
Recurrent blistering in the distal finger may result in soft tissue and bone reabsorption, with bending of the nail around the shortened fingertip. Satter[18] has reported this deformity in a 9-year-old boy with the AR Kindler syndrome, now recognized as a form of EB caused by mutations in *FERMT1*.

SUMMARY

Nail involvement is a very common feature of EB. The spectrum of clinical severity is large, and nail abnormalities may cause severe disability or just be a mild cosmetic problem.

There are families with DEB in which mild nail involvement without blistering may be present for generations before a family member develops blisters in the skin. Physicians should be aware that pachyonychia of the toenails in a child may be a sign of DEB. Ask about nail abnormalities in family members, and when possible, perform

Table 1
Classification of EB and the nail involvement in the different subtypes of EB

Major Type of EB	Subtypes	Frequency of Nail Involvement	Nail Signs
EBS (simplex)	EBS superficialis AD	70%	Dystrophic nails
	Lethal acantholytic EBS AR	100%	Nail loss
	Plakophilin deficiency AR	100%	Thickened dystrophic nail
	EBS localized AD	Uncommon	Blistering may cause onycholysis and onychomadesis, with normal regrowth or thickened dystrophic nails
	Dowling-Meara AD	>75%	Onychomadesis, pachyonychia, onychogryphosis, pincer nails or absent nails
	EBS other generalized AD (previously called Koebner)	14%	Onychomadesis with normal regrowth, pachyonychia, thickened great toenail
	AR EBS		Hyperkeratotic nails, horizontal ridging, anonychia
	EBS-Ogna AD		Onychogryphosis
	EBS migratory circinate	Absent	None
	EBS with mottled pigmentation	Uncommon	Dystrophic nails, small toenail
	EBS with muscular dystrophy	50%	Onychomadesis, pachyonychia, onychogryphosis, pincer nails, anonychia
	EBS with pyloric atresia	Absent	None
JEB	Herlitz AR	>75%	Pachyonychia, exuberant granulation tissue, nail erosion, anonychia
	Non-Herlitz AR (generalized and localized)	>75%	Anonychia, dystrophic nails
	With pyloric atresia AR		Nail thinning and atrophy or absent nails
	Inversa JEB	>50%	Dystrophic or absent nails
	Late-onset JEB		Onycholysis, nail loss, Beau's lines
	LOC syndrome	100%	Nail thickening, nail erosions with granulation tissue, anonychia
DEB (dystrophic EB)	DDEB generalized	>75%	Nail thickening, onychogryphosis, anonychia, pseudosyndactyly
	RDEB severe generalized	>75%	Anonychia, pseudosyndactyly
	RDEB generalized other	>75%	Dystrophic or absent nails
	Acral DDEB and RDEB	>75%	Nail thickening anonychia
	Pretibial DDEB and RDEB,	>75%	Nail thickening
	Pruriginous DEB, AD or AR	>75%	Nail thickening, anonychia
	DDEB nails only	100%	Pachyonychia, thickened dystrophic nails anonychia
	DEB-BDN	25–50%	Nail thickening, anonychia pseudosyndactyly
	RDEB inversa	>75%	Nail thickening
	RDEB centripetalis	>75%	Dystrophic or absent nails
Kindler syndrome	AR		Nail dystrophy, parrot beak nail deformity, absent nails

Abbreviations: AD, autosomal dominant; AR, autosomal recessive; DDEB-BDN - bullous dermolysis of the newborn; LOC, laryngo-onycho-cutaneous.
Scale: absent or none, rare, 1+, 2+, 3+, 4+.

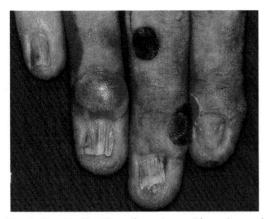

Fig. 4. Non-Herlitz EB: nail erosions with periungual granulation tissue.

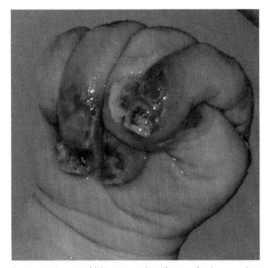

Fig. 5. Periungual blisters and nail atrophy in a patient with Herlitz JEB.

a genetic analysis of *COL7A1* in families with AD nail dystrophy.

REFERENCES

1. Sinclair RD, Wojnarowska F, Leigh IM, et al. The basement membrane zone of the nail. Br J Dermatol 1994;131(4):499–505.
2. Cameli N, Picardo M, Pisani A, et al. Characterization of the nail matrix basement membrane zone: an immunohistochemical study of normal nails and of the nails in Herlitz junctional epidermolysis bullosa. Br J Dermatol 1996;134(1):182–4.
3. Moss C, Wong A, Davies P. The Birmingham Epidermolysis Bullosa Severity score: development and validation. Br J Dermatol 2009;160(5):1057–65.
4. Bruckner-Tuderman L, Schnyder UW, Baran R. Nail changes in epidermolysis bullosa: clinical and pathogenetic considerations. Br J Dermatol 1995;132: 339–44.
5. Rizzo C, Anandasabapathy N, Walters RF, et al. Pretibial epidermolysis bullosa. Dermatol Online J 2008; 14(10):26.
6. Dharma B, Moss C, McGrath JA, et al. Dominant dystrophic epidermolysis bullosa presenting as familial nail dystrophy. Clin Exp Dermatol 2001;26: 93–6.
7. Sato-Matsumura KC, Yasukawa K, Tomita Y, et al. Toenail dystrophy with COL7A1 glycine substitution mutations segregates as an autosomal dominant trait in 2 families with dystrophic epidermolysis bullosa. Arch Dermatol 2002;138(2):269–71.
8. Tosti A, Piraccini BM, Scher RK. Isolated nail dystrophy suggestive of dominant dystrophic epidermolysis bullosa. Pediatr Dermatol 2003;20(5): 456–7.
9. Fine JD, Eady RAJ, Bauer EA, et al. The classification of inherited epidermolysis bullosa (EB): report of the third international consensus on diagnosis and classification of EB. J Am Acad Dermatol 2008;58:931–50.
10. Horn HM, Tidman MJ. The clinical spectrum of epidemolysis bullosa simplex. Br J Dermatol 2000; 142:468–72.
11. Figueira EC, Crotty A, Challinor CJ, et al. Granulation tissue in the eyelid margin and conjunctiva in junctional epidermolysis bullosa with features of LOC syndrome. Clin Experiment Ophthalmol 2007;35(2):163–6.
12. Shabbir G, Hassan M, Kazmi A. Laryngo-onychocutaneous syndrome: a study of 22 cases. Biomedica 1986;2:15–25.
13. McLean WH, Irvine AD, Hamill KJ, et al. An unusual N-terminal deletion of the laminin alpha3a isoform leads to the chronic granulation tissue disorder laryngo-onycho-cutaneous syndrome. Hum Mol Genet 2003;12(18):2395–409.
14. Parsapour K, Reep MD, Mohammed L, et al. Herlitz junctional epidermolisys bullosa presenting at birth with anonychia. Pediatr Dermatol 2001;18(3): 217–22.
15. Fritsch A, Loeckermann S, Kern JS, et al. A hypomorphic mouse model of dystrophic epidermolysis bullosa reveals mechanisms of disease and response to fibroblast therapy. J Clin Invest 2008; 118(5):1669–79.
16. Kim CC, Liang MG, Pfendner E, et al. What syndrome is it? Pediatr Dermatol 2007;24(3):306–8.
17. Phillips RJ, Atherton DJ, Gibbs ML, et al. Laryngo-onycho-cutaneous syndrome: an inherited epithelial defect. Arch Dis Child 1994;70:319–26.
18. Satter EK. A presumptive case of Kindler Syndrome with a new clinical finding. Pediatr Dermatol 2008; 25(6):646–7.

Oral Manifestations in the Epidermolysis Bullosa Spectrum

J. Timothy Wright, DDS, MS

KEYWORDS

- Mucosa • Enamel • Odontogenic • Dental caries
- Periodontal • Enamel hypoplasia • Microstomia
- Ankyloglosia

Epidermolysis bullosa (EB) represents a spectrum of conditions characterized by blistering and mechanical fragility of the skin. There is tremendous genetic heterogeneity and marked variation in clinical phenotypes in the multiple EB disorders. The most recent classification recognizes four major EB groupings and more than 30 EB subtypes.[1] The four major EB groups include intraepidermal EB (simplex), junctional EB, dermolytic EB (dystrophic), and mixed EB (Kindler syndrome). The molecular basis is now known for 13 of EB subtypes.[1] Depending on the specific EB type there can be significant morbidity involving the soft and hard tissues of the craniofacial complex (**Table 1**).

Individuals with EB display tremendous diversity in the various tissues and body systems involved and phenotypic severity.[2–4] Similarly, the craniofacial and oral manifestations of the different EB types vary markedly in character and severity depending largely on the EB type.[5,6] The tissues affected and the phenotypes displayed in affected individuals are closely related to the specific abnormal or absent proteins resulting from the causative genetic mutations for these disorders. For example, type VII collagen is critical for maintaining the integrity of the oral mucosa in the same manner it is in skin. It is not essential for normal development in the forming tooth bud. Consequently individuals with type VII collagen mutations typically have a developmentally normal dentition but can have severely affected oral soft tissues. In contrast, laminin 332 is highly expressed during tooth development so individuals

with mutations that affect laminin 332 function have defects in the enamel of their teeth.[7–9] In this article, the major oral manifestations are reviewed for different EB subtypes and related to the causative genetic mutations and gene expression.

INTRAEPIDERMAL EPIDERMOLYSIS BULLOSA

The EB simplex subtypes are caused by mutations in the *PKP1*, *DSP*, *KRT5*, *KRT14*, *PLEC1*, and *ITGA6* genes.[1] These genes all cause intraepidermal cleavage in the skin and are all expressed by the oral mucosa which, like skin, is comprised of a stratified epithelium.[10–12] Not surprisingly, individuals with EB simplex also exhibit an increased fragility of the oral mucosa with a high percentage of individuals experiencing blistering and ulceration of the oral mucosa.[5] In most cases, these are localized and occur most often secondary to trauma or tissue manipulation; however, some individuals can experience significant oral blistering and severe mucosal involvement. Typically, oral soft tissue lesions heal without scarring although some severely affected EB simplex subtypes (eg, Dowling-Meara) can display some oral scarring (**Fig. 1**).

Although many of the causative genes for EB simplex are known to be expressed in the odontogenic epithelium of developing teeth, the dentition in EB simplex tends to form normally.[9] These genes are also known to be expressed by the epithelial glands of the salivary tissues. Salivary function seems normal in people with

Department of Pediatric Dentistry, School of Dentistry, Brauer Hall # 7450, The University of North Carolina, Chapel Hill, NC 27599-7450, USA
E-mail address: tim_wright@dentistry.unc.edu

Dermatol Clin 28 (2010) 159–164
doi:10.1016/j.det.2009.10.022

Table 1
Oral manifestations in common epidermolysis bullosa subtypes

EB Type	OMIM no.	Oral Blistering	Oral Scarring	Microstomia	Enamel Defects
Simplex					
Localized	#131800	+	−	−	−
Generalized	#131900	+	−	−	−
Dowling-Meara	#131760	+	±	−	−
Junctional					
Non-Herlitz	#226650	+	−	−	++
Herlitz	#226700	+	−*	+	++
Dystrophic					
Dominant	#131750	+	±	−	±
Recessive	#226600	++	++	++	−
Kindler					
Kindler Syndrome	#173650	+	+	+	

Abbreviations: OMIM, Online Mendelian Inheritance in Man; +, frequently present; ++, always present; ±, variably present or absent; −, not present.

the EB simplex subtypes who have been tested.[13] The limited intraoral soft tissue morbidity in EB simplex and the normal tooth formation are likely the primary reasons that individuals with these EB subtypes have a prevalence of dental caries similar to unaffected populations.[14]

JUNCTIONAL EPIDERMOLYSIS BULLOSA

The junctional forms of EB are caused by mutations in *LAMA3*, *LAMB3*, *LAMC3*, *COL17A1*, *ITG6A*, and *ITGB4*, which are important in basement membrane–mediated cell adhesion.[1,15,16] The proteins transcribed from these genes are important in epithelial cell adhesion in the oral mucosa and the developing tooth bud.[8,17] The tissue fragility resulting from these mutations is

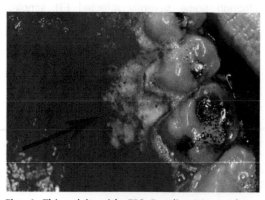

Fig. 1. This adult with EBS Dowling-Meara shows a normal soft tissue palatal architecture and a localized area of gingival hyperkeratosis (*arrow*).

variable but almost all individuals with the junctional forms of EB have an increased fragility of the oral mucosa that is accompanied by blister formation and ulceration.[5,18] In some individuals this can be severe. Despite the high prevalence of oral soft tissue lesions in the different junctional EB subtypes, most affected individuals do not have significant oral scarring. The soft tissue mobility and architecture remain relatively normal. One exception to this is the Herlitz EB subtype that is characterized by exuberant perioral granulation tissue (**Fig. 2**). This frequently results in a reduction in the oral opening (microstomia) and some loss of tissue mobility in the lips and perioral tissues.[5]

The genes that are causative of the junctional EB subtypes are all critical for normal tooth formation.[8,17] Specifically, these genes produce proteins that are involved in cell adhesion of the odontogenic epithelium, which gives rise to the cells that produce the dental enamel, the ameloblasts. Ameloblasts secrete an extracellular matrix and maintain contact and adhesion to the adjacent ameloblasts and thereby control the microenvironment that is critical for allowing normal mineralization of the enamel. When cell adhesion between ameloblasts is lost, then enamel defects are created. Dysfunctional ameloblast adhesion can result in leaking of serum fluids into the developing enamel, resulting in a retention of albumin and decreased mineralization.[19] In cases of individuals with junctional EB, the enamel lesions can vary from generalized pitting to a generalized hypoplasia, leaving only a very thin layer of enamel on the tooth surface (see **Fig. 2**). Some cases of Herlitz EB subtype also exhibit abnormal tooth

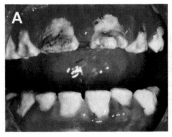
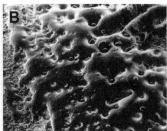
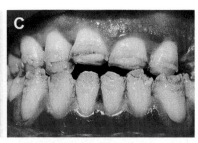

Fig. 2. The Herlitz junctional EB subtype is characterized by generalized enamel hypoplasia that results in yellow brown coloration of the teeth that frequently are spaced as seen in this child (*A*). Scanning electron microscopy of the tooth surfaces demonstrates the severe pitting that is often seen with junctional EB (*B*). Individuals who are heterozygous for junctional EB–associated genes can have enamel defects as seen in this male heterozygous for a *COL17A1* mutation (*C*). (*Courtesy of* Dr Dedee Murrell and Dr Richard Widmer.)

eruption.[20] This is often most notable in the molar regions but also can affect anterior teeth. Abnormal tooth eruption could occur due to dysfunction of the odontogenic epithelium that is known to play an important role in tooth eruption. Heterozygous carriers of *COL17A1* mutations have been shown to have enamel defects that range from horizontal hypoplastic bands to white mottled enamel.[21]

Individuals with junctional EB are at increased risk for developing dental caries.[14] This is thought to be primarily a function of their having marked enamel defects. The presence of extensive pitting over the tooth surface creates noncleansable areas that are ideal for microbial growth and substrate retention that are known to cause dental caries. Generalized thin enamel that is frequently rough in nature also reduces the tooth's primary resistance to the development and progression of caries. Salivary function seems normal in most individuals with junctional EB subtypes.[13] Occasional affected individuals can develop lesions resulting in transient occlusion of a salivary duct. These episodes typically self-correct with no specific treatment.

DERMOLYTIC EPIDERMOLYSIS BULLOSA

The dystrophic EB types are caused by mutations in *COL7A1* gene that codes for anchoring fibril protein that are located below the basal lamina at the dermal-epidermal basement membrane zone.[22] The dominant subtype tends to be less severe than the generalized recessive subtype with severity related to the amount and functionality of the anchoring fibril protein that is present. Type VII collagen is present in the basement membrane zone of the oral mucosa and is present during the early stages of tooth formation.[23] The *COL7A1* gene is not expressed by the ameloblasts.

The soft tissue manifestations of dystrophic EB range from mild to extremely severe.[5,24–27] For example, in dominant dystrophic EB, the oral manifestations can involve an increased tissue fragility but infrequent blistering. Blistering often can be induced easily, and dental treatments in even mildly affected dominant dystrophic EB should be approached with extra diligence to reduce soft tissue trauma. Individuals with severe generalized recessive dystrophic EB typically have extreme fragility of their oral and perioral mucosa. This is usually evident shortly after birth and can interfere with a neonate's ability to suckle. The oral ulcerations can affect all areas of the oral mucosa, including the tongue. The lesions heal with scarring. The continual process of blister formation and healing with scarring results in marked changes in the oral architecture. The tongue looses the lingual papillae and becomes bound down to the floor of the mouth, known as ankyloglossia (**Fig. 3**). Anatomic structures, such as the palatal rugae, are ablated (**Fig. 4**). The oral

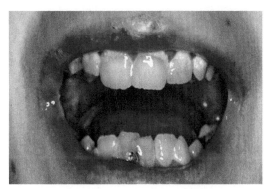

Fig. 3. Severe generalized recessive dystrophic EB is associated with ankyloglossia and a loss of the normal lingual papillae that cover the dorsal surface of the tongue, leaving a smoothed appearance that is frequently decorated with ulcerations.

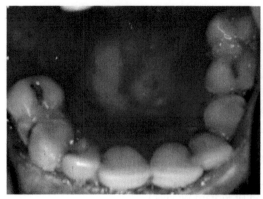

Fig. 4. Continual blistering and healing associated with severe generalized recessive dystrophic EB results in loss of normal anatomic oral features, such as the palatal rugae, leaving a smooth and ulcerated roof of the mouth.

vestibules that normally form corridors for food clearance between the teeth and lips and cheeks become obliterated with the soft tissue attachment advancing until it is just below the crowns of the teeth. The soft tissues defining the oral opening fail to grow normally due to scarring, resulting in a typically markedly restricted oral aperture. The presence of severe microstomia can impede the degree to which affected individuals can open their mouth, dramatically limiting the distance between the teeth even when they are fully open (**Fig. 5**).

Milia are frequently observed on the skin of individuals with EB and these also can occur intraorally. These intraoral keratocysts occur most commonly in the dermolytic forms of EB, with approximately 50% of individuals with dominant and recessive forms having milia compared with

approximately 10% to 20% of individuals with EB simplex.[5]

Individuals with certain forms of EB are at increased risk for developing squamous cell carcinomas and this is the case in severe generalized recessive dystrophic EB.[28,29] Although carcinomas occur with far greater frequency on the skin in individuals with EB, they can occur intraorally.[5,18,29,30] Individuals with severe generalized recessive dystrophic EB are at increased risk of oral squamous cell carcinoma formation and should, therefore, be extravigilant in monitoring changes in oral ulcerations, such as the development of raised, indurated borders.

Type VII collagen is not expressed by ameloblasts and the enamel seems to generally form normally in individuals with the dermolytic forms of EB.[9,31] Despite having relatively normal tooth formation, the prevalence of dental caries and resulting dental morbidity in severe generalized recessive dystrophic EB can be severe.[14,32,33] The tremendous oral soft tissue involvement results in the need to consume soft diets that are frequently high in calories to meet the nutritional needs of individuals. In the presence of marked oral blistering, affected individuals frequently eat slowly and with increased frequency. The loss of normal tongue mobility and obliteration of the oral vestibule decrease the normal food clearance, causing additional prolongation of the dental surfaces to potentially cariogenic substrates. Despite normal salivary secretion in most people with dermolytic EB subtypes, the oral cavity tends to be inoculated with high numbers of bacteria and there tends to be excessive tooth plaque formation that further promotes the formation of dental caries.[33] Taken together, these factors produce an extremely high risk for dental caries in individuals with severe generalized recessive dystrophic EB that can be challenging to prevent and difficult to treat. Many severely affected individuals have tremendous difficulty performing normal oral hygiene due to their extreme soft tissue fragility, and the use of anticariogenic mouth rinses can be unpleasant due to the presence of alcohol or strong flavoring agents.[34]

MIXED EPIDERMOLYSIS BULLOSA (KINDLER SYNDROME)

Kindler syndrome is an autosomal recessive genodermatosis caused by mutations in the *KIND1* gene that encodes for kindlin-1, which is a component of focal contacts in basal keratinocytes.[35] Kindlin-1 is known to be expressed by the oral epithelium, including the surface of the tongue.[4,6] It is not known whether or not it is expressed by

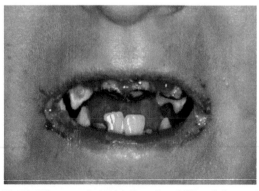

Fig. 5. Microstomia and reduced mobility of the oral tissues are typical features of severe generalized recessive dystrophic EB that limits oral access and can contribute to the formation of rampant dental caries, as seen in this child.

the odontogenic epithelium. Oral blistering in neonates and infants can be severe in Kindler syndrome.[1] The severity of the oral involvement regarding tissue fragility diminishes with age. Individuals affected with Kindler syndrome are at risk for developing marked periodontal disease that can have its onset during the teenage years. The kindlin-1 protein is expressed by the epithelium that attaches the oral mucosa to the tooth.[36] The abnormal functioning of kindlin-1 in forming normal focal adhesion in the basal keratinocytes seems to cause abnormal attachment and a predisposition to early-onset periodontal disease. Inflammation and gingival hyperplasia have been noted in young children with Kindler syndrome, suggesting that periodontal health may be compromised well before clinical signs of periodontal disease and alveolar bone loss.[37]

It is not known if kindlin-1 is expressed by the odontogenic epithelium; however, the dentition of affected individuals seems normal. Similarly, salivary function and risk of dental caries are unknown in this rare syndrome.

SUMMARY

The diverse conditions classified as EB share skin fragility and blistering and can have marked oral involvement. The genes that cause EB are also involved in development and maintenance of a variety of oral tissues. The specific oral manifestations and their severity are defined by the expression of genes that are important in cell adhesion and integrity. Some of the EB-associated proteins are critical for normal enamel formation (eg, laminin 332) and, when abnormal, result in varying degrees of enamel hypoplasia. Other proteins, such as kindlin-1, are important in maintaining mucosal integrity but seem not to affect tooth formation. Some of the oral morbidity associated with the EB conditions results from secondary effects of the condition, such as dental caries in the severe generalized recessive dystrophic EB subtype. Phenotype-genotype studies evaluating specific EB subtypes and their allelic mutations are complicated by the multitudes of mutations in the different genes known to cause EB and the many variable resulting phenotypes.[38,39] Although much has been learned over the past 30 years regarding the molecular basis of these conditions and their association with specific phenotypes, further phenotype-genotype studies regarding the oral manifestations of these conditions would advance not only understanding of EB but also the role of these genes and yet to be discovered EB-associated genes in oral development and health.

REFERENCES

1. Fine JD, Eady RA, Bauer EA, et al. The classification of inherited epidermolysis bullosa (EB): report of the Third International Consensus Meeting on Diagnosis and Classification of EB. J Am Acad Dermatol 2008; 58(6):931–50.
2. Gedde-Dahl T Jr. Sixteen types of epidermolysis bullosa. On the clinical discrimination, therapy, and prenatal diagnosis. Acta Derm Venereol Suppl (Stockh) 1981;95(Suppl):74–87.
3. Fine J-D, Wright JT. Epidermolysis bullosa. In: Demis JD, editor, Clinical dermatology, vol. 2. Philadelphia: Lippincott-Raven; 1995. p. 1–35.
4. Lai-Cheong JE, Tanaka A, Hawche G, et al. Kindler syndrome: a focal adhesion genodermatosis. Br J Dermatol 2009;160(2):233–42.
5. Wright JT, Fine J-D, Johnson LB. Oral soft tissues in hereditary epidermolysis bullosa. Oral Surg Oral Med Oral Pathol 1991;71:440–6.
6. Wiebe CB, Petricca G, Hakkinen L, et al. Kindler syndrome and periodontal disease: review of the literature and a 12-year follow-up case. J Periodontol 2008;79(5):961–6.
7. Meneguzzi B, Marinkovich MP, Aberdam D, et al. Kalinin is abnormally expressed in epithelial basement membranes of Herlitz's Junctional epidermolysis bullosa patients. Exp Dermatol 1992;1:221–9.
8. Aberdam D, Aguzzi A, Baudoin C, et al. Developmental expression of nicein adhesion protein (laminin-5) subunits suggests multiple morphogenic roles. Cell Adhes Commun 1994;2:115–29.
9. Wright JT, Fine J-D, Johnson LB. Developmental defects of enamel in humans with hereditary epidermolysis bullosa. Arch Oral Biol 1993;38:945–55.
10. Pelissier A, Ouhayoun JP, Sawaf MH, et al. Evolution of cytokeratin expression in developing human tooth germ. J Biol Buccale 1990;18:99–108.
11. Modolo F, Martins MT, Loducca SV, et al. Expression of integrin subunits alpha2, alpha3, alpha5, alphav, beta1, beta3 and beta4 in different histological types of ameloblastoma compared with dental germ, dental lamina and adult lining epithelium. Oral Dis 2004;10(5):277–82.
12. Kieffer-Combeau S, Meyer JM, Lesot H. Cell-matrix interactions and cell-cell junctions during epithelial histo-morphogenesis in the developing mouse incisor. Int J Dev Biol 2001;45(5–6):733–42.
13. Wright JT, Childers NK, Evans KL, et al. Salivary function of persons with hereditary epidermolysis bullosa. Oral Surg Oral Med Oral Pathol 1991;71: 553–9.
14. Wright JT, Fine J-D, Johnson L. Dental caries risk factors in hereditary epidermolysis bullosa. Pediatr Dent 1994;16:427–32.
15. Uitto J, Pulkkinen L, Christiano AM. Molecular basis of the dystrophic and junctional forms of

epidermolysis bullosa: mutations in the type VII collagen and kalinin (Laminin 5) genes. J Invest Dermatol 1994;103:39S–46S.

16. McGrath JA, Gatalica B, Christiano AM, et al. Mutations in the 180-kD bullous pemphigoid antigen (BPAG2), a hemidesmosomal transmembrane collagen (COL17A1), in generalized atrophic benign epidermolysis bullosa. Nat Genet 1995;11(1):83–6.

17. Asaka T, Akiyama M, Domon T, et al. Type XVII collagen is a key player in tooth enamel formation. Am J Pathol 2009;174(1):91–100.

18. Sedano HO, Gorlin RJ. Epidermolysis bullosa. Oral Surg Oral Med Oral Pathol 1989;67:555–63.

19. Kirkham J, Robinson C, Strafford SM, et al. The chemical composition of tooth enamel in junctional epidermolysis bullosa. Arch Oral Biol 2000;45(5):377–86.

20. Brooks JK, Bare LC, Davidson J, et al. Junctional epidermolysis bullosa associated with hypoplastic enamel and pervasive failure of tooth eruption: oral rehabilitation with use of an overdenture. Oral Surg Oral Med Oral Pathol Oral Radiol Endod 2008;105(4):e24–28.

21. Murrell DF, Pasmooij AM, Pas HH, et al. Retrospective diagnosis of fatal BP180-deficient non-Herlitz junctional epidermolysis bullosa suggested by immunofluorescence (IF) antigen-mapping of parental carriers bearing enamel defects. J Invest Dermatol 2007;127(7):1772–5.

22. Christiano AM, Greenspan DS, Hoffman GG, et al. A missense mutation in type VII collagen in two affected siblings with recessive dystrophic epidermolysis bullosa. Nat Genet 1993;4(1):62–6.

23. Heikinheimo K, Morgan PR, Happonen R-P, et al. Distribution of extracellular matrix proteins in odontogenic tumours and developing teeth. Virchows Arch B Cell Pathol Incl Mol Pathol 1991;61:101–9.

24. Album MM, Gaisin A, Lee KWT, et al. Epidermolysis bullosa dystrophica polydysplastica. Oral Surg Oral Med Oral Pathol 1977;43:859–72.

25. Crawford E, Burkes EJ, Briggaman R. Hereditary epidermolysis bullosa: oral manifestations and dental therapy. Oral Surg Oral Med Oral Pathol 1976;42:490–500.

26. Winter G. Dental problems in epidermolysis bullosa. In: Priestley GC, Tidman MJ, Weiss JB, et al, editors. Epidermolysis bullosa: a comprehensive review of classification, management and laboratory studies. Berkshire (UK): D.E.B.R.A; 1990. p. 21–7.

27. Wright JT, Fine J-D, Johnson LB, et al. Oral involvement of recessive dystrophic epidermolysis bullosa inversa. Am J Med Genet 1993;47:1184–8.

28. Schwartz RA, Birnkrant AP, Rubenstein DJ, et al. Squamous cell carcinoma in dominant type epidermolysis bullosa dystrophica. Cancer 1981;47:615–20.

29. Fine JD, Johnson LB, Weiner M, et al. Epidermolysis bullosa and the risk of life-threatening cancers: the National EB Registry experience, 1986–2006. J Am Acad Dermatol 2009;60(2):203–11.

30. Reed WB, College J, Francis MJO, et al. Epidermolysis bullosa dystrophica with epidermal neoplasms. Arch Dermatol 1974;110:894–902.

31. Kirkham J, Robinson C, Strafford SM, et al. The chemical composition of tooth enamel in recessive dystrophic epidermolysis bullosa: significance with respect to dental caries. J Dent Res 1996;75:1672–8.

32. De Benedittis M, Petruzzi M, Favia G, et al. Orodental manifestations in Hallopeau-Siemens-type recessive dystrophic epidermolysis bullosa. Clin Exp Dermatol 2004;29(2):128–32.

33. Harris JC, Bryan RA, Lucas VS, et al. Dental disease and caries related microflora in children with dystrophic epidermolysis bullosa. Pediatr Dent 2001;23(5):438–43.

34. Wright JT, Fine J-D, Johnson LB. Hereditary epidermolysis bullosa: oral manifestations and dental management. Pediatr Dent 1993;15:242–8.

35. Jobard F, Bouadjar B, Caux F, et al. Identification of mutations in a new gene encoding a FERM family protein with a pleckstrin homology domain in Kindler syndrome. Hum Mol Genet 2003;12(8):925–35.

36. Abdallah BM, Jensen CH, Gutierrez G, et al. Regulation of human skeletal stem cells differentiation by Dlk1/Pref-1. J Bone Miner Res 2004;19(5):841–52.

37. Wiebe CB, Penagos H, Luong N, et al. Clinical and microbiologic study of periodontitis associated with Kindler syndrome. J Periodontol 2003;74(1):25–31.

38. Varki R, Sadowski S, Pfendner E, et al. Epidermolysis bullosa. I. Molecular genetics of the junctional and hemidesmosomal variants. J Med Genet 2006;43(8):641–52.

39. Varki R, Sadowski S, Uitto J, et al. Epidermolysis bullosa. II. Type VII collagen mutations and phenotype-genotype correlations in the dystrophic subtypes. J Med Genet 2007;44(3):181–92.

Alopecia in Epidermolysis Bullosa

Antonella Tosti, MD[a],*, Bruna Duque-Estrada, MD[b],
Dédée F. Murrell, MA, BMBCh, FAAD, MD[c]

KEYWORDS

• Epidermolysis bullosa • Alopecia • Hair loss • Scalp

The expression of the basement membrane zone (BMZ) components in the anagen hair follicles of the human scalp is similar to that of interfollicular epidermis, with expression of plectin, 180-kD bullous pemphigoid antigen (BP180), 230-kD bullous pemphigoid antigen (PB230), $\alpha 6\beta 4$ integrin, laminin 311, laminin 332, and type 4 and type 7 collagen.[1,2] Expression of the BMZ components, however, varies according with the different follicular portions. In particular, the upper and middle portions of the hair follicle (infundibulum and isthmus), including the bulge region, show expression of all BMZ components with a labeling intensity under immunofluorescence similar to that found in the interfollicular epidermis. In the lower part of the follicle and in the hair bulb, expression of laminin 311 and collagen 4 is continuous, but labeling for other BMZ components shows a gradual decrease with discontinuous expression of $\alpha 6\beta 4$ integrin and laminin 332, particularly outside the hair bulb. Between the dermal papilla and the epithelial cells inside the hair bulb, all of the BMZ components are evident, with the exception of the BP230.[1,2] The reduced expression of all BMZ components outside the hair bulb and the complete absence of BP230 at the dermal papilla junction seem to be responsible for the incomplete ultrastructure of hemidesmosomes in these regions. Desmosomes are also important in hair structure and function. These components include the desmogleins 1 and 3 (involved in pemphigus foliaceus and vulgaris, respectively, where alopecia can result from an autoimmune mechanism), desmoplakins, plakophilin, and plakoglobin.

Taken together, these findings show that in normal conditions the BMZ components are expressed to a lesser degree in the transient regions of the hair follicles as compared with the permanent region (the upper portion of the follicle). The complete structure of the hemidesmosomes is then responsible for the stabilization of the upper follicle to the surrounding connective tissues, while the incomplete hemidesmosome structure may facilitate the movement of the transient region.

Blistering of the scalp involving the lamina lucida and below, as in junctional and dystrophic forms of epidermolysis bullosa (EB), usually leads to cicatricial alopecia secondary to the inflammatory process in the interfollicular epidermis and in the upper portion of the hair follicle. As the BMZ components are similar at these sites, absence or anomalous formation of the specifically affected proteins increases hair and skin fragility secondary to trauma.[3–5] In this way, blister formation in the occipital area is very common, as it is an important support area of the scalp. The occurrence of alopecia in different forms of EB is summarized in **Table 1**.

Funding Sources: None.

The authors have no conflict of interest to disclose.

The authors declare that this manuscript represents original and valid work and has not been published elsewhere.

[a] Department of Dermatology, University of Bologna, Via Massarenti, 1. 40138, Bologna, Italy

[b] Instituto de Dermatologia Azulay, Av. Sernambetiba 3300, bloco 01, apt.1802, CEP: 22630–010, Rio de Janeiro, Brazil

[c] Department of Dermatology, St George Hospital, University of New South Wales, Sydney, NSW 2217, Australia

* Corresponding author.

E-mail address: antonella.tosti@unibo.it (A. Tosti).

doi:10.1016/j.det.2009.10.018

derm.theclinics.com

Table 1
Classification of EB and hair abnormalities in the different subtypes of EB

	Subtypes	Hair/Scalp Involvement
EB simplex	EBS superficialis AD	None
	Lethal acantholytic EBS AR	Alopecia universalis
	Plakophilin deficiency AR	Sparse, dry, wiry hair; loss of eyelashes/eyebrows
	EBS localized AD	None
	Dowling-Meara AD	None
	EBS other generalized AD (previously called Koebner)	None
	Autosomal recessive EBS	None
	EBS-Ogna AD	None
	EBS migratory circinate	None
	EBS with mottled pigmentation	None
	EBS with muscular dystrophy	Occasional congenital alopecia
	EBS with pyloric atresia	None
JEB (junctional EB)	Herlitz AR	May occur, particularly if there is survival long term to develop cicatricial alopecia
	Non-Herlitz AR (generalized and localized)	Patchy or diffuse cicatricial alopecia; partial absence of eyelashes, eyebrows, and pubic and axillary hair
	With pyloric atresia AR	Scarring alopecia if scalp affected
	Inversa JEB	None reported
	Late-onset JEB	None
	LOC syndrome	Scalp erosions
DEB (dystrophic EB)	DDEB generalized	Telogen effluvium if anemic
	RDEB severe generalized (previously called RDEB, Hallopeau-Siemens)	Sparse scalp hair; scarring alopecia around hairline
	RDEB generalized other	As for RDEB-GS but less pronounced
	Acral DDEB and RDEB	None
	Pretibial DDEB and RDEB	None
	Pruriginous DEB, AD, or AR	Scalp folliculitis
	DDEB nails only	None
	DEB-BDN	None
	RDEB inversa	None
	RDEB centripetalis	None
Kindler syndrome	AR	None

Abbreviations: AD, autosomal dominant; AR, autosomal recessive; DDEB, dominant dystrophic EB; DDEB-BDN, bullous dermolysis of the newborn; EBS, epidermolysis bullosa simplex; LOC, laryngo-onycho-cutaneous; RDEB, recessive dystrophic EB.

HAIR CHANGES IN EB
EB simplex

Most cases of autosomal dominant EBS are caused by dominant negative mutations in either KRT5 or KRT14. These keratins are different than those expressed in the hair shaft and, as blistering occurs in the basal layer of the skin, generally there is no scarring unless there is secondary infection.

Even patients with recessive EBS caused by keratin 14 null mutations do not get a specific alopecia. If these patients become anemic because of blistering or are very sick from sepsis, they may develop a telogen effluvium, which is reversible if the cause is reversed.

Complete absence of hair, eyebrows, eyelashes, and vellus hairs is a distinctive feature of lethal acantholytic EB, which is caused by truncation mutations in the desmoplakin gene, removing the C terminus of the protein. Currently there is one published case,[6] but another case recently presented with similar alopecia (Amy Paller and Dedee Murrell, personal communication, July 2009).

In patients with suprabasal EB caused by plakophilin 1 deficiency (previously described as ectodermal dysplasia–skin fragility syndrome), the hair is sparse, short, dry and curly; eyebrows and eyelashes may be absent. Some patients just have woolly hair, while others have hypotrichosis.[7–9] The hair loss that develops is permanent (John McGrath, personal communication, June 2009). Recently, a knockout mouse for desmoglein 3 was created that displayed telogen hair loss and blistering, but as yet there is no human corollary as a form of EB.[10]

EBS with muscular dystrophy (EBS-MD) generally is regarded as not causing alopecia, although there have been two reports of EBS-MD with congenital alopecia.[11]

Junctional EB

Localized or diffuse scarring alopecia may be observed in Herlitz JEB (**Fig. 1**),[12] but most patients do not survive beyond 1 year. The reason why it is not often reported is likely that other symptoms occur before the alopecia manifests itself.

Non-Herlitz JEB is genetically heterogeneous. When caused by defects in Lm332, in some patients the alopecia may be very severe because of exuberant granulation tissue formation and scarring (**Fig. 2**). In others, however, it may cause more subtle alopecia and loss of eyebrows. In non-Herlitz JEB caused by type XVII collagen deficiency, previously known as generalized atrophic benign EB (GABEB), patchy or even diffuse scarring alopecia has been reported as a hallmark. Alopecia usually develops in early childhood as a consequence of scalp erosions and blistering. Partial absence of eyelashes, eyebrows, and pubic and axillary hair also has been reported.[5,13,14] In some patients, the scarring alopecia has a typical male baldness pattern. The degree of hair involvement can vary considerably between patients with type XVII collagen deficiency.

Because of the thinning of the skin and loss of hair follicles, this type of alopecia has been referred to as atrophic. For some reasons yet not fully understood, female patients may develop a male pattern of diffuse alopecia. By the third or fourth decade, this may be so severe that female patients opt to wear a wig.[13,15,16]

According to Pasmooij and colleagues,[17] patients with reduced staining with 1A8C and 1D1 caused by COL17A1 mutations have normal primary hair and sparse secondary hair, whereas patients with lack of staining of the type XVII collagen antibodies 1A8C and 1D1 caused by COL17A1 mutations have sparse primary and absent secondary hair and even nonscarring universal alopecia with almost complete absence of vellus hair, eyelashes, eyebrows, and secondary hairs. This fits with COL17A1 knock-out mice that developed sparse nonpigmented hair and subsequently alopecia.[18]

JEB with pyloric atresia (PA) or due to reduced integrin beta 4 may result in scarring alopecia if the affected area of the scalp is eroded, but it does not appear to cause a primary alopecia (**Fig. 3**).[19] Interestingly the only case of JEB, reported with

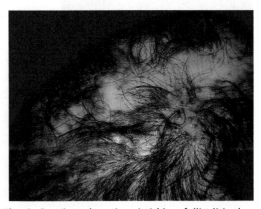

Fig. 2. Scarring alopecia mimicking folliculitis decalvans in non-Herlitz JEB caused by heterozygous laminin B3 defects.

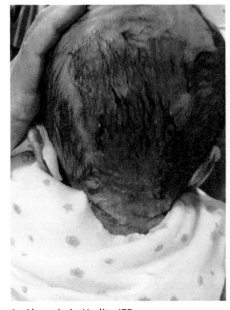

Fig. 1. Alopecia in Herlitz JEB.

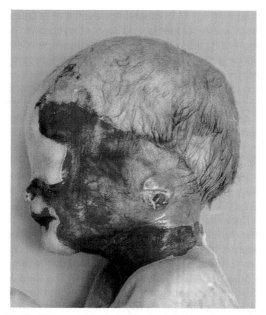

Fig. 3. JEB caused by integrin B4 deficiency from aplasia cutis congenita.

alopecia and absence of axillary and pubic hair, was a long-term survivor without PA, who had homozygous missense mutations in ITGB4.[20]

Dystrophic EB

Recessive DEB generalized severe

Gradual onset of scarring alopecia in areas of trauma from rubbing and blistering is very common (**Fig. 4**A, B). Puberty is usually very delayed or absent in these patients. Three adults with recessive DEB (RDEB) of generalized severe subtype had very sparse scalp hair, and none had experienced puberty.[21] Generally, the authors have observed that the hair loss in RDEB is worse in female patients who choose to plait their hair or tie it up in a pony tail, compared with males with short hair or females who do not regularly put their hair under tension. (**Fig. 4**C, D).

Folliculitis-like lesions were reported in one case patient with DEB pruriginosa. Scalp lesions of the 18-year-old boy consisted of multiple, nonpainful, red follicular papules and pustules.

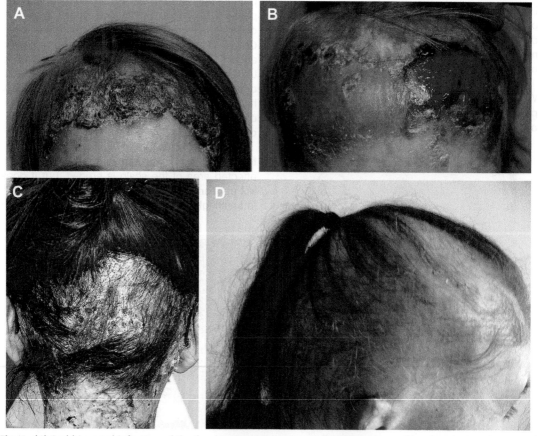

Fig. 4. (*A*) Scabbing and infection of the forehead and frontal scalp in RDEB-GS, resulting in scarring alopecia of the frontal scalp 6 months later (*B*). (*C*) Occipital scabbing and hair loss in RDEB-GS in a female patient with long hair and traction. (*D*) Diffuse alopecia in RDEB-GS after longstanding traction.

Histopathological sections demonstrated hyperkeratosis within the folliculitis-like lesion, with a flattened rete ridge near the orifice of the hair follicle, and a subepidermal cleft. Fibrosis was present, as well as mild perivascular and perifollicular lymphohistiocytic infiltrate in the papillary dermis. Interestingly, no infiltration of neutrophils was observed in the orifice of the hair follicles.[22]

Kindler Syndrome

Interestingly, Kindler syndrome has not been associated with alopecia. Perhaps this is because the defective protein, kindlin or FHH1 (fermitin family homolog 1), is in focal contacts rather than hemidesmosomes and not expressed in hair follicles.

REFERENCES

1. Chuang YH, Dean D, Allen J, et al. Comparison between the expression of basement membrane zone antigens of human interfollicular epidermis and anagen hair follicle using indirect immunofluorescence. Br J Dermatol 2003;149:274–81.

2. Joubeh S, Mori O, Hashimoto K, et al. Immunofluorescence analysis of the basement membrane zone components in human anagen hair follicles. Exp Dermatol 2003;12:365–70.

3. Jonkman MF, De Jong MC, Heeres K, et al. 180-kD bullous pemphigoid antigen (BP180) is deficient in generalized atrophic benign epidermolysis bullosa. J Clin Invest 1995;95:1345–52.

4. Schumann H, Hammami-Hauasli N, Pulkkinen L, et al. Three novel homozygous point mutations and a new polymorphism in the COL17A1 gene: relations to biological and clinical phenotypes of junctional epidermolysis bullosa. Am J Hum Genet 1997;60:1344–53.

5. Swensson O, Christophers E. Generalized atrophic benign epidermolysis bullosa in 2 siblings complicated by multiple squamous cell carcinomas. Arch Dermatol 1998;1334:199–203.

6. Jonkman MF, Pasmooij AM, Pasmans SG, et al. Loss of desmoplakin tail causes lethal acantholytic epidermolysis bullosa. Am J Hum Genet 2005;77(4):653–60.

7. McGrath JA, McMillan JR, Shemanko CS, et al. Mutations in the plakophilin 1 gene result in ectodermal dysplasia/skin fragility syndrome. Nat Genet 1997;17:241–4.

8. McGrath JA, Hoeger PH, Christiano AM, et al. Skin fragility and hypohidrotic ectodermal dysplasia resulting from ablation of plakophilin 1. Br J Dermatol 1999;140:297–307.

9. Hamada T, South AP, Mitsuhashi Y, et al. Genotype-phenotype correlation in skin fragility–ectodermal dysplasia syndrome resulting from mutations in plakophilin 1. Exp Dermatol 2002;11:107–14.

10. Ghoreski K, Huenefeld C, Glocova I, et al. Functional restoration of inherited epidermolysis bullosa after adult bone marrow-derived adult stem cells. J Invest Dermatol 2009;129:47 [Abstract 270].

11. Chiaverini C, Charlesworth A, Meneguzzi G, et al. Epidermolysis bullosa simplex with muscular dystrophy. Derm Clin N Am, in press.

12. Laimer M, Lanschuetzer CM, Diem A, et al. Herlitz junctional EB. Derm Clin N Am, in press.

13. Hintner H, Wolff K. Generalized atrophic benign epidermolysis bullosa. Arch Dermatol 1982;118: 375–84.

14. Hashimoto I, Schnyder UW, Anton-Lamprecht I. Epidermolysis bullosa hereditaria with junctional blistering in an adult. Dermatologica 1976;152: 72–86.

15. Yancey KB, Hintner H. Derm Clin N Am, in press.

16. Jonkman MF, Jong MC, Heeres K, et al. Generalized atrophic benign epidermolysis bullosa: either the 180-kD bullous pemphigoid antigen or laminin 5 is deficient. Arch Dermatol 1996;132:145–50.

17. Pasmooij AM, Pas HH, Jansen GH, et al. Localized and generalized forms of blistering in junctional epidermolysis bullosa due to COL17A1 mutations in the Netherlands. Br J Dermatol 2007;156:861–70.

18. Nishie W, Sawamura D, Goto M, et al. Humanization of autoantigen. Nat Med 2007;13(3):378–83.

19. Dang NN, Klingberg S, Rubin AI, et al. Differential expression of pyloric atresia in junctional epidermolysis bullosa with novel ITGB4 mutations. Acta Derm Venereol 2008;88(5):438–48.

20. Inoue M, Tamai K, Shimizu H, et al. A homozygous missense mutation in the cytoplasmic tail of beta4 integrin, G931D, that disrupts hemidesmosome assembly and underlies non-Herlitz junctional epidermolysis bullosa without pyloric atresia? J Invest Dermatol 2000;114(5):1061–4.

21. Horn HM, Tidman MJ. The clinical spectrum of dystrophic epidermolysis bullosa. Br J Dermatol 2002;146(2):267–74.

22. Fan YM, Yang YP, Li SF. Medical genetics: sporadic dystrophic epidermolysis bullosa with albopapuloid and prurigo- and folliculitis-like lesions. Int J Dermatol 2009;48(8):855–7.

Understanding the Pathogenesis of Recessive Dystrophic Epidermolysis Bullosa Squamous Cell Carcinoma

Andrew P. South, PhD[a],*, Edel A. O'Toole, MB, PhD, FRCP, FRCPI[b]

KEYWORDS

- Epidermolysis bullosa • Cancer • Metastasis
- *COL7A1* • Type VII collagen

It has been apparent since 1974 that patients suffering from recessive dystrophic epidermolysis bullosa (RDEB) are at increased risk of developing life-threatening skin cancers.[1] Comprehensive analysis of epidermolysis bullosa patients in the continental United States over a 20-year period has now translated this risk into figures pertaining to incidence, mortality, and morbidity.[2] The data are shocking and clear: The cumulative risk of developing squamous cell carcinoma (SCC) and subsequent death in patients with generalized severe RDEB (gs-RDEB) at age 55 is greater than 90% and 78%, respectively. Such frequency of SCC development in a genetic disease is only exceeded by patients suffering from xeroderma pigmentosum, where mutations in DNA repair machinery result in dramatic hypersensitivity to sunlight and a greater than 2000-fold increase in skin cancers. The comparison with xeroderma pigmentosum is interesting, though. Although an increase in incidence is seen, with a frequency of 50% for all nonmelanoma skin cancer in patients under 10 years, metastatic disease is comparable to spontaneous SCC: Metastasis in xeroderma pigmentosum is reported at 4% compared to 2% to 4% for the general population.[3–5] In xeroderma pigmentosum, internal malignancies are also increased (20-fold increase in brain tumors for instance), which is not the case in RDEB.[2] Therefore, clear differences exist in the pathogenesis of SCC between xeroderma pigmentosum and RDEB.

A number of studies have tried to explore the reasons for such an unrivalled high incidence of aggressive SCC in RDEB patients. This review summarizes what is currently known about the pathogenesis of RDEB-associated SCC and speculates as to what the true causes of this phenomenon may be.

DYSTROPHIC EPIDERMOLYSIS BULLOSA

Dystrophic epidermolysis bullosa (DEB) is caused exclusively by mutations in *COL7A1*, the gene that encodes type VII collagen. The generally accepted dogma is that patients with the most severe form of the disease, gs-RDEB, harbor premature termination codon mutations in *COL7A1*. This means there is less type VII collagen present in the patients' skin, with decreased or absent anchoring fibril formation, resulting in more severe disease. However, there are exceptions: In patients with gs-RDEB, 9.4% of identified mutated alleles were missense substitutions[6] and 2.4% of this series of patients harbored missense substitutions on both alleles.

[a] Centre For Oncology and Molecular Medicine, Ninewell's Hospital and Medical School, Dundee, DD1 9SY, UK
[b] Centre for Cutaneous Research, Blizard Institute of Cell and Molecular Science, Barts and the London School of Medicine and Dentistry, Queen Mary, University of London, 4 Newark Street, Whitechapel, London E1 2AT, UK
* Corresponding author.
E-mail address: a.p.south@dundee.ac.uk (A.P. South).

Dermatol Clin 28 (2010) 171–178
doi:10.1016/j.det.2009.10.023
0733-8635/09/$ – see front matter © 2010 Elsevier Inc. All rights reserved.

CANCER IN EPIDERMOLYSIS BULLOSA

The first comprehensive review of the literature brought together a number of case reports and summarized that over two thirds of RDEB patients eventually die from SCC.[1] Since this publication, additional cases have been generally reported on a case-by-case basis, although in some instances up to 10 patients have been described.[7] Reports have also identified patients suffering from dominant DEB (DDEB) and junctional epidermolysis bullosa (JEB) who have developed SCC, although few details of metastasis or death were observed. In the largest cohort of epidermolysis bullosa patients studied to date, Fine and colleagues[2] demonstrated solid statistics for RDEB and that SCC does occur with an increased incidence in JEB patients but not in DDEB patients. Some reports suggest that DDEB patients develop aggressive SCC. However, this evidence does not represent a comprehensive cohort study.[7–9] One report of malignant melanoma in a child with RDEB can be found in the literature[10] and three cases of melanoma were reported by Fine and colleagues[2] in 2009, suggesting possible increased risk in childhood (2.5% in RDEB by age 12 compared to 1.35%–2.7% lifetime risk in the general population). Other tumors were reported by Fine and colleagues[2] but not in a frequency significant enough to suggest any difference in the RDEB population; clearly cutaneous SCC is the principle cancer.

OPEN QUESTIONS IN RECESSIVE DYSTROPHIC EPIDERMOLYSIS BULLOSA

A number of unanswered questions remain concerning the pathology of RDEB-associated SCC: Is it the SCC keratinocyte itself that is tumorigenic? Is COL7A1 a tumor suppressor? Or is it the microenvironment of RDEB that predisposes to SCC alone? Other key questions need to be answered: What is the mutagen in RDEB? Why do other blistering or proliferative skin diseases not show such high incidence of SCC? And why is SCC the major cancer to affect this patient group? No single experiment or investigation has provided clear-cut answers to these questions and the data can be conflicting and controversial.

CLINICAL-PATHOLOGICAL STUDIES

Clinically, the risk of developing SCC appears to parallel the severity and extent of ulceration and scarring of the skin, which in turn correlates with loss of type VII collagen expression and decreased or absent anchoring fibrils.[11,12] However, no data are available and no detailed analysis has been carried out of the COL7A1 mutation spectrum in a large cohort of RDEB patients who have gone on to develop SCC. Such clinical, genetic, and immunohistology data could potentially shed light into the matter. Reported RDEB SCCs generally occur over joints and on the distal extremities in areas of chronic wounding and scarring, paralleling what is seen in cases of Marjolin ulcer and other genetic skin diseases predisposing to scar formation. Marjolin ulcer (reviewed by Ogawa and colleagues[13]) and SCC arising in burn scars (reviewed by Kowal-Vern and Criswell[14]) do recur and are typically more aggressive than UV-induced SCC: A mortality rate of 21% is seen in all burn-scar cancers.[14] Burn-scar malignancies also include melanoma, but the frequency, like in RDEB, is much less than SCC. SCCs have been observed in various other chronic skin disorders, such as lupus vulgaris, discoid lupus erythematosus, necrobiosis lipoidica, and chronic radiodermatitis (reviewed by Kaplan[15]). Clearly however, there is a shorter latency period in RDEB (tumors developing in second decade of life as opposed to 30–50 years in Marjolin ulcer) and increased mortality is also seen in RDEB.[2,14] One might speculate that this shorter latency could be due to the extent and persistence of chronic wounds and scarring in RDEB. Certainly this clinical parallel exists and has yet to be fully explored.

Other genetic skin diseases have been associated with cutaneous SCC. Anecdotal reports have linked nonbullous congenital ichthyosiform erythroderma[16] and Darier disease, with aggressive SCC,[17] as well as with Huriez[18] and KID (keratitis, ichtyosis, deafness) syndromes.[19] Up to 10% of Kindler syndrome patients, another condition associated with chronic scarring, suffer from SCC[20] and reports of recurrence and metastatic SCC exist,[21,22] but the numbers are too small for statistical analysis and incidence in these reported cases are much lower than that for RDEB.

Goldberg and colleagues[23] postulated that repetitive tissue stress leads to tumor promotion and that this was likely to be relevant for RDEB. In support of this theory, Smoller and colleagues[24] observed growth-activated keratinocytes in biopsies from RDEB scarred skin based on the expression of protein markers similarly regulated in psoriatic skin, such as intense suprabasal expression of K16, involucrin, and filaggrin. Six RDEB patients and four patients with epidermolysis bullosa simplex (EBS) were studied. RDEB biopsies from clinically normal, unwounded skin did not show a growth-activated pattern of antibody immunoreactivity. The investigators speculated as to whether this growth activation could be a reason for SCC development.

Such a study in RDEB patients asks: Are observed phenomena a result of the phenotype rather than a factor predisposing to SCC? The answer has not been determined; many factors related to wound healing, tissue stress, and remodeling have been shown to promote tumorigenicity in other experimental systems. To follow up on a single line of enquiry would certainly require increased numbers, more controls, and good experimental data. Demonstrating a similar scenario in other non–tumor bearing skin diseases would suggest that indeed these observations are a result and not a cause. The same logic can be applied to studies investigating the presence of natural killer cells, fibroblast growth factor (FGF), and metalloproteinase (MMP) proteins in patients with RDEB. The activity of natural killer cells, which play a key role in immune response to certain viruses and cancers, was analyzed in a cohort of 11 RDEB, 6 DDEB, 7 JEB, and 10 EBS patients, as well as in 20 normal and 12 malabsorption control subjects. Reduced activity was seen in RDEB, DDEB, and JEB patients, and in malabsorption controls.[25] As junctional and dystrophic EB patients are frequently malnourished this could well explain the observation. Nevertheless, a reduction in circulating immune cells may well be an important compounding factor in SCC development.

Are increased levels of urine FGF–2 observed in RDEB patients[26] a result of repetitive tissue injury or the distinct pathology of RDEB generated by mutations in COL7A1? Indeed, elevated FGF–2 was seen in 51% of 39 RDEB patients but also in 21% of 33 unaffected family members and 13% of 30 EBS patients. No elevated levels were seen in 12 JEB patients ruling out a response to blister formation but the identification of variation in the unaffected family members and EBS patients suggest the absence of a direct link to SCC formation. Similarly in wound healing, matrix MMPs are expressed during keratinocyte, fibroblast, and inflammatory cell migration and during connective tissue remodeling.[27] The increase in MMP in some RDEB patients[28,29] should come as no surprise given the extent of tissue remodeling that occurs. However, a polymorphism increasing the activity of the MMP1 promoter has been recently shown to modify the severity of disease in a French RDEB cohort.[30] Whether patients developing SCC have higher levels of MMP1 expression has yet to be determined. One study has identified the expression of MMP in RDEB-associated SCC.[31] The investigators looked at expression of MMP7, MMP13, and MMP9 using immunohistochemistry in archival samples (25 RDEB SCC, 61 UV SCC, 29 Bowens disease). MMP7 and MMP13 were present in the majority of SCCs

studied and MMP9 was present in infiltrating stromal cells in all SCCs studied (RDEB and non-RDEB). The report suggests there was an increase in intensity of MMP7 staining in RDEB SCC, particularly within the invasive edge of tumors, yet distribution and incidence remained comparable to UV-induced SCC.[31]

Expression of MUC1 (mucin-1), a cell surface protein associated with breast cancer, has been observed in 25 of 25 RDEB SCCs, 5 of 5 JEB SCCs, and 52 of 55 UV-induced SCCs, suggesting that this glycoprotein is a marker of SCC similarly expressed in epidermolysis bullosa and non–epidermolysis bullosa cancers.[32]

In the only study of its kind to date, gene expression analysis was carried out in three RDEB patients presenting with SCC. RNA from tumor and peritumoral skin was compared with three spontaneous SCC patients. For the most part, an identical pattern of gene expression was observed except for the lack of IGFBP-3 (insulin growth factor-binding protein 3, a mediator of apoptosis) expression in RDEB SCC tumors, findings which were corroborated with protein expression in 7 of 11 RDEB SCCs compared with 1 of 21 non-RDEB SCCs.[33] The gene expression platform used for this experiment was a nylon array spotted with around 4000 skin-related genes. This made it possible to relate the lack of discernible differences to the number of genes present. Another problem that will be experienced by such in vivo expression profiling experiments is the heterogeneity seen in SCC tumors from both RDEB and non-RDEB patients: The degree of differentiation, the degree of infiltrating cells, and the size of invading tumor keratinocyte islands will add numerous confounding factors to the expression profiles of tumor cells at the time of RNA isolation, which could well mask true differences between RDEB and non-RDEB SCC.

COL7A1, TYPE VII COLLAGEN, AND CANCER

Since the identification of type VII collagen and development of monoclonal antibodies,[34,35] a number of studies have looked for expression in a wide range of tumors. The resulting data have been variable and in some cases contrasting. Initially, a study of a wide range of tumors concluded that, in general, invasive and metastatic tumors do not express extensively type VII collagen. However, exceptions to this rule exist in bladder cancer, squamous carcinomas of the lung, tumors of the head and neck region, female genital tract tumors, and in some adenocarcinomas of the breast.[36]

In a separate study of head and neck SCC, Wetzels and colleagues[37] noted that type VII collagen was localized to the basement membrane in all 42 SCCs studied and was also present in the cytoplasm of 36% of tumors. This finding was later confirmed by an independent group.[38] Type VII collagen expression was reported in well-differentiated or moderately differentiated colon cancer and one study concluded that this expression was transiently involved in the progression from dysplastic epithelia to colon cancer.[39] Conflicting data were later published identifying no type VII collagen expression in colon cancer.[40] Type VII collagen expression was observed in neoplastic nervous system tissues and cell lines[41] and in thyroid tumors.[42] In prostate cancer, early stromal invasion is associated with the loss of a number of hemidesmosome-associated adhesive elements, such as laminin 5, type VII collagen, and α6 and β4 integrins.[43] Invasive tumor cells then go on to produce basement membrane–like matrices and express related integrin receptors.[44] In addition, anticancer drugs shown to be effective against prostate cancer down-regulate COL7A1 expression in vitro.[45] Decreased type VII collagen has been observed in cutaneous SCC[46] and dissolution of type VII collagen was associated with more invasive melanoma cell lines,[47] which parallels in vivo observations.[48] More recently, a study of esophageal SCC identified a direct correlation with type VII collagen and increased aggressiveness in tumors.[49] Studying 109 patients, 35% presented with intracellular type VII collagen expression and patients with negative type VII collagen had an increased 5-year survival rate. This year, Kita and colleagues[50] have confirmed these findings using messenger RNA analysis, demonstrating an increased 5-year survival rate in patients with low levels of COL7A1 (22 patients) versus those with high levels of COL7A1 messenger RNA (44 patients[50]). A similar study examining the messenger RNA expression of COL7A1 in colorectal cancer (n = 33), adenoma (n = 29), and normal tissue from the same patient and healthy volunteers (n = 20) noted that COL7A1 was up-regulated in both adenoma and cancer and concluded that this was an early event.[51]

This histological and messenger RNA expression data are very difficult to distil into any conclusive statement as to the role of type VII collagen in cancer. It seems apparent that certain cancers will up- or down-regulate type VII collagen in a seemingly opposing manner. The observations in prostate cancer are interesting in that initial loss of type VII collagen leads to dysplasia while up-regulation leads to metastasis.[43,44] The lack of prostate cancer in RDEB patients and the obvious metastasis of RDEB SCC would suggest this mechanism is not relevant to RDEB SCC. One explanation

from all the in vivo expression data could be that there is no definitive relationship in non-RDEB cancers, and type VII collagen expression is inconsequential. To complicate matters, COL7A1 has recently been identified as a gene with a high rate of methylation silencing in breast cancer cell lines.[52] In this study, COL7A1 was identified as being methylated in 10 of 11 and mutated in 1 of 11 breast cancer lines. Analysis of publicly available expression array data sets identified decreasing COL7A1 expression to correlate with increasing tumor grade in breast cancer.[52] Interestingly, no COL7A1 methylation (or mutation) was identified in colon cancer lines, even though the colon cancer lines had an overall increase in genomic methylation.[52]

Intracellular expression of type VII collagen is reported in RDEB SCC[53] and in wounded RDEB skin,[54] suggesting that either intracellular expression is associated with cancerous and precancerous lesions or is a transient response to wound healing. Again, whether this is truly a mechanism or a consequence remains an open question.

WHAT IS KNOWN ABOUT NON–RECESSIVE DYSTROPHIC EPIDERMOLYSIS BULLOSA SQUAMOUS CELL CARCINOMA?

Can what is known about SCC in the general population help in understanding the pathogenesis of RDEB-associated SCC? Unlike the mechanisms and pathways basal cell carcinoma, the mechanisms and pathways implicated in SCC development are still unknown. The two main experimental human SCC models rely on the expression of oncogenic Ras. Boukamp and colleagues have expressed oncogenic RasV12 in benign HaCat cells to produce aggressive tumors in mice (reviewed by Boukamp[55]), while normal primary keratinocytes can be malignantly converted by the expression of RasV12 coupled with suppression of nuclear factor kappa B (NFKappa-B) signaling through the expression of IKBaM.[56] It is clear that oncogenic Ras is extremely important in murine models of SCC,[57] but the data on Ras mutations in human cutaneous SCC are variable. The highest figure of 67% comes from 12 of 18 SCCs in a study of North African xeroderma pigmentosum patients,[58] yet a separate study in a Japanese xeroderma pigmentosum cohort identified only 1 mutation in 26 SCCs and this mutation was not in the activating codons 12, 13, or 61.[59] Reported Ras mutations in SCC from the general population vary from 0% to 22% and seemingly higher in keratoacanthomas (30%), a well-differentiated variant of SCC.[60] A proportion of this positive data is derived from classical tumorigenicity assays where human tumor DNA is transfected into mouse 3T3 fibroblasts. These cells are then selected and injected into mice. The resulting tumors are isolated and human DNA and *Ras* mutations are subsequently identified. Such a process of transfection, selection, and propagation could theoretically result in culture artifacts and indeed tumorigenic basal cell carcinoma DNA has been identified through this technique.[61] We have demonstrated lack of *Ras* mutations in six RDEB SCC patients and four non-RDEB SCC patients.[62]

Other molecules have been implicated in SCC development. These molecules include p53, p16, c-myc, PI3-kinase, and STAT3. However, in each case, heterogeneity is observed. No clear pathway or molecule has been identified.[63] The heterogeneity is also seen at the level of chromosomal rearrangements with 9p and 3p loss being the biggest identified abnormality.[64] *P16* resides on 9p and could represent an important early event in SCC. A number of tumor suppressor genes reside on 3p, but as yet no definitive data exist to implicate these loci implicitly.

P53 mutation and *p16* methylation (responsible for transcriptional silencing) have been identified in a proportion of RDEB-associated SCCs (three of eight and two of eight samples respectively),[65] demonstrating a similar pattern of mutation and silencing as non-RDEB SCC.

WHAT HAS BEEN DONE EXPERIMENTALLY TO MODEL RECESSIVE DYSTROPHIC EPIDERMOLYSIS BULLOSA SQUAMOUS CELL CARCINOMA?

Unfortunately, *COL7A1*-null mice die too early to initiate cancer studies.[66] Recently, however, a hypomorphic *COL7A1* mouse exhibiting many features of human RDEB has survived longer and could represent a feasible model for cancer studies.[67] To date, no cancer experiments have been reported in these mice or in an inducible knockout mouse. However, such experiments promise to generate valuable information eventually.

Controversy exists in the literature as to the action of type VII collagen on keratinocyte migration and invasion. In 1992, Chen and colleagues[68] reported that by reexpressing type VII collagen using a lentiviral system, a phenotypic reversion and reduction in colloidal gold migration with increased cell attachment was observed in both RDEB keratinocytes and RDEB fibroblasts, suggesting that lack of type VII increases adhesion and migration in RDEB skin cells. The same group later showed that type VII collagen improved wound healing of human skin grafted onto athymic mice[69] and went on to report this to be a result of increased migration in normal keratinocytes and fibroblasts in response to type VII collagen, dependent on the alpha-helical domain of type VII collagen.[70] These data demonstrate that, when present, wild-type *COL7A1* increases the migratory capacity of normal human keratinocytes and fibroblasts.

In 2005, Ortiz-Urda and colleagues[71,72] demonstrated that the NC1 domain of type VII collagen was required for increased migration and tumor formation when primary keratinocytes are transduced with oncogenic Ras and the NFKappaB super-repressor, IKBaM. Interestingly, this model also represents one of the only in vivo models of SCC formation where metastasis is seen and in addition to type VII collagen, laminin 332 and β4 integrin are also required. Therefore, in this metastatic setting, it seems that *COL7A1* is required. This does not reflect what is happening clinically in RDEB though, as patients without detectable *COL7A1* and presenting with early premature termination codon mutations still go on to develop life-threatening SCC.[62,73]

We recently demonstrated that by knocking down type VII collagen expression in cutaneous SCC lines, an increase in migration and invasion coupled with disorganized and reduced differentiation and promotion of epithelial-mesenchymal transition is seen.[74] In addition, loss of type VII collagen increased CXCL10-CXCR3 and downstream phospholipase activity, mediated through transforming growth factor (TGF)–beta signaling. The relationship between type VII collagen and disorganized and reduced cellular differentiation in RDEB is curious, given that the majority of RDEB SCC tumors are in fact well differentiated and indeed well-differentiated tumors will go on to metastasize in RDEB patients.[11] Perhaps the process of loss of differentiation and metastasis are indeed linked and this is missed when looking at primary tumor material. Disorganized epithelial differentiation is a major feature of cutaneous and mucosal dysplasia (a precursor of SCC) and is known to be mediated through the TGF–beta pathway.[75] The RDEB hypomorphic mouse dermis has increased TGF–beta1 and connective tissue growth factor expression, suggesting that this mechanism is relevant in vivo.[67] In the knockdown model, increased migration in type VII collagen knock-down cells was shown to be dependent on MMP2 and CXCR3 expression. The relationship between phospholipase activity and RDEB SCC remains to be investigated but certainly promising leads have been identified through this well-controlled approach.

SUMMARY

In summary, the picture is clear that RDEB patients develop numerous life-threatening SCCs. A slight increase in melanoma is seen but overall SCC is likely the only tumor these patients will encounter and, what is more likely, SCC will develop and will cause death. The reasons for this remain unclear. In other tumor types and patient groups, the expression of type VII collagen can either be a good prognostic indicator, such as in melanoma and breast cancer, or can be a bad prognostic indicator, such as in esophageal SCC and colon cancer. The expression of type VII collagen can influence the migration and invasion in either a positive or negative manner, depending on cell type and cellular assay used. Again, the reasons for this are not clear.

The production of a hypomorphic mouse model of DEB[67] or the development of an inducible knockout mouse presents the opportunity to ask questions regarding host and tumor cells deficient or competent in COL7A1 expression. It will be interesting to see whether cancers are more frequent or more aggressive when induced or xenografted in these animals. In addition to these studies, more focused research using clinical human RDEB material will no doubt assist in our understanding of the pathogenesis of RDEB.

REFERENCES

1. Reed WB, College J Jr, Francis MJ, et al. Epidermolysis bullosa dystrophica with epidermal neoplasms. Arch Dermatol 1974;110(6):894–902.
2. Fine JD, Johnson LB, Weiner M, et al. Epidermolysis bullosa and the risk of life-threatening cancers: the National EB Registry experience, 1986–2006. J Am Acad Dermatol 2009;60(2):203–11.
3. Daya-Grosjean L, Sarasin A. The role of UV induced lesions in skin carcinogenesis: an overview of oncogene and tumor suppressor gene modifications in xeroderma pigmentosum skin tumors. Mutat Res 2005;571(1-2):43–56.
4. Brantsch KD, Meisner C, Schonfisch B, et al. Analysis of risk factors determining prognosis of cutaneous squamous-cell carcinoma: a prospective study. Lancet Oncol 2008;9(8):713–20.
5. Veness MJ, Porceddu S, Palme CE, et al. Cutaneous head and neck squamous cell carcinoma metastatic to parotid and cervical lymph nodes. Head Neck 2007;29(7):621–31.
6. Varki R, Sadowski S, Uitto J, et al. Epidermolysis bullosa. II. Type VII collagen mutations and phenotype-genotype correlations in the dystrophic subtypes. J Med Genet 2007;44(3):181–92.
7. McGrath JA, Schofield OM, Mayou BJ, et al. Epidermolysis bullosa complicated by squamous cell carcinoma: report of 10 cases. J Cutan Pathol 1992;19(2):116–23.
8. Song IC, Dicksheet S. Management of squamous cell carcinoma in a patient with dominant-type epidermolysis bullosa dystrophica: a surgical challenge. Plast Reconstr Surg 1985;75(5):732–6.
9. Christiano AM, Crollick J, Pincus S, et al. Squamous cell carcinoma in a family with dominant dystrophic epidermolysis bullosa: a molecular genetic study. Exp Dermatol 1999;8(2):146–52.
10. Chorny JA, Shroyer KR, Golitz LE. Malignant melanoma and a squamous cell carcinoma in recessive dystrophic epidermolysis bullosa. Arch Dermatol 1993;129(9):1212.
11. Mallipeddi R. Epidermolysis bullosa and cancer. Clin Exp Dermatol 2002;27(8):616–23.
12. McGrath JA, Ishida-Yamamoto A, O'Grady A, et al. Structural variations in anchoring fibrils in dystrophic epidermolysis bullosa: correlation with type VII collagen expression. J Invest Dermatol 1993; 100(4):366–72.
13. Ogawa B, Chen M, Margolis J, et al. Marjolin's ulcer arising at the elbow: a case report and literature review. Hand (NY) 2006;1(2):89–93.
14. Kowal-Vern A, Criswell BK. Burn scar neoplasms: a literature review and statistical analysis. Burns 2005;31(4):403–13.
15. Kaplan RP. Cancer complicating chronic ulcerative and scarifying mucocutaneous disorders. Adv Dermatol 1987;2:19–46.
16. Brown VL, Farrant PB, Turner RJ, et al. Multiple aggressive squamous skin cancers in association with nonbullous congenital ichthyosiform erythroderma. Br J Dermatol 2008;158(5):1125–8.
17. Alexandrescu DT, Dasanu CA, Farzanmehr H, et al. Development of squamous cell carcinomas in Darier disease: a new model for skin carcinogenesis? Br J Dermatol 2008;159(6):1378–80.
18. Hamm H, Traupe H, Brocker EB, et al. The scleroatrophic syndrome of Huriez: a cancer-prone genodermatosis. Br J Dermatol 1996;134(3):512–8.
19. Madariaga J, Fromowitz F, Phillips M, et al. Squamous cell carcinoma in congenital ichthyosis with deafness and keratitis. A case report and review of the literature. Cancer 1986;57(10):2026–9.
20. Lai-Cheong JE, Tanaka A, Hawche G, et al. Kindler syndrome: a focal adhesion genodermatosis. Br J Dermatol 2009;160(2):233–42.
21. Lotem M, Raben M, Zeltser R, et al. Kindler syndrome complicated by squamous cell carcinoma of the hard palate: successful treatment with high-dose radiation therapy and granulocyte-macrophage colony-stimulating factor. Br J Dermatol 2001;144(6):1284–6.
22. Emanuel PO, Rudikoff D, Phelps RG. Aggressive squamous cell carcinoma in Kindler syndrome. Skinmed 2006;5(6):305–7.

23. Goldberg GI, Eisen AZ, Bauer EA. Tissue stress and tumor promotion. Possible relevance to epidermolysis bullosa. Arch Dermatol 1988;124(5):737–41.

24. Smoller BA, McNutt NS, Carter DM, et al. Recessive dystrophic epidermolysis bullosa skin displays a chronic growth-activated immunophenotype. Implications for carcinogenesis. Arch Dermatol 1990;126(1):78–83.

25. Tyring SK, Chopra V, Johnson L, et al. Natural killer cell activity is reduced in patients with severe forms of inherited epidermolysis bullosa. Arch Dermatol 1989;125(6):797–800.

26. Arbiser JL, Fine JD, Murrell D, et al. Basic fibroblast growth factor: a missing link between collagen VII, increased collagenase, and squamous cell carcinoma in recessive dystrophic epidermolysis bullosa. Mol Med 1998;4(3):191–5.

27. Mott JD, Werb Z. Regulation of matrix biology by matrix metalloproteinases. Curr Opin Cell Biol 2004;16(5):558–64.

28. Bruckner-Tuderman L, Winberg JO, Anton-Lamprecht I, et al. Anchoring fibrils, collagen VII, and neutral metalloproteases in recessive dystrophic epidermolysis bullosa inversa. J Invest Dermatol 1992;99(5):550–8.

29. Bodemer C, Tchen SI, Ghomrasseni S, et al. Skin expression of metalloproteinases and tissue inhibitor of metalloproteinases in sibling patients with recessive dystrophic epidermolysis and intrafamilial phenotypic variation. J Invest Dermatol 2003;121(2):273–9.

30. Titeux M, Pendaries V, Tonasso L, et al. A frequent functional SNP in the MMP1 promoter is associated with higher disease severity in recessive dystrophic epidermolysis bullosa. Hum Mutat 2008;29(2):267–76.

31. Kivisaari AK, Kallajoki M, Mirtti T, et al. Transformation-specific matrix metalloproteinases (MMP)-7 and MMP-13 are expressed by tumour cells in epidermolysis bullosa-associated squamous cell carcinomas. Br J Dermatol 2008;158(4):778–85.

32. Cooper HL, Cook IS, Theaker JM, et al. Expression and glycosylation of MUC1 in epidermolysis bullosa-associated and sporadic cutaneous squamous cell carcinomas. Br J Dermatol 2004;151(3):540–5.

33. Mallipeddi R, Wessagowit V, South AP, et al. Reduced expression of insulin-like growth factor-binding protein-3 (IGFBP-3) in squamous cell carcinoma complicating recessive dystrophic epidermolysis bullosa. J Invest Dermatol 2004;122(5):1302–9.

34. Sakai LY, Keene DR, Morris NP, et al. Type VII collagen is a major structural component of anchoring fibrils. J Cell Biol 1986;103(4):1577–86.

35. Leigh IM, Eady RA, Heagerty AH, et al. Type VII collagen is a normal component of epidermal basement membrane, which shows altered expression in recessive dystrophic epidermolysis bullosa. J Invest Dermatol 1988;90(5):639–42.

36. Wetzels RH, Robben HC, Leigh IM, et al. Distribution patterns of type VII collagen in normal and malignant human tissues. Am J Pathol 1991;139(2):451–9.

37. Wetzels RH, van der Velden LA, Schaafsma HE, et al. Immunohistochemical localization of basement membrane type VII collagen and laminin in neoplasms of the head and neck. Histopathology 1992;21(5):459–64.

38. Kainulainen T, Grenman R, Oikarinen A, et al. Distribution and synthesis of type VII collagen in oral squamous cell carcinoma. J Oral Pathol Med 1997;26(9):414–8.

39. Visser R, Arends JW, Leigh IM, et al. Patterns and composition of basement membranes in colon adenomas and adenocarcinomas. J Pathol 1993;170(3):285–90.

40. Tani T, Karttunen T, Kiviluoto T, et al. Alpha 6 beta 4 integrin and newly deposited laminin-1 and laminin-5 form the adhesion mechanism of gastric carcinoma. Continuous expression of laminins but not that of collagen VII is preserved in invasive parts of the carcinomas: implications for acquisition of the invading phenotype. Am J Pathol 1996;149(3):781–93.

41. Paulus W, Baur I, Liszka U, et al. Expression of type VII collagen, the major anchoring fibril component, in normal and neoplastic human nervous system. Virchows Arch 1995;426(2):199–202.

42. Lohi J, Leivo I, Owaribe K, et al. Neoexpression of the epithelial adhesion complex antigens in thyroid tumours is associated with proliferation and squamous differentiation markers. J Pathol 1998;184(2):191–6.

43. Nagle RB, Knox JD, Wolf C, et al. Adhesion molecules, extracellular matrix, and proteases in prostate carcinoma. J Cell Biochem Suppl 1994;19:232–7.

44. Bonkhoff H. Analytical molecular pathology of epithelial-stromal interactions in the normal and neoplastic prostate. Anal Quant Cytol Histol 1998;20(5):437–42.

45. Hurst R, Elliott RM, Goldson AJ, et al. Se-methylselenocysteine alters collagen gene and protein expression in human prostate cells. Cancer Lett 2008;269(1):117–26.

46. Dumas V, Kanitakis J, Charvat S, et al. Expression of basement membrane antigens and matrix metalloproteinases 2 and 9 in cutaneous basal and squamous cell carcinomas. Anticancer Res 1999;19(4B):2929–38.

47. Bechetoille N, Haftek M, Staquet MJ, et al. Penetration of human metastatic melanoma cells through an authentic dermal-epidermal junction is associated with dissolution of native collagen types IV and VII. Melanoma Res 2000;10(5):427–34.

48. Kirkham N, Price ML, Gibson B, et al. Type VII collagen antibody LH 7.2 identifies basement

membrane characteristics of thin malignant melanomas. J Pathol 1989;157(3):243–7.

49. Baba Y, Iyama K, Honda S, et al. Cytoplasmic expression of type VII collagen is related to prognosis in patients with esophageal squamous cell carcinoma. Oncology 2006;71(3-4):221–8.

50. Kita Y, Mimori K, Tanaka F, et al. Clinical significance of LAMB3 and COL7A1 mRNA in esophageal squamous cell carcinoma. Eur J Surg Oncol 2009;35(1):52–8.

51. Skovbjerg H, Anthonsen D, Lothe IM, et al. Collagen mRNA levels changes during colorectal cancer carcinogenesis. BMC Cancer 2009;9:136.

52. Chan TA, Glockner S, Yi JM, et al. Convergence of mutation and epigenetic alterations identifies common genes in cancer that predict for poor prognosis. PLoS Med 2008;5(5):e114.

53. Kanitakis J, Barthelemy H, Faure M, et al. Intracellular expression of type VII collagen in squamous cell carcinoma complicating dystrophic epidermolysis bullosa. Br J Dermatol 1997;137(2):310–3.

54. McGrath JA, Leigh IM, Eady RA. Intracellular expression of type VII collagen during wound healing in severe recessive dystrophic epidermolysis bullosa and normal human skin. Br J Dermatol 1992;127(4):312–7.

55. Boukamp P. Non-melanoma skin cancer: what drives tumor development and progression? Carcinogenesis 2005;26(10):1657–67.

56. Dajee M, Lazarov M, Zhang JY, et al. NF-kappaB blockade and oncogenic Ras trigger invasive human epidermal neoplasia. Nature 2003;421(6923):639–43.

57. Balmain A, Ramsden M, Bowden GT, et al. Activation of the mouse cellular Harvey-ras gene in chemically induced benign skin papillomas. Nature 1984;307(5952):658–60.

58. Daya-Grosjean L, Robert C, Drougard C, et al. High mutation frequency in ras genes of skin tumors isolated from DNA repair deficient xeroderma pigmentosum patients. Cancer Res 1993;53(7):1625–9.

59. Sato M, Nishigori C, Lu Y, et al. Far less frequent mutations in ras genes than in the p53 gene in skin tumors of xeroderma pigmentosum patients. Mol Carcinog 1994;11(2):98–105.

60. Corominas M, Kamino H, Leon J, et al. Oncogene activation in human benign tumors of the skin (keratoacanthomas): is HRAS involved in differentiation as well as proliferation? Proc Natl Acad Sci U S A 1989;86(16):6372–6.

61. Ananthaswamy HN, Price JE, Goldberg LH, et al. Detection and identification of activated oncogenes in human skin cancers occurring on sun-exposed body sites. Cancer Res 1988;48(12):3341–6.

62. Pourreyron C, Cox G, Mao X, et al. Patients with recessive dystrophic epidermolysis bullosa develop squamous-cell carcinoma regardless of type VII collagen expression. J Invest Dermatol 2007;127(10):2438–44.

63. Green CL, Khavari PA. Targets for molecular therapy of skin cancer. Semin Cancer Biol 2004;14(1):63–9.

64. Purdie KJ, Harwood CA, Gulati A, et al. Single nucleotide polymorphism array analysis defines a specific genetic fingerprint for well-differentiated cutaneous SCCs. J Invest Dermatol 2009;129(6):1562–8.

65. Arbiser JL, Fan CY, Su X, et al. Involvement of p53 and p16 tumor suppressor genes in recessive dystrophic epidermolysis bullosa-associated squamous cell carcinoma. J Invest Dermatol 2004;123(4):788–90.

66. Heinonen S, Mannikko M, Klement JF, et al. Targeted inactivation of the type VII collagen gene (Col7a1) in mice results in severe blistering phenotype: a model for recessive dystrophic epidermolysis bullosa. J Cell Sci 1999;112(Pt 21):3641–8.

67. Fritsch A, Loeckermann S, Kern JS, et al. A hypomorphic mouse model of dystrophic epidermolysis bullosa reveals mechanisms of disease and response to fibroblast therapy. J Clin Invest 2008;118(5):1669–79.

68. Chen M, Kasahara N, Keene DR, et al. Restoration of type VII collagen expression and function in dystrophic epidermolysis bullosa. Nat Genet 2002;32(4):670–5.

69. Woodley DT, Remington J, Huang Y, et al. Intravenously injected human fibroblasts home to skin wounds, deliver type VII collagen, and promote wound healing. Mol Ther 2007;15(3):628–35.

70. Chen M, Hou Y, Wang X, et al. A 684 helical domain of type VII collagen promotes in vivo skin wound closure by enhancing fibroblast and keratinocyte migration. J Invest Dermatol 2008;128:S48.

71. Ortiz-Urda S, Garcia J, Green CL, et al. Type VII collagen is required for Ras-driven human epidermal tumorigenesis. Science 2005;307(5716):1773–6.

72. Tran M, Rousselle P, Nokelainen P, et al. Targeting a tumor-specific laminin domain critical for human carcinogenesis. Cancer Res 2008;68(8):2885–94.

73. Rodeck U, Uitto J. Recessive dystrophic epidermolysis bullosa-associated squamous-cell carcinoma: an enigmatic entity with complex pathogenesis. J Invest Dermatol 2007;127(10):2295–6.

74. Martins VL, Vyas JJ, Chen M, et al. Increased invasive behaviour in cutaneous squamous cell carcinoma with loss of basement-membrane type VII collagen. J Cell Sci 2009;122(Pt 11):1788–99.

75. Guasch G, Schober M, Pasolli HA, et al. Loss of TGFbeta signaling destabilizes homeostasis and promotes squamous cell carcinomas in stratified epithelia. Cancer Cell 2007;12(4):313–27.

Epidermolysis Bullosa Nevi

Christoph Michael Lanschuetzer, MD*, Martin Laimer, MD,
Elke Nischler, MD, Helmut Hintner, MD

KEYWORDS

- Epidermolysis bullosa nevi • Melanocytic lesions
- Digital dermoscopy • ABCD rule of dermoscopy

Epidermolysis bullosa nevi (EB nevi)[1–9] are large, eruptive, asymmetrical, often irregularly pigmented melanocytic lesions (**Boxes 1** and **2**). Such nevi may give rise to small satellite nevi surrounding the primary nevus, and thus frequently manifest clinical features suggestive of melanoma (**Fig. 1**). They usually arise in sites of previous bullae or erosions (**Fig. 2**). The nevi were initially reported in generalized atrophic benign EB (now classified as non-Herlitz junctional EB).[10,11] Today it is well accepted that the occurrence of EB nevi is a frequent phenomenon in patients suffering from all variants of EB, which, however, are apparently only recessively inherited.

Two pathogenic theories about the development of EB nevi have been proposed. According to one theory, the repetitive disruption of the basement membrane primes local nevus cell nests or single melanocytes to break senescence and undergo proliferation.[8,12] According to the second theory, viable melanocytes/nevus cells, probably deriving from incipient nevi or subclinical nests of nevus cells, free-float in the fluid-filled cavity of an EB blister and, after settling down at random (often at the edge of the blister), proliferate excessively in the microenvironment of epidermal regeneration.[1,2,13] We detected such "flocking-bird" melanocytes histologically in the blister cavity (produced by the biopsy trauma) in a histologic section of an EB nevus of a patient with junctional EB. Furthermore, we found melanocytic cells in a cytospin specimen prepared from a blister located on top of a large EB nevus. We detected in addition cytokines and growth factors, such as hepatocyte growth factor, interleukin 8, granulocyte-macrophage colony-stimulating factor, prostaglandin E2, and leukotriene B4 in such fluid,[13] which might potentiate melanocytic proliferation.[1,12–14] Interestingly, eruptive nevi have been reported to develop following various other bullous diseases as well.[15,16]

EB nevi mature as most common acquired melanocytic nevi: They begin as flat, pigmented lesions, and later, while acquiring dermal components, lose their pigment. More precisely, EB nevi gradually appear in infancy or adolescence as stippled maculae, and over years develop papular areas resulting in dermal shagreen-nevi (see **Fig. 2, Fig. 3**).[1]

Melanocytic nevi are considered to be benign hamartomatous proliferations of melanocytes. They can be of clinical significance because they are risk markers, simulants, and potential precursors of malignant melanoma.[17] To distinguish benign from malignant lesions, clinical criteria have been established describing asymmetry, border irregularity, color variegation, and diameter larger than 6 mm (the ABCD rule).[18] EB nevi are clinically highly suspect for cutaneous melanoma if one applies the ABCD rule.[2,7,13,19] Moreover, the continuous (over years!), sometimes explosive growth with the frequent appearance of satellite lesions reinforces the impression of malignant transformation.[7,13]

We recently demonstrated that digital dermoscopy is useful in differentiating EB nevi from melanoma.[19] In this study, 23 EB nevi of 11 patients were analyzed with a dermoscope. Clinically, all 23 EB nevi were asymmetrical, most of them in two axes. Many lesions (especially older

Department of Dermatology, Paracelsus Medical University, Müllner Hauptstr. 48, Salzburg 5020, Austria
* Corresponding author.
E-mail address: c.lanschuetzer@salk.at (C.M. Lanschuetzer).

Dermatol Clin 28 (2010) 179–183
doi:10.1016/j.det.2009.10.024

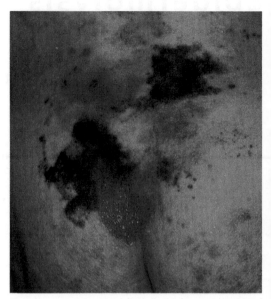

Fig. 1. Large EB nevi with protrusions and satellite lesions in an area of extensive blistering are highly suggestive of melanoma.

ones) showed random papillomatous portions. On dermoscopic inspection, 21 of 23 pigmented lesions showed a pigment network or pigmentary dots/globules and streaks and were hence classified as being of melanocytic origin. Ten lesions were classified according to the classification of atypical nevi by Hofmann-Wellenhof and colleagues[20] as reticular (2 of 23), reticular-globular (3 of 23), reticular-homogeneous (4 of 23), and globular-homogeneous (1 of 23), while most lesions (13 of 23) were unclassifiable.

With regard to pigmentation, 17 EB nevi showed multifocal hypo- or hyperpigmentation.

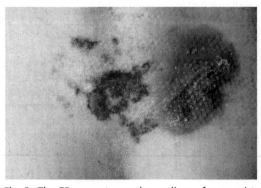

Fig. 2. The EB nevus traces the outlines of a preexisting blister on the left and mirrors the healing blister with erosions on the right. Taken together, these two lesions are evocative of a butterfly, which is represented in the logo of the EB support organization DebRA-Austria.

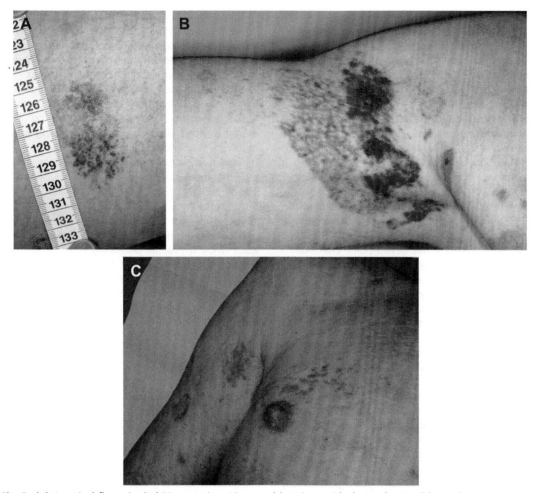

Fig. 3. (A) A typical flat, stippled EB nevus in a 13-year-old patient with dystrophic EB. (B) Papular portions arise within an EB nevus in a 35-year-old patient with junctional EB. (C) Two unpigmented "shagreen" EB nevi on the chest and the upper arm in a 65-year-old patient with junctional EB.

With regard to structure, the global patterns of 20 EB nevi were classified as having a multicomponent pattern[21,22] or showed a "three-structure type" pattern (**Fig. 4**).[23] Both such patterns are highly suggestive for malignant melanoma. An atypical pigment network with irregular meshes and thick lines (17 of 23), irregular dots and globules of different size (16 of 23) haphazardly dispersed, and homogeneous areas (23 of 23) were the predominant primary structures seen in EB nevi.[19] Milky red areas, a vascular pattern highly suggestive of cutaneous melanoma,[24] were present in 5 lesions. So-called "comma vessels," which are stereotypical for benign papillomatous nevi, were seen in the elevated portions of 2 EB nevi. Peculiar "glomerular clumps" of vessels were detected in 5 lesions. Such a vascular pattern has never been reported so far in any other kind of nevi. An atypical vascular

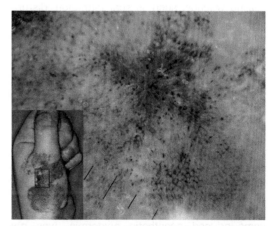

Fig. 4. The EB nevus on the thumb of a 5-year-old boy with recessive "EB simplex with muscular dystrophy" features an atypical pigment network, irregular dots and globules, and homogeneous white and reddish areas (ie, a multicomponent pattern).

pattern as defined by the seven-point checklist[24] (ie, linear, dotted, globular red) was present in only 2 lesions.

In addition to these pattern analysis criteria, criteria of the ABCD rule of dermoscopy[25] were applied to all EB nevi. The 23 lesions showed structural asymmetry in two axes. However, an abrupt border cut-off was documented in only 3 lesions and in 1 segment, respectively. The colors white (23 of 23), light brown (23 of 23), dark brown (13 of 23), blue-gray (12 of 23), and red (11 of 23) dominated, while black and blue were almost absent.

The combination of dermoscopic features found in EB nevi resulted in a high total dermoscopy score for the ABCD rule of dermoscopy[25] as well as a high score for the seven-point checklist.[24] Thus a total dermoscopy score greater than 5.45 (ABCD rule of dermoscopy) was achieved in 17 lesions and a score greater than 3 (seven-point checklist) was recognized in 16 lesions. Such dermoscopy scores are highly suggestive for melanoma.

Interestingly, EB nevi also show an analogy to recurrent nevi (pseudomelanoma, persistent nevus), which occur after incomplete surgical excision or trauma of an intradermal nevus. Upon wound healing and scar formation, such previously traumatized moles also frequently mimic cutaneous melanoma clinically, histologically, and dermoscopically.[26]

We believe that the asymmetry, irregular shape, multifocal hyper- or hypopigmentation, and structural variegation of EB nevi revealed by dermoscopy can be attributed to the arbitrary arrangement of independently proliferating melanocytic clones. Further changes taking place in healing wounds, such as scar formation, disruption of rete ridges, and neovascularization, enhance the irregular appearance of these moles.

Nevertheless, strong morphologic indicators for invasive cutaneous melanoma (ie, tumor progression, such as steel-blue areas caused by melanin pigment in the papillary dermis, and black dots, which represent melanin in the stratum corneum and which are indicative for a vertical, upward "pagetoid" spread of melanocytes) were typically not seen in EB nevi, as melanocytes usually stay in the level of clefting and, unlike melanoma cells, do not penetrate into other cutaneous layers. Also, a blue-whitish veil, which represents a melanoma-induced acanthotic epidermis, was not found in the EB nevi investigated.

Taking all the above listed arguments into consideration, an unequivocal differentiation from cutaneous melanoma is not always possible.

Although we have never seen a malignant melanoma develop within an EB nevus, the number of EB nevi studied so far is certainly not large enough to completely rule out the possibility that EB nevi might also be a melanoma precursor lesion.[1,2,19] The state of chronic skin wounding and regeneration in EB patients, however, seems to promote cancerogenesis, as demonstrated by the extremely high incidence of metastasizing squamous cell carcinomas in young patients with recessive dystrophic EB.[27–29] Moreover, these patients have also been reported to be at an elevated risk for the development of malignant melanomas.[30]

Therefore, we recommend a regular clinical, photographic and dermoscopic follow-up. At least twice a year all persisting wounds and EB nevi should be evaluated with a low threshold for histopathological examination if warranted. Our practice is to punch biopsy EB nevi showing dermoscopic features of concern as well as dermoscopically featureless lesions. Given the skin fragility and potentially impaired wound healing in EB patients, we avoid prophylactic total excision of large EB nevi, but rather use the dermoscope to select appropriate sites for punch biopsies within giant EB nevi.

REFERENCES

1. Grubauer G, et al. [Acquired, surface giant nevus cell nevi in generalized, atrophic, benign epidermolysis bullosa]. Hautarzt 1989;40(8):523–6 [in German].
2. Bauer JW, et al. Large melanocytic nevi in hereditary epidermolysis bullosa. J Am Acad Dermatol 2001; 44(4):577–84.
3. Natsuga K, et al. Two cases of atypical melanocytic lesions in recessive dystrophic epidermolysis bullosa infants. Clin Exp Dermatol 2005;30(6):636–9.
4. Gallardo F, et al. Large atypical melanocytic nevi in recessive dystrophic epidermolysis bullosa: clinicopathological, ultrastructural, and dermoscopic study. Pediatr Dermatol 2005;22(4):338–43.
5. Stavrianeas NG, et al. Eruptive large melanocytic nevus in a patient with hereditary epidermolysis bullosa simplex. Dermatology 2003;207(4):402–4.
6. Bichel J, et al. [Large melanocytic nevi in generalized atrophic benign epidermolysis bullosa (epidermolysis bullosa nevi)]. Hautarzt 2001;52(9):812–6 [in German].
7. Cash SH, et al. Epidermolysis bullosa nevus: an exception to the clinical and dermoscopic criteria for melanoma. Arch Dermatol 2007;143(9):1164–7.
8. Hoss DM, et al. Atypical melanocytic lesions in epidermolysis bullosa. J Cutan Pathol 1994;21(2):164–9.

9. Lanschuetzer CM. Epidermolysis bullosa naevi. In: Fine J-D, Hintner H, editors. Life with epidermolysis bullosa (EB). NewYork: Springer: Wien; 2009. p. 107–15.

10. Hintner H, Wolff K. Generalized atrophic benign epidermolysis bullosa. Arch Dermatol 1982;118(6): 375–84.

11. Darling TN, et al. Generalized atrophic benign epidermolysis bullosa. Adv Dermatol 1997;13:87–119 [discussion: 120].

12. Soltani K, et al. Large acquired nevocytic nevi induced by the Koebner phenomenon. J Cutan Pathol 1984;11(4):296–9.

13. Lanschuetzer CM, et al. Pathogenic mechanisms in epidermolysis bullosa naevi. Acta Derm Venereol 2003;83(5):332–7.

14. Herlyn M, et al. Biology of tumor progression in human melanocytes. Lab Invest 1987;56(5):461–74.

15. Kirby JD, Darley CR. Eruptive melanocytic naevi following severe bullous disease. Br J Dermatol 1978;99(5):575–80.

16. Kopf AW, et al. Eruptive nevocytic nevi after severe bullous disease. Arch Dermatol 1977;113(8):1080–4.

17. Elder DE, et al. The early and intermediate precursor lesions of tumor progression in the melanocytic system: common acquired nevi and atypical (dysplastic) nevi. Semin Diagn Pathol 1993;10(1):18–35.

18. Friedman RJ, Rigel DS, Kopf AW. Early detection of malignant melanoma: the role of physician examination and self-examination of the skin. CA Cancer J Clin 1985;35(3):130–51.

19. Lanschuetzer CM, et al. Epidermolysis bullosa naevi reveal a distinctive dermoscopic pattern. Br J Dermatol 2005;153(1):97–102.

20. Hofmann-Wellenhof R, et al. Dermoscopic classification of atypical melanocytic nevi (Clark nevi). Arch Dermatol 2001;137(12):1575–80.

21. Pehamberger H, Steiner A, Wolff K. In vivo epiluminescence microscopy of pigmented skin lesions. I. Pattern analysis of pigmented skin lesions. J Am Acad Dermatol 1987;17(4):571–83.

22. Steiner A, Pehamberger H, Wolff K. In vivo epiluminescence microscopy of pigmented skin lesions. II. Diagnosis of small pigmented skin lesions and early detection of malignant melanoma. J Am Acad Dermatol 1987;17(4):584–91.

23. Blum A, et al. The dermoscopic classification of atypical melanocytic naevi (Clark naevi) is useful to discriminate benign from malignant melanocytic lesions. Br J Dermatol 2003;149(6):1159–64.

24. Argenziano G, et al. Epiluminescence microscopy for the diagnosis of doubtful melanocytic skin lesions. Comparison of the ABCD rule of dermatoscopy and a new 7-point checklist based on pattern analysis. Arch Dermatol 1998;134(12): 1563–70.

25. Nachbar F, et al. The ABCD rule of dermatoscopy. High prospective value in the diagnosis of doubtful melanocytic skin lesions. J Am Acad Dermatol 1994;30(4):551–9.

26. Marghoob AA, Kopf AW. Persistent nevus: an exception to the ABCD rule of dermoscopy. J Am Acad Dermatol 1997;36(3 Pt 1):474–5.

27. Pellicano R, Fabrizi G, Cerimele D. Multiple keratoacanthomas and junctional epidermolysis bullosa. A therapeutic conundrum. Arch Dermatol 1990; 126(3):305–6.

28. Swensson O, Christophers E. Generalized atrophic benign epidermolysis bullosa in 2 siblings complicated by multiple squamous cell carcinomas. Arch Dermatol 1998;134(2):199–203.

29. Weber F, et al. Squamous cell carcinoma in junctional and dystrophic epidermolysis bullosa. Acta Derm Venereol 2001;81(3):189–92.

30. Fine JD, Bauer EA, McGuire J, et al, editors. Epidermolysis bullosa. Baltimore (MD): The Johns Hopkins University Press; 1999.

Quality of Life Measurements in Epidermolysis Bullosa: Tools for Clinical Research and Patient Care

John W. Frew, MBBS[a,b],
Dédée F. Murrell, MA, BMBCh, FAAD, MD[a,b],*

KEYWORDS

- Quality of life • Epidermolysis bullosa
- Questionnaires • QOLEB • Measurement tools

Quality of life (QOL) is an abstract, multidimensional construct reflecting the physical, psychological, and social aspects of an individual's well-being. Commonly, QOL is equated with burden of disease; however, they have subtle differences that have important consequences in the clinical setting. The World Health Organization (WHO) defines *health* as "total physical, mental and social well-being,"[1] with this holistic view very similar to the traditional view of QOL. Burden of disease, however, is regarded as a measurement of the negative impact a disease or condition has on an individual.

Therefore, the holistic nature of QOL measurements (as opposed to merely the burden of disease) provides a more accurate representation of the overall physical, psychological, and social state of an individual.[2,3] This holistic approach to medicine is extremely important in dermatology, because many dermatologic conditions have not only physical but also pronounced psychological and social consequences. Epidermolysis bullosa (EB) is a prime example of a dermatologic condition with profound impacts across all aspects of health. In dermatologic medicine, assessing a patient's overall health also involves an informal evaluation of their QOL.

Although the use of formal QOL measurement tools in dermatology is somewhat recent, the dermatologist's concern for the overall welfare of the patient is not. The development of new, formal, clinically useful QOL tools is driven by the expectations of patients and the wider medical community regarding therapeutic modalities. Dermatologists strive to provide timely, effective treatments with minimal adverse effects while minimizing social and economic impacts on individuals and the community. As stated by Halioua and colleagues,[4] "effectiveness alone is no longer sufficient." QOL tools allow dermatologists to quantitatively measure the dimensions of the WHO's definition of health, and use these measurements in several different areas, including health advocacy, clinical research, and evaluation of new therapeutic modalities.

WHY MEASURE QUALITY OF LIFE?

Although QOL measurement is justifiable in its own right, results from QOL studies can be used

[a] University of New South Wales, Sydney 2052, Australia
[b] Department of Dermatology, St George Hospital, James Laws House, Gray Street, Kogarah, NSW 2217, Sydney, Australia
* Corresponding author. Department of Dermatology, St George Hospital, James Laws House, Gray Street, Kogarah, NSW 2217, Sydney, Australia.
E-mail address: d.murrell@unsw.edu.au (D.F. Murrell).

Dermatol Clin 28 (2010) 185–190
doi:10.1016/j.det.2009.10.019

several different ways. QOL evaluation simply can be seen as a formalized version of the holistic care that countless dermatologists provide daily. The critical difference is that most QOL measurement tools are developed using a rigorous process and statistically validated, thereby ensuring that the results gleaned by these tools are accurate and reliable when compared across cohorts, or between different intervals.[2,3]

QOL evaluation can have great uses in assessing the efficacy of new therapeutic modalities, particularly in EB. These therapies may range from new forms of dressings to more recent developments, such as cellular therapies. Because EB can have such profound clinical manifestations (eg, in generalized severe recessive dystrophic [RDEB]), even if the clinical outcome of a particular novel therapy may indicate improvement but the overall change in QOL is negligible or in fact decreases (eg, from the invasiveness of the procedure), patients may not consider continuation of this therapy as the most beneficial course of action.

Because EB is a rare condition, many patient advocacy and support groups, such as DebRA (Dystrophic EB Research Association), are challenged with the task of obtaining funding, both for patient support and research. Quantitative evaluation of the QOL of individuals who have EB compared with other chronic skin conditions, such as psoriasis or atopic eczema, may support gathering private or public sector funding for continuing treatments and research support. From a health economics perspective, the same quantitative data can be used to evaluate or determine resource allocation (ie, money) based on measurements such as the Disability Adjusted Life Years (DALY).[3]

Because of the chronic nature of EB, many adult patients who have widespread blistering tend to underreport symptoms and exhibit a high level of resilience. This behavior can lead to more inexperienced clinicians potentially undertreating these patients, with potentially disastrous consequences, particularly for patients who have RDEB exhibiting locally recurrent squamous cell carcinoma or regional metastases.[5]

This issue is particularly pertinent in palliative settings, and QOL evaluation, including assessments of pain levels, can be of great value. However, even among the general EB population, the restrictions on social interaction and increased incidence of depression[5,6] may cause patients (particularly adolescents) to be shy and introverted. When this situation occurs, or when parents and caregivers tend to speak for older patients, QOL scores and other measurement tools can help elucidate a patient's perception of pain, depression, or other concerns. Eliminating this "caregiver-bias"

can be especially useful in building rapport with adolescent patients.

PREVIOUS QUALITY OF LIFE STUDIES IN EPIDERMOLYSIS BULLOSA

Generic QOL tools are useful in evaluating patients who have EB, although these tools have their shortcomings. Content validity issues and ceiling effects restrict the usefulness of several of these questionnaires.

The Dermatology Life Quality Index (DLQI)[7] is a widely used QOL instrument that has been used in EB and other bullous diseases. In 2002, Horn and Tidman[5] undertook a QOL evaluation of 115 individuals in Scotland who had various forms of EB. The results indicated that patients who had generalised severe RDEB (GS-RDEB) scored significantly higher on most questions than patients who had epidermolysis bullosa simplex (EBS). However, those who had GS-RDEB scored paradoxically low on a small number of questions gauging the impact of disease on activities such as shopping and gardening.[8–12] This trend is believed to be because the DLQI asks patients to report the impact of their condition "in the past week," and because EB is lifelong, patients have never been able to participate in these activities and therefore the impact is minimized. As a result, QOL is overestimated in several patients who have EB because of the poor content validity of these questions regarding this population.[8–12]

Overall, the DLQI is seen to be accurate in assessing QOL in milder subtypes of EBS and dominant dystrophic EB,[8–12] although its usefulness in more severe subtypes is questioned. This finding is mainly caused by the content validity issues outlined above, although significant ceiling effects were also seen among the GS-RDEB cohort in the review by Horn and Tidman.[5]

Fine and associates[12] conducted a QOL study focused on mobility and pain levels using an activities of daily living (ADL) score. This study contains data from a large cohort of 425 patients and provides useful quantitative data on the level of independence and levels of pain for adults and children within stratified subtypes of EB. However, as a general QOL tool, no results are presented encompassing psychosocial aspects of health. Also, the questionnaire contains 109 questions and is therefore a formidable survey to be used on a repeated basis in a study, let alone a clinical setting.

Another article by Fine and colleagues[13] comments on the psychosocial impact of EB, not only on individuals but also on their families. This report gave solid quantitative data on the impact that having a child who has EB has on parental relationships and the birth of subsequent children.

These data illuminate what impact the birth of a child who has EB has on the wider family unit and, in a clinical context, other issues such as family separation and psychological issues that clinicians may encounter in the future. In a more recent qualitative study on the impact of EB on parents, Scheppingen and colleagues[14] showed similar results to those of Fine and colleagues.[13]

Scheppingen and colleagues[6] also undertook a second qualitative study focusing on the impact of EB in children. Of the 48 eligible children in their Dutch database, 11 children aged 6 to 17 from 9 families were recruited for interviewing. Because their sample size was small compared with that of the two studies mentioned earlier,[14,15] the content validity of the responses may be restricted. Nevertheless, their qualitative results, which concur with comments made independently in the development of an EB-specific QOL tool,[7-11] illustrate how their results and study methodology (specifically their use of the "cloud ranking scale") may be used in future developments of a quantitative QOL tool specifically for children who have EB.

However, because of their qualitative nature, the results by Scheppingen and colleagues[14] may not be perceived as the most appropriate form of QOL analysis to use as evidence for sourcing funding or clinical measurement because of the preference for quantitative data in these situations. Their results found itch and pain to be the most significant factors in EB, which are parameters usually best assessed with visual analog scales and frequency scales because they are physical symptoms.[2,3]

Since obtaining ethical approval in 2005, the authors' Sydney-based clinical research team has worked to produce an EB-specific QOL tool applicable not only for research but also as an accurate, easy-to-use questionnaire for use in a clinical context.[7-11] To develop content validity, the initial 25-item Quality of Life in Epidermolysis Bullosa (QOLEB) questionnaire was developed from in-depth interviews with 70 adults and children and their families and five experts in EB. After further standard methodologies were used to reduce the questions to an essential core, the QOLEB was distributed to a cohort of 130 individuals from the Australasian EB Registry, representing all forms of EB, and was shown to be a valid, reliable tool for evaluating QOL in patients who had EB. Redundant questions were then removed from the QOLEB after factor analysis, resulting in a final 17-item QOLEB (**Box 1**). It encompasses physical, psychological, and social aspects of the disease and is designed to be used alongside other disease tools, such as visual analog scales for pain and itch evaluation. It is free of the ceiling effects that affect other questionnaires, such as

the DLQI, and is versatile enough to be used in various settings.[7-11] One disadvantage is the lack of a children-specific version of the QOLEB. Although the DLQI has an illustrated children's version,[15] the QOLEB currently does not. Future work must focus on an accurate adaptation of the QOLEB for evaluating QOL in children.

Quality of Life in Epidermolysis Bullosa Scoring

Throughout the literature concerning QOL in EB, a fair consensus is maintained in line with general clinical opinion concerning the subtypes of EB, which show higher impact on QOL than others. As illustrated in **Fig. 1**, EBS subtypes score at the lower end of QOL impact, with GS-RDEB and Herlitz junctional epidermolysis bullosa at the high end of QOL impact. Discrepancies arise only when phenotypic heterogeneity is expected, such as in patients who have EBS, with cohorts in some studies containing a larger or smaller numbers of patients who have Dowling-Meara EBS, who generally have a more severe clinical phenotype than patients who have localized EBS.

When separated into different dimensions, interesting results were found during development of the QOLEB concerning the psychological impact (depression and anxiety) of EB on patients who have RDEB. Levels of depression and anxiety scores were lower than anticipated, which was attributed to the resilience phenomenon, although further research is required to ascertain the validity of these results.

When comparing the usefulness of existing QOL measurement tools for patients who have EB, the purpose of the QOL evaluation and the specific cohort of patients who will be participating must be considered.

The QOL measurement tool with the most content validity for quantitatively evaluating QOL among a wide variety of EB subtypes is the QOLEB questionnaire. However, if a cohort mostly consists of patients mildly affected with EBS, then the DLQI may also be appropriate. For clinical settings, the most concise, valid questionnaires are the most useful (QOLEB and DLQI); however, in the setting of clinical research specifically evaluating specific dimensional constructs (functional, psychosocial, psychosexual), a specialist specific questionnaire may be more appropriate.

Since completion of the QOLEB, the authors learned of another study of QOL in EB conducted in March 2008 in Italy,[16] which performed a cross-sectional survey of southern Italian patients who had EB using the SF-36, Skindex-29, GHQ-12, and EQ-5D. This study presented some interesting

Box 1
QOLEB questionnaire

Quality of Life in Epidermolysis Bullosa (QOLEB) Questionnaire

Please answer these questions about how EB affects your life. Please choose an option from the right hand column that most closely matches your situation. Please note how long it took you to complete this questionnaire at the end.

1) Does your EB affect your ability to move around at home?	❏ Not at all ❏ A little ❏ A lot ❏ Severely
2) Does your EB affect your ability to bath or shower?	❏ No, No impact ❏ Yes, I sometimes need assistance ❏ Yes, need assistance most of the time ❏ Yes, I need assistance every time I bath/shower
3) Does your EB cause you physical pain?	❏ No pain ❏ Occasional pain ❏ Frequent pain ❏ Constant pain
4) How does your EB affect your ability to write?	❏ It does not interfere with writing ❏ I find it difficult to grip the pen ❏ I find it easier to type than write ❏ I cannot write due to my EB
5) Does your EB affect your ability to eat?	❏ No, I eat normally ❏ A little ❏ A lot ❏ I rely on my gastrostomy tube for nutrition
6) Does your EB affect your ability to go shopping?	❏ No, not at all ❏ A little ❏ A lot ❏ I need assistance all the time.
7) How does EB affect your involvement in sports?	❏ No impact. ❏ I need to be cautious in sports ❏ I need to avoid some sports ❏ I need to avoid all sports
8) How frustrated do you feel about your EB?	❏ No frustration ❏ A little ❏ A lot
9) Does your EB affect your ability to move around outside of your home?	❏ Not at all ❏ A little ❏ A lot ❏ Severely
10) How does your EB affect your relationships with family members?	❏ No impact at all ❏ A small impact ❏ A large impact ❏ A very large impact
11) How embarrassed do people make you feel about your EB?	❏ No embarrassment ❏ A little ❏ A lot ❏ Extremely
12) Have you needed to, or do you need to modify your home (installing ramps etc) due to your EB?	❏ No, not at all ❏ A few ❏ A lot ❏ Extensive
13) Does your EB affect your relationships with friends?	❏ No, Not at all ❏ A little ❏ A lot ❏ It severely restricts my social interaction

14) How worried or anxious do you feel because of your EB?	❏ Not anxious at all ❏ A little ❏ A lot ❏ Extremely
15) How are you or your family affected financially by your EB?	❏ No financial impact ❏ Slightly Affected ❏ Greatly Affected ❏ Severely Affected
16) How depressed do you feel because of your EB?	❏ Not depressed at all ❏ A little ❏ A lot ❏ Constantly very depressed
17) How uncomfortable are you made to feel by others (eg-teasing or staring) because of your EB?	❏ Not at all ❏ A little ❏ A lot ❏ So much that I don't go out socially

How long did it take you to complete this questionnaire? .... Minutes

Thank you.

From Frew JW, Martin LK, Nijsten T, Murrell DF. Quality of life evaluation in epidermolysis bullosa (EB) through the development of the QOLEB questionnaire: an EB-specific quality of life instrument. Br J Dermatol 2009 Aug 13 [Epub ahead of print]; with permission.

findings that support the conclusions of this article's authors. One similar observation was the psychological resilience displayed by severely affected patients compared with their reported level of physical impairment. Ceiling effects were shown in the general health scale and Skindex-29, because these did not distinguish among EB types or subtypes, justifying the need for an EB-specific scale. Limiting factors were the inclusion of only 6 of 125 patients who had EBS, and a 64% response rate among patients who had already agreed to participate by phone, with a bias toward the more severe forms. The study showed the heavy burden that EB imposes on the caregiver and family.

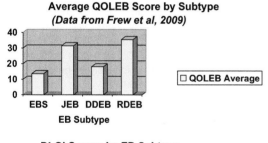

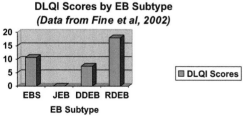

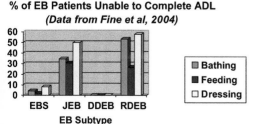

Fig. 1. Quality of life results adapted from various studies

FUTURE ENDEAVORS FOR QUALITY OF LIFE MEASUREMENT IN EPIDERMOLYSIS BULLOSA

The development of QOL tools in EB is barely in its infancy; the hope is that the future will see not only the development but also the widespread application of QOL measurement in EB cohorts. Its responsiveness across time in the same patients during interventions will need to be assessed. Necessary developments for the near future include an appropriate pediatric QOL measurement tool and further exploration of the psychosocial impacts of EB on individuals and families. With the advent of new therapeutic modalities, experts recognize that QOL, not just the absence of disease, is important in patient outcomes and that the best standard of care must be achieved for individuals who have EB.

ACKNOWLEDGMENTS

The authors would like to thank all patients who have EB and their families who have contributed to clinical research, particularly with our QOL studies; Sr Lesley Rhodes, RN, for her help with compiling and collecting QOLEB questionnaires; Dr Linda Martin and Dr Tamar Nijsten as coinvestigators, and DebRA Australia and DebRA New Zealand for their ongoing support.

REFERENCES

1. World Health Organisation (WHO). Preamble to the Constitution of the World Health Organization as adopted by the International Health Conference. New York: WHO; June 19–22, 1946. Official records of the WHO no. 2. p. 100.
2. Kerr C, Taylor R, Heard G. Handbook of public health methods unit 24: questionnaires. Sydney: McGraw-Hill; 1998: p. 156–61.
3. ÓConnor R. Measuring quality of life in health. Sydney: Churchill Livingstone; 2004.
4. Halioua B, Beumont M, Lunel F. Quality of life in dermatology. Int J Dermatol 2000;39:801–6.
5. Horn H, Tidman M. Quality of life in epidermolysis bullosa. Clin Exp Dermatol 2002;27:707–10.
6. Scheppingen C, Lettinga AT, Duipmans JC, et al. Main problems experienced by children with epidermolysis bullosa: a qualitative study with semi-structured interviews. Acta Derm Venereol 2008;88:143–50.
7. Finlay A, Khan K. Dermatology Life Quality Index (DLQI)—a simple practical measure for routine clinical use. Clin Exp Dermatol 1994;19:210–6.
8. Frew J, Martin L, Murrell DF. Quality of life evaluation in epidermolysis bullosa. Presented at the Australasian College of Dermatologists, 40th Annual Scientific Meeting; Adelaide, Australia; May 13–16, 2007.
9. Frew JW, Martin LK, Murrell DF. Development of the quality of life questionnaire for epidermolysis bullosa. Presented at the 66th Annual Meeting of the American Academy of Dermatology; San Antonio, Texas; February 1–5, 2008.
10. Frew JW, Martin LK, Murrell DF. Development of a quality of life instrument for epidermolysis bullosa. Presented at the 2008 International Investigative Dermatology Meeting; Kyoto, Japan; May 14–17, 2008.
11. Frew JW, Martin LK, Nijsten T, Murrell DF. Development of a quality of life index for epidermolysis bullosa (EB) through the development of the QOLEB questionnaire, an EB-specific quality of life instrument. Br J Dermatol 2009, in press. DOI: 10.111/j.1365–2133.2009.09347.x
12. Fine JD, Johnson LB, Weiner M, et al. Assessment of mobility, activities and pain in different subtypes of epidermolysis bullosa. Clin Exp Dermatol 2004;29:122–7.
13. Fine JD, Johnson LB, Weiner M, et al. Impact of inherited epidermolysis bullosa on parental interpersonal relationships, marital status and family size. Br J Dermatol 2005;152:1009–14.
14. Scheppingen C, Lettinga AT, Duipmans JC, et al. The main problems of parents of a child with epidermolysis bullosa. Qual Health Res 2008;18(4):545–56.
15. Holme SA, Man I, Sharpe SL, et al. The children's dermatology life quality index: validation of the cartoon version. Br J Dermatol 2003;148:285–90.
16. Tabolli S, Sampogna F, Di Pietro C, et al. Quality of life in patients with epidermolysis bullosa. Br J Dermatol 2009;161(4):869–77.

Index

Note: Page numbers of article titles are in **boldface** type.

Dermatol Clin 28 (2010) 191–195
doi:10.1016/S0733-8635(09)00117-X

Moving?

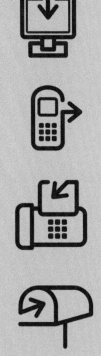